Essential Practice Guidelines in Primary Care

CURRENT ◊ CLINICAL ◊ PRACTICE

NEIL S. SKOLNIK, MD • SERIES EDITOR

Essential Practice Guidelines in Primary Care

Edited by

Neil S. Skolnik, MD

Abington Memorial Hospital, Abington, PA
and Temple University School of Medicine, Philadelphia, PA

Associate Editors
Doron Schneider, MD
Abington Memorial Hospital, Abington, PA

Richard Neill, MD
University of Pennsylvania, Philadelphia, PA

Lou Kuritzky, MD
University of Florida, Gainesville, FL

HUMANA PRESS ✳ TOTOWA, NEW JERSEY

MT

Due diligence has been taken by the publishers, editors, and authors of this book to assure the accuracy of the information published and to describe generally accepted practices. The contributors herein have carefully checked to ensure that the drug selections and dosages set forth in this text are accurate and in accord with the standards accepted at the time of publication. Notwithstanding, as new research, changes in government regulations, and knowledge from clinical experience relating to drug therapy and drug reactions constantly occurs, the reader is advised to check the product information provided by the manufacturer of each drug for any change in dosages or for additional warnings and contraindications. This is of utmost importance when the recommended drug herein is a new or infrequently used drug. It is the responsibility of the treating physician to determine dosages and treatment strategies for individual patients. Further it is the responsibility of the health care provider to ascertain the Food and Drug Administration status of each drug or device used in their clinical practice. The publisher, editors, and authors are not responsible for errors or omissions or for any consequences from the application of the information presented in this book and make no warranty, express or implied, with respect to the contents in this publication.

This publication is printed on acid-free paper. ∞
ANSI Z39.48-1984 (American Standards Institute) Permanence of Paper for Printed Library Materials.

Production Editor: Robin B. Weisberg

Cover design by Patricia F. Cleary

For additional copies, pricing for bulk purchases, and/or information about other Humana titles, contact Humana at the above address or at any of the following numbers: Tel.: 973-256-1699; Fax: 973-256-8314; E-mail: orders@humanapr.com, or visit our Website: http://humanapress.com

Printed in the United States of America. 10 9 8 7 6 5 4 3 2 1
eISBN: 1-59745-313-7
Library of Congress Cataloging-in-Publication Data

Essential practice guidelines in primary care / edited by Neil S. Skolnik ; associate editors, Doron Schneider, Richard Neill, Lou Kuritzky.
    p. ; cm. -- (Current clinical practice)
 Includes bibliographical references and index.
 ISBN-13: 978-1-58829-508-8
 ISBN-10: 1-58829-508-7 (alk. paper)
 1. Evidence-based medicine--Handbooks, manuals, etc. 2. Primary care (Medicine)--Handbooks, manuals, etc. 3. Family medicine--Handbooks, manuals, etc. I. Skolnik, Neil S. II. Series.
 [DNLM: 1. Evidence-Based Medicine--Handbooks. 2. Evidence-Based Medicine--Practice Guideline.
 3. Primary Health Care--Handbooks. 4. Primary Health Care--Practice Guideline. WB 39 H2359 2007]
 R729.G4H36 2007
 616--dc22
                                                           2006022682

11/9/09

Introduction

Wisdom is the principal thing; therefore
get wisdom and with all thy getting
get understanding.
—Proverbs 4:7

In addition to wisdom, physicians need information—in many different settings—when learning new and reviewing previously learned material, during case conferences, and at the point-of-care while taking care of patients. Numerous studies have shown that physicians regularly encounter questions that need an answer while they are seeing patients (1). Unfortunately, only about one-third of those questions are eventually pursued to find an answer, likely because of the difficulty of finding answers and the time constraints under which physicians find themselves (2–4). It is important to understand that when information is readily available, physicians utilize that information, and that information impacts on patient care and can alter the clinical decisions that occur (5–7). National clinical guidelines have been increasingly recognized as a potential way of improving the quality of medical care by giving physicians clear, evidence-based guidance on how to treat complex diseases where an abundance of literature may exist.

The evolution of medical knowledge proceeds along a predictable route. It starts with careful observation. Next comes the generation of hypotheses. The hypotheses are then tested through studies. These studies are eventually synthesized into evidence-based guidelines developed through a rigorous process that includes a comprehensive review of the literature combined with expert opinion. Guidelines should be constructed with the clinician in mind so that they are understandable and easy to implement. In order for guidelines to be useful, they must then be disseminated so that physicians are familiar with their content, and tools and resources must be made available to clinicians so the guidelines can be implemented at the point-of-care and referred to wherever and whenever information is needed (8). *Essential Practice Guidelines in Primary Care* puts the most important evidence-based, nationally recognized, clinical guidelines together in one place so that busy clinicians can go to one source when, in the care of a patient, a question arises that is best answered by an existing clinical guideline.

The increasing amount and complexity of medical information has led to new strategies being developed to allow physicians to access current information from the medical literature in order to continue to provide excellent, up-to-date medical care. Electronic handheld references, which have emerged over the last few years, provide an opportunity for physicians to answer important clinical questions during the time those questions are most meaningful, that is, when patients are being taken care of and decisions are being made. Currently, about half of all primary care physicians are using handheld computers. In March 2004, the Institute of Medicine issued a report that stated, "Personal digital assistants [PDAs] are increasingly being used to support safety and quality in point-of-care applications. These technologies have the potential for widespread adoption because of their greater flexibility, convenience, and mobility relative to wired network communication systems. Many physicians and other health care providers are already incorporating handheld devices into their day-to-day functioning to better manage the care of their patients while at the same time reduce medical errors" *(9)*.

With the busy clinician in mind, *Essential Practice Guidelines in Primary Care* has been constructed from its origin to have a companion PDA resource, with summaries of the guidelines in this book, and additional summaries of guidelines not included in the book. In fact, the PDA version of *Essential Practice Guidelines in Primary Care* was developed first. Shortly after being published, an *Annals of Internal Medicine* book review stated that the PDA-based *Clinical Guidelines Handbook* was "an important tool for bringing evidence-based medicine to the point-of-care." That review was an important impetus to develop the print edition. In our opinion, the print edition is best used as a single resource where a clinician can read through a large selection of guidelines to gain an overview and understanding of any given guideline and the PDA version is best used to look up information that is needed quickly either at the point-of-care or during a conference. Together, these complimentary textbooks, in print and electronic, should facilitate the implementation of nationally recognized clinical guidelines by primary care physicians. (To order the PDA version of this title [ISBN 1-934115-47-9], please contact the publisher, Humana Press, at www.humanapress.com.)

A book, like a plant, grows best in the right environment. The development of a book works best when it occurs with the cooperation of many people, both personal and professional. That cooperation merits thanks. First of all I would like to thank the three associate editors of this book—Lou Kuritzky, Richard Neill, and Doron Schneider. Their contributions were integral to the evolution of the book.

Richard Lansing deserves praise and thanks as both a friend and as the editor at Humana Press with whom I first discussed the concept of this book and who recognized the value of practice guidelines to primary care physicians. Many thanks to Robin Weisberg for her insightful editing as this book was coming together.

I would like to thank my fellow faculty in the Family Medicine Residency Program at Abington Memorial Hospital. I feel lucky to be a part of such an outstanding and caring faculty—Matthew Clark, Amy Clouse, Pam Fenstemacher, Trip Hansen, and John Russell—where we all challenge each other daily and share an excitement and joy in teaching and learning. I also owe thanks to our superb residents who stand shoulder to shoulder with us in providing excellent evidence-based, compassionate care to our patients and who regularly, and at times respectfully, ask the tough questions that keep us attending physicians going back to the literature and keep us on our toes. I am also filled with appreciation for being a part of Abington Memorial Hospital where the administration strongly supports excellence in patient care and residency education, and where the excellent relationships between departments lead to the collaboration between the departments of Internal Medicine and Family Medicine that helped to make this book. Specifically within the hospital I would like to mention Dick Jones, Meg McGoldrick, Gary Candia, Jack Kelly, and Warren Matthews, all of whom provide our academic Family Medicine Residency Program with the resources and guidance we need to carry out our mission.

Finally, and of highest importance, no person, no plant, and no book grows to its fullest without the love and support of family. My eternal gratitude and love belong to my wife, Alison, who puts up with my foibles and shares my joys and dreams and is my partner in this journey that is our life; my ongoing wonder and love goes to my son, Aaron, whose intelligence, sharp observational skills, and appreciation of nature have taken us on fishing trips on lakes throughout northeastern United States and Canada; and my ongoing wonder and love goes to my daughter Ava, whose singing and wonderful dancing I tremendously enjoy and who constantly amazes me with her beauty, intelligence, and humor.

Neil S. Skolnik, MD

REFERENCES

1. Schilling, LM, Anderson RJ. Answering patient-specific questions using information resources available in an outpatient clinic. Semin Med Prac 2000;3(4):11–21.
2. Ely JW, Osheroff JA, Ebell MH, et al. Analysis of questions asked by family doctors regarding patients' care. BMJ 1999;319:358–361.
3. Gorman PN. Information needs of physicians. J Am Soc Inform Sci 1995;46:729–736.
4. Green ML, Ciampi MA, Ellis PJ. Residents' medical information needs in clinic: are they being met? Am J Med 2000;109:218–223.
5. Covell DG, Uman GC, Manning PR. Information needs in office practice: are they being met? Ann Intern Med 1985;103:596–599.
6. Sacket DL, Straus SE. Finding and applying evidence during clinical rounds: the "evidence cart." JAMA 1998;280:1336–1338.
7. Gundersen L. The effect of clinical practice guidelines on variations in care. Ann Intern Med 2000;133:317.

8. Weingarten S. Using practice guideline compendiums to provide better preventive care. Ann Intern Med 1999;130:454–458.

9. Aspeden P, Corrigan JM, Wolcott J, Erickson SM (eds.). Patient Safety: Achieving a New Standard for Care (Institute of Medicine report). Washington, DC: National Academies Press, 2004, p. 70.

Contents

Contributors

ROSS ALBERT, MD, PhD • Family Medicine Residency Program, Abington Memorial Hospital, Abington, PA

MARGOT BOIGON, MD • Associate Program Director, Internal Medicine Residency Program, Abington Memorial Hospital, Abington, PA

AMY CLOUSE, MD • Associate Director, Family Medicine Residency, Abington Memorial Hospital, Abington, PA

MATTHEW CLARK, MD • Associate Director, Family Medicine Residency, Abington Memorial Hospital, Abington, PA

ANDREW COHEN, MD • Family Medicine Residency, Abington Memorial Hospital, Abington, PA

TINA H. DEGNAN, MD • Family Medicine Residency, Abington Memorial Hospital, Abington, PA

DIANE DIETZEN, MD, FACP • Director, Palliative Care; Associate Program Director, Internal Medicine Residency Program, Abington Memorial Hospital, Abington, PA

BENJAMIN J. EPSTEIN, PharmD, BCPS • Assistant Professor, Department of Pharmacy Practice, College of Pharmacy, University of Florida, Gainesville, FL

PAM FENSTEMACHER, MD • Associate Director, Family Medicine Residency, Abington Memorial Hospital, Abington, PA

BRETT FISSELL, MD • Gwynedd Family Practice, North Wales, PA

MICHAEL GAGNON, MD • Family Medicine Residency, Abington Memorial Hospital, Abington, PA

MARY HOFMANN, MD, FACP • Chief, Section of Geriatric Medicine, Abington Memorial Hospital, Abington, PA

LOUIS KURITZKY, MD • Clinical Assistant Professor, Department of Community Health and Family Medicine, University of Florida, Gainesville, FL

WILLIAM McCARBERG, MD • Founder, Pain Management Program, Kaiser Permanente San Diego, and Assistant Clinical Professor, University of California San Diego, San Diego, CA

MARIO NAPOLETANO, MD • Gwynedd Family Practice, North Wales, PA

RICHARD NEILL, MD • Assistant Professor of Family Medicine and Community Health; Residency Director, Family Medicine Residency, Department of Family Medicine and Community Health, University of Pennsylvania, Philadelphia, PA

ANN PEFF, MD • Director, Medical Student Program, Abington Memorial Hospital, Abington, PA

JOHN RUSSELL, MD • Associate Director, Family Medicine Residency, Abington Memorial Hospital, Abington, PA

GEORGE P. N. SAMRAJ, MD • Associate Professor, Department of Family Medicine, University of Florida, Gainesville, FL

DORON SCHNEIDER, MD • Associate Program Director, Internal Medicine Residency Program; and Associate Patient Safety Officer, Abington Memorial Hospital, Abington, PA

NEIL S. SKOLNIK, MD • Associate Director, Family Medicine Residency Program, Abington Memorial Hospital, Abington, PA and Professor of Family and Community Medicine, Temple University School of Medicine, Philadelphia, PA

DAVID GARY SMITH, MD, FACP • Program Director, Internal Medicine Residency Program, Abington Memorial Hospital, Abington, PA and Associate Professor of Medicine, Temple University School of Medicine, Philadelphia, PA

JOHN E. SUTHERLAND, MD • Executive/Program Director, NE Iowa Medical Education Foundation/FM Residency, Waterloo, IA

JAYA UDAYASANKAR, MD • Diabetes and Endocrine Fellow, Division of Metabolism, Endocrinology, and Nutrition, University of Washington, Seattle, WA

DAVID WEBNER, MD • Assistant Professor, Departments of Family Medicine and Orthopaedic Surgery, Sports Medicine, Team Physician, University of Pennsylvania, Philadelphia, PA

I   CARDIOLOGY

1

Seventh Report of the Joint National Committee on Prevention, Detection, Evaluation, and Treatment of High Blood Pressure

Benjamin J. Epstein, PharmD, BCPS

INTRODUCTION

Cardiovascular disease (CVD) is the leading cause of death in the industrialized world. It is present in approx 50 million Americans, but afflicts close to 1 billion persons worldwide. Increasingly, societies with lesser socioeconomic privilege suffer cardiovascular end points, accounting for as much as 80% of the worldwide CVD burden. The presence of hypertension increases the risk of disease in all atherosclerotic beds by several orders of magnitude. Data from the Framingham Heart Study revealed that among men and women who are normotensive at the age of 55 or 65, the lifetime risk of hypertension is 90%. As the population continues to grow, the number of patients with hypertension will also increase. Consequently, effective management of hypertension is of paramount importance for dampening the imminent growth of CVD during the next century.

From: *Current Clinical Practice: Essential Practice Guidelines in Primary Care*
Edited by: N. S. Skolnik © Humana Press, Totowa, NJ

The implications of blood pressure (BP) control are tremendous, thus, it is not surprising that correspondingly prodigious efforts have been devoted to the increasing awareness and effective treatment of hypertension. The National High Blood Pressure Education Program, a coalition of 39 major professional, public, and voluntary organizations and 7 federal agencies, has been fundamental in this effort. For more than 30 yr, the organization, which is overseen by the National Heart, Lung, and Blood Institute, has prepared and disseminated guidelines and advisories focused on increasing awareness, prevention, treatment, and control of hypertension. The Seventh Report of the Joint National Committee on Prevention, Detection, Evaluation, and Treatment of High Blood Pressure (JNC 7) was constructed to address four issues: (1) publication of new landmark clinical trials and observational data in patients with hypertension have reshaped best practice regarding hypertension; (2) previous guidelines have been perceived as unwieldy, hence preparation of a clearer and more concise guideline was in order; (3) simplification of BP definitions was needed; and (4) suboptimal implementation of prior JNC recommendations demanded reinvigorating clinician energy toward hypertension *(1–3)*.

CLASSIFICATION OF BP

The JNC 7 BP categorization system has been reorganized and modified with the goal of simplifying the classification of BP for adults over the age of 18 yr (Table 1). Patients with a systolic BP (SBP) below 120 mmHg and a diastolic BP (DBP) below 80 mmHg are classified as "normal." This differs from the previous nomenclature, which identified this level of BP as "optimal." This distinction is important as it underscores the relationship between BP and cardiovascular risk, which is continuous and linear (i.e., there does not appear to be a BP lesser than which CVD risk increases). Although there is still some debate on this issue, most clinical trial data do not confirm a "*J*-curve" depiction of treated BP vs outcomes. This is a concern based on limited data that persons who have BP lowered "too much" might demonstrate an increase in adverse outcomes. This finding has generally not been borne out in clinical trials. Obviously, a threshold must exist, but it appears to be low levels of BP readily achievable in most patients. One possible exception is patients with significant coronary artery disease (CAD), in whom excessive reduction of BP (especially diastolic) may provoke myocardial ischemia *(4,5)*.

Hypertension is defined as an SBP of 140 mmHg or higher or a DBP of 90 mmHg or higher. Recently, JNC created a new classification, prehypertension, for those patients with an SBP between 120 and 139 mmHg or a DBP between 80 and 89 mmHg. In previous classification, patients with this level of BP were classified as "normal" (120–129/80–84 mmHg) or "borderline" (130–139/85–89 mmHg). Given that prehypertension clearly heralds frank

Table 1
Blood Pressure (BP) Classification and Management

BP classification	Systolic and diastolic[a] (mmHg)	Lifestyle modification	Initial drug therapy	
			Without compelling indications	With compelling indications
Normal	<120 and <80	Encourage	—	—
Prehypertension	120–139 or 80–89	Yes	No antihypertensive drug indicated	Drug(s) for compelling indications[b]
Stage 1	140–159 or 90–99	Yes	Thiazide-type diuretics for most. May consider ACEI, ARB, BB, CCB, or combination	Drug(s) for the compelling indications[b]
Stage 2	≥160 or ≥100	Yes	Two-drug combination for most[c] (usually thiazide-type diuretic and ACEI or ARB or BB or CCB)	Other antihypertensive drugs (diuretics, ACEI, ARB, BB, CCB) as needed

[a]Classification and treatment should be based on the highest BP category. For instance, if DBP is 76 mmHg and SBP is 147 mmHg, the patient should be classified as and treated for stage I hypertension.

[b]Treat patients with chronic kidney disease or diabetes to BP goal of <130/80 mmHg.

[c]Initial combined therapy should be used cautiously in those at risk for orthostatic hypotension.
DBP, diastolic blood pressure; SBP, systolic blood pressure; ACEI, angiotensin-converting enzyme inhibitor; ARB, angiotensin receptor blocker; BB, β-blocker; CCB, calcium channel blocker.
Compiled from refs. 1–3.

5

hypertension, this category was established to underscore the importance of implementing strategies that are capable of curtailing the progression of pre-hypertension to hypertension during the early stages of high BP. The staging process for hypertension adopted by JNC 7 differs from previous editions in that stages 2 and 3 hypertension are now combined to simplify the schema. The rational for this change is that patients with stages 2 and 3 hypertension are treated similarly. It is important to note that if a patient's SBP and DBP are in different stages, the higher of the two should be used to classify the patient (e.g., a BP of 145/85 mmHg would be stage 1 hypertension, not prehypertension). Hypertension is no longer stratified on the presence or absence of target organ damage because this dichotomy complicates the staging process but does not significantly modify treatment strategy.

BP AND CARDIOVASCULAR DISEASE RISK

The risk of myocardial infarction (MI), heart failure (HF), and stroke increases at all levels of BP higher than 115/75 mmHg and CVD risk doubles for each increment of 20/10 mmHg over this value. When evaluating individual patients, SBP should be considered as the primary determinant of cardiovascular risk. Although the concept of concentrating efforts on control of SBP has only been recently been popularized, actuarial tables have demonstrated, for the last four to five decades, that SBP is a better predictor of adverse outcome than DBP.

Based on the aforementioned definitions, the National Health and Examination Survey (NHANES) III has reported that 31% of Americans are prehypertensive, 29% are hypertensive, and just 39% are normotensive. Perhaps more alarming is the insidious nature of the disease—among those with hypertension, 30% are unaware; among those who are aware, 11% are not being treated pharmacologically, and 25% are on medication but do not have their BP controlled.

BP MEASUREMENT AND FOLLOW-UP

Accurate BP measurement in the office is requisite to successful management. Clinicians are should ensure that not only are the BP monitoring devices maintained in appropriate calibration, but that the personnel recording BP are consistently providing accurate results.

The auscultatory method of BP measurement is preferred. Patients should be sufficiently rested (≥ 5 min in a chair) and caffeine intake and smoking should have been avoided in the preceding 30 min. The appropriate size cuff (i.e., cuff bladder encircling at least 80% of the arm) should be selected in order to avoid over- or underestimation of BP. It is recommended that clinicians initially estimate a target BP for cuff inflation by palpating the radial pulse during cuff inflation. This is done until the pulse disappears. At this the point, the cuff should be inflated by an additional 20–30 mmHg. However, not all clinicians

Table 2
Recommendations for Follow-Up Based on Initial Office Blood Pressure (BP) in Patients Without Target Organ Damage

BP classification	Recommended follow-up[a]
Normal	Recheck in 2 yr[a]
Prehypertension	Recheck in 1 yr[a]
Stage 1 hypertension	Confirm within 2 mo
Stage 2 hypertension	Evaluate or refer to source of care within 1 mo. For patients with more severe hypertension (e.g., >180/110 mmHg), evaluate and treat immediately or within 1 wk depending on clinical situation or complications.

[a]Modify the scheduling of follow-up according to reliable information about past BP measurements, other cardiovascular risk factors, and/or target organ disease. Provide advice about lifestyle modifications.
Adapted from ref. *1*.

perform this task in clinical practice. Instead, many clinicians arbitrarily inflate the cuff to levels well more than the anticipated BP (e.g., 220 mmHg) prior to deflation. The cuff should not be deflated faster than 2 mmHg/s. Auscultation of the first Korotkoff sound is representative of the systolic value and disappearance of Korotkoff sound reflects the diastolic value. The average of the two measurements should be recorded. A multitude of other factors are capable of influencing BP measurement. For a more thorough discussion of appropriate BP measurement and factors that can influence it, *see* the most recent recommendations endorsed by the American Heart Association *(6)*.

In adults with normal BP, follow-up is recommended every 2 yr to re-evaluate BP and the associated risk factors (Table 2). If prehypertension is present, patients should be re-evaluated on a yearly basis. Both normotensive and prehypertensive patients benefit from lifestyle modification; therefore, patients should receive written and verbal advice at these stages. Stage 1 hypertension should be confirmed within 2 mo. The presence of stage 2 hypertension mandates evaluation or referral within 1 mo and depending on the clinical situation, treatment may be in indicated within 1 wk or immediately. A shorter follow-up interval may be prudent, irrespective of BP, in patients with cardiovascular risk factors, evidence of target organ damage, or when clinical judgment so dictates.

Ambulatory BP monitoring (ABPM) may be desirable in some situations (Table 3). ABPM provides the clinician with a 24-h view of the patient's BP, which may be helpful, for example, when a white-coat effect is suspected. It is important to recognize that ABPM values are typically lower than clinic readings, with hypertensive patients displaying an average BP of more than 135/85 mmHg during waking hours and more than 120/75 mmHg during sleep.

Table 3
Ambulatory BP Monitoring

Ambulatory BP may be helpful in the following contexts
   Suspected white-coat hypertension and no target organ damage
   Apparent drug resistance
   Hypotensive symptoms with antihypertensive medication
   Episodic hypertension
   Autonomic dysfunction

Adapted from ref. *1.*

There is convincing evidence that ABPM correlates better with target organ damage, provides a more complete measure of the percentage of BP readings that are elevated, the overall BP load, and the degree to which the BP falls at night (i.e., "dippers" vs "nondippers"). An intermediate alternative to office and ABPM is patient self-monitoring. Self-monitoring is a practical approach to assess differences between actual and office BP, and it may also be useful in evaluating the merit of ABPM. For example, if a patient with elevated office BP has out-of-office BPs that are consistently less than 130/80 mmHg, then ABPM can be avoided. Before accepting self-measured BP records as the final decision point, the clinician should corroborate the accuracy of the equipment with which the patient is measuring BP, and appropriateness of the patient's technique.

PATIENT EVALUATION

Evaluation of the hypertensive patient should address three primary objectives: (1) assess lifestyle and identify other cardiovascular risk factors (Table 4) or concomitant disorders that may modify prognosis; (2) uncover secondary causes of elevated BP (Table 5); and (3) assess the presence of target organ damage (Table 4) and CVD. An effective patient evaluation requires an accurate compilation of medical history, physical examination, laboratory test results, and diagnostic procedures. Table 6 lists the components of a thorough physical examination and the diagnostic procedures recommended prior to initiating therapy. More extensive evaluation can usually be overlooked unless there is suspicion of secondary causes of high BP. Not strong evidence base exists to guide physicians as to which patients should be evaluated for secondary causes; however, it is usually recommended for patients in whom age (e.g., onset before age 35), family history (e.g., a very strong family history of hypertension), physical examination (e.g., signs of thyroid disease, abdominal bruit, disparate timing of cardiac pulse with peripheral pulse as in aortic coarctation), severity of hypertension (e.g., very labile BP or BP >220/140), or initial laboratory results (e.g., unprovoked hypokalemia, hypercalcemia, abnormal urinalysis, and abnormal thyroid function tests) suggest

Table 4
Risk Factors for Cardiovascular Disease

Major risk factors	*Target organ damage*
Modifiable	Heart
Hypertension	Left ventricular hypertrophy
Diabetes mellitus	Angina or prior myocardial infarction
Elevated LDL or low HDL	Prior coronary revascularization
Obesity (BMI >30 kg/m^2)	Heart failure
Physical inactivity	Brain
Tobacco use	Stroke or transient ischemic attack
Renal insufficiency (GFR < 60 mL/min)	Dementia
Microalbuminuria or proteinuria	Chronic kidney disease
Nonmodifiable	Peripheral artery disease
Age (older than 55 for men, 65 for women)	Retinopathy
Family history of premature CVD	
(men <55 yr of age or women <65 yr of age)	

BMI, body mass index; CVD, cardiovascular disease; GFR, glomerular filtration rate; HDL, high-density lipoprotein; LDL, low-density lipoprotein.

Table 5
Secondary Causes of Hypertension

Diagnosis	*Diagnostic test*
Chronic kidney disease (GFR <60 mL/min or proteinuria 300 mg/d)	Estimated GFR[a]
Renovascular hypertension	Doppler flow study or magnetic resonance angiography
Sleep apnea	Sleep study
Primary aldosteronism and other mineralocorticoid-induced states	24-h urinary aldosterone level
Cushing syndrome and other glucocorticoid-induced states	History, dexamethasone suppression test
Thyroid or parathyroid disease	TSH, serum PTH
Coarctation of the aorta	CT angiography
Pheochromocytoma	24-h urinary catecholamines
Drugs (*see* Table 9)	History, drug screening

[a]GFR can be estimated by the Cockroft-Gault or MDRD methods.
CT, computed tomography; GFR, glomerular filtration rate; PTH, parathyroid hormone; TSH, thyroid-stimulating hormone.
Adapted from ref. *1.*

such a possibility. Similarly, if BP responds poorly to pharmacological therapy (requires more than three drugs for control); BP increases after initially being well controlled; or the onset of hypertension is abrupt, the clinician may wish to investigate for secondary causes (Table 5).

Table 6
Components of Thorough Physical and Diagnostic Evaluation

Physical examination
  Measurement of BP, including verification in the contralateral arm
  Examination of the optic fundi;
  Assessment of BMI (kg/m^2)
  Auscultation for carotid, abdominal, and femoral bruits
  Palpation of the thyroid gland
  Examination of the heart and lungs
  Examination of the abdomen for enlarged kidneys, masses, and abnormal
    aortic pulsation
  Palpation of the lower extremities for edema and pulses
  Neurological assessment
Diagnostic procedures
  12-lead ECG
  Blood glucose
  Hematocrit
  Potassium
  Calcium
  Creatinine
  Fasting lipid panel
  Urinalysis

BP, blood pressure; BMI, body mass index; ECG, electrocardiogram.

TREATMENT

Pharmacological

The vast majority of patients will satisfy their DBP goal if the SBP goal is achieved. Hence, control of SBP might be viewed as the "rate-limiting factor" in achieving optimal BP control, and it is the most effective predictor of CVD. Antihypertensive therapy has been definitively shown to reduce the incidence of stroke by 35–40%, MI by 20–25%, and HF by more than 50%. The majority of patients with hypertension can achieve adequate BP control; however, as many as two-thirds will require treatment with two or more antihypertensives from different classes. The threshold for initiation of therapy and general recommendations for management are presented in Table 1. Lifestyle modifications should serve as the foundation of any BP treatment strategy (Table 7).

There is convincing evidence that thiazide-type diuretics, angiotensin-converting enzyme (ACE) inhibitors, angiotensin receptor blockers (ARBs), β-blockers, and calcium channel blockers (CCBs) reduce the complications associated with hypertension. The totality of evidence suggests that these classes of drugs foster similar cardiovascular protection. However, individual clinical trials have reported conflicting results, suggesting that there may be

Table 7
Recommended Lifestyle Modifications and Expected Blood Pressure Response[a]

Intervention	Recommendation	Expected decrease in SBP mmHg[b]
Weight loss	Implement strategies that achieve or maintain ideal body weight (body mass index 18.5–24.9 kg/m^2)	5–20
DASH eating plan	Plan consists of fruits, vegetables, and low-fat dairy products, and minimizes consumption of saturated and total fat	8–14
Restrict dietary sodium intake	Reduce dietary sodium intake not more than 2.4 g sodium or 6 g sodium chloride (approx 3/4 tsp salt per day)	2–8
Increase physical activity	Regular aerobic physical activity (e.g., brisk walking) at least 30 min/d, most days of the week	4–9
Restrict alcohol consumption	Limit consumption to not more than two drinks (e.g., 24 oz beer, 10 oz wine, or 3 oz 80-proof whiskey) daily in men and one drink daily in women	2–4

[a]For overall cardiovascular risk reduction, encourage smoking cessation.
[b]The effects of implementing these modifications are dose- and time-dependent and could be greater for some individuals.
SBP, systolic blood pressure; DASH, Dietary Approaches to Stop Hypertension.
Adapted form refs. 1,16,17.

differences among these agents when individual outcomes or specific patient populations are considered. These disparities provide the framework for the "compelling indications" section (see the Compelling Indications section).

Thiazide-type diuretics are the preferred initial agent in most patients with hypertension in the absence of a compelling indication for another agent (see Fig. 1). The rationale for this hierarchy rests on evidence from multiple clinical trials, which have been confirmed most recently by the Antihypertensive and Lipid-Lowering Treatment to Prevent Heart Attack Trial (ALLHAT). In ALLHAT, treatment with chlorthalidone, lisinopril, or amlodipine resulted in equivalent outcomes with respect to coronary heart disease in more than 33,000 high-risk hypertensive patients. Indeed, ALLHAT established that if the ultimate goal in hypertension treatment is to reduce mortality, all three classes of drugs (CCBs, ACE inhibitors, and diuretics), produced equally favorable results, with no clear "winner." However, several of the secondary outcomes in ALLHAT, such as HF and stroke, favored patients treated with chlorthalidone. It is unclear whether this advantage was the result of an inherent attribute of chlorthalidone or more favorable BP control in chlorthalidone-treated

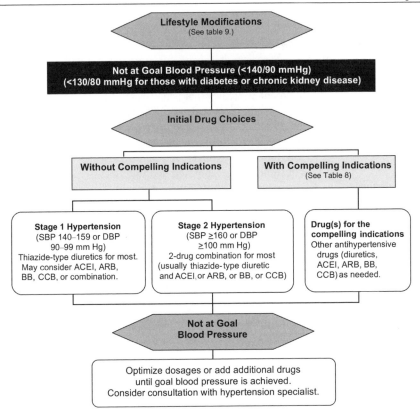

Fig. 1. Treatment algorithm for patients with hypertension. (Adapted from ref. *1.)*

subjects, which was especially prominent among the black cohort of the study population. Chlorthalidone was as effective as other strategies despite provoking a higher incidence of metabolic derangements, including treatment-emergent diabetes mellitus and lipoprotein disturbances. Patients with diabetes at baseline also benefited from chlorthalidone.

Thiazide-type diuretics are relatively well tolerated at doses applied in clinical trials that reduced cardiovascular end points, such as cardiovascular death, MI, and stroke (12.5–25 mg of chlorthalidone or 25–50 mg of hydrochlorothiazide). Finally, thiazide-type diuretics are available generically and are less expensive than other agents. Collectively, the safety, efficacy, and low cost of thiazide-type diuretics justify their role as first-line antihypertensives.

ACE inhibitors, ARBs, CCBs, and β-blockers can be considered as part of combination therapy for patients who require a second agent to achieve target BP. Alternatively, these agents are reasonable for initial monotherapy if a diuretic cannot be taken or if there is another reason that a nondiuretic would be preferred (*see* the next section). The starting dose of most antihypertensives is lower than the dose utilized in many intervention trials; consequently, the dose should be titrated upward before adding a second agent. However, if the SBP is more than 20 mmHg above goal or DBP is more than 10 mmHg above goal, two medications can be started simultaneously, because monotherapy is unlikely to produce sufficient BP reduction. In addition, combination therapy may achieve the BP goal more rapidly and at lower doses of individual agents, which may translate into improved tolerability.

It is recommended that once antihypertensive therapy is initiated, follow-up and dose adjustment should occur at intervals of 1 mo or less until target BP is reached. More vigilant monitoring is required in patients with stage 2 hypertension or comorbidities. Once BP is at goal, follow-up visits can be extended to 3- to 6-mo intervals. It is prudent that serum creatinine and potassium are monitored at least once or twice a year and even more frequently following dose adjustment, especially in patients treated with ACE inhibitors, ARBs, or diuretics.

Compelling Indications

Hypertension often coexists with other disease entities, which on the basis of clinical trial data may serve as compelling indications for certain classes of antihypertensives. For example, the presence of HF in hypertensive patients will often entail using multiple classes of an antihypertensive (i.e., diuretic, β-blocker, and ACE inhibitor). Table 8 summarizes the compelling indications recognized by JNC 7 and the antihypertensive therapies that have been associated with positive outcomes in these patient populations in clinical trials. When considering one of these agents for initial therapy, it is prudent to integrate safety, efficacy, and cost into the decision-making process.

Coronary Disease

In patients with ischemic heart disease, lowering BP attenuates the imbalance in myocardial oxygen supply and demand by decreasing the impedance to left ventricular outflow, which helps reduce ischemia and cardiovascular events. Some, but not all, studies have suggested that cardiovascular events may increase in patients with CAD. No such threshold has been observed for SBP if DBP falls to below 55–60 mmHg (i.e., *J*-curve). For patients with stable angina, appropriate initial antihypertensive therapy could rationally include a β-blocker that, in addition to having a favorable impact on anginal symptoms, will reduce BP, cardiac output, and heart rate, thereby reducing myocardial oxygen demand. If angina is suboptimally controlled on an adequate dose of a β-blocker, a long-acting dihydropyridine CCB (e.g., amlodipine, felodipine) can be added to existing therapy. If contraindications to β-blocker therapy exist, a nondihydropyridine CCB (e.g., verapamil and diltiazem) should be considered because these agents also exert an antianginal effect, improve the balance

Table 8
Compelling Indications for Individual Drug Classes

Recommended drugs	Heart failure	Postmyocardial infarction	High coronary risk	Diabetes	Chronic kidney disease	Recurrent stroke prevention
Diuretic	✓	—	✓	✓	—	✓
β-blocker	✓	✓	✓	✓	—	—
ACE inhibitor	✓	✓[a]	✓	✓	✓	✓[b]
ARB	✓	—[a]	—	✓	✓	✓[b]
CCB	—	—	✓	✓	—	—
Aldo. antagonist	✓	✓	—	—	—	—

[a]ARBs are not endorsed in JNC 7 for this population. However, data published after release of JNC 7 suggest equivalence between captopril 50 mg three times daily and valsartan 160 mg twice daily in patients with postmyocardial infarction and left ventricular dysfunction.

[b]The Food and Drug Administration has approved the ARB losartan for the prevention of stroke in patients with hypertension and LVH, except in black patients.

Aldo, aldosterone; ARB, angiotensin receptor blocker; ACE, angiotensin-converting enzyme; CCB, calcium channel blocker; LVH, left ventricular hypertrophy.

Adapted from ref. 2.

14

between myocardial oxygen supply and demand, and lower BP. When combination therapy is indicated, long-acting dihydropyridine CCBs are preferred over nondihydropyridine agents because the combination of a β-blocker plus a nondihydropyridine CCB can result in bradycardia and atrioventricular block. It is prudent to avoid short-acting dihydropyridine CCBs (e.g., immediate-release nifedipine); these agents may precipitate cardiovascular events in this setting owing to profound vasodilatation and resultant reflex tachycardia.

Since publication of JNC 7, the Comparison of Amlodipine vs Enalapril to Limit the Occurrences of Thrombosis (CAMELOT) study has been reported *(7)*. CAMELOT also showed that in patients with angiographically documented CAD and normal BP (average BP, 129/78 mmHg), amlodipine significantly reduced adverse cardiovascular outcomes. It is defined as a composite of cardiovascular death, nonfatal MI, resuscitated cardiac arrest, coronary revascularization, hospitalization for angina pectoris, hospitalization for congestive HF, fatal or nonfatal stroke or transient ischemic attack, and any new diagnosis of peripheral vascular disease. The results suggest that the optimal level for SBP may be less than 140 mmHg, perhaps in the 120 mmHg range *(8)*.

Heart Failure

HF mandates the consideration of several classes of antihypertensives in order to address multiple neurohormonal and hemodynamic derangements. Left ventricular dysfunction is a compelling indication for ACE inhibitors at all stages of the disease. ARBs represent an alternative to ACE inhibitors for patients unable to take an ACE inhibitor owing to intolerable cough, and based on the results of CHARM-Alternative, possibly angioedema (this data was not available at the time JNC 7 was prepared) *(9)*.

Multiple clinical trials have determined that β-blockers reduce morbidity and mortality in the setting of HF and, thus, should be considered in this population. Carvedilol, metoprolol, and bisoprolol have been proven effective in clinical trials of patients with HF. It is imperative that β-blockers are initiated at doses shown to be safe in clinical trials and titrated to the dose proven to prolong survival.

The aldosterone antagonist, spironolactone, confers an incremental survival benefit in patients with advanced (stage C, New York Heart Association class III–IV) HF when administered in low doses (12.5–25 mg daily) with standard background therapy. Eplerenone, a selective aldosterone antagonist, decreases mortality when added to standard background therapy following MI in patients with a left ventricular ejection fraction (LVEF) of 40% or more and symptoms of HF. Aldosterone antagonists increase the risk for hyperkalemia, especially if background therapy includes an ACE inhibitor or ARB. Meticulous monitoring of potassium is indicated when aldosterone antagonists are used in clinical practice; studies of their use have typically excluded patients with serum creatinine greater than 2.5 mg/dL, hence clinicians should be wary of aldosterone antagonist use in persons with such reduction in renal function.

Diuretics play a critical role in the management of patients with HF. Although they have not been clearly shown to influence survival, they do reduce morbidity by modulating fluid retention associated with HF. Paradoxically, thiazide-type diuretics decrease the risk for developing HF in patients at risk for the disease, but do not alter its progression once it is established (i.e., they do not decrease mortality). Thiazide-type diuretics may be sufficient to control BP and to alleviate symptoms of congestion in the early stages of HF assuming renal function is adequate (creatinine clearance >30 mL/min), but eventually loop diuretics (i.e., furosemide, torsemide, and bumetanide) are required to manage volume overload.

Diabetes

When diabetes and hypertension coexist, they elicit an additive effect on the risk for coronary, cerebrovascular, renal, and retinal disease. Few clinical trials have enrolled diabetics exclusively, but many trials have consist of substantial subpopulations of diabetics. Collectively, these data demonstrate that aggressive BP control in diabetes reduces cardiovascular events. Remarkably, hypertension control in diabetics is superior to glucose control, even in reduction of microvascular end points (nephropathy, retinopathy, and neuropathy) *(10)*. In addition, the presence of proteinuria (either microalbuminuria or overt proteinuria) or renal insufficiency (estimated glomerular filtration rate [GFR] <60 mL/min), hallmarks of diabetes, is an independent predictor of increased cardiovascular risk. JNC 7 recommendations for BP control in diabetics are now in accord with guidelines endorsed by the American Diabetes Association: both recommend that BP should be lowered to less than 130/80 mmHg with an antihypertensive regimen that includes ACE inhibitor or ARB.

Thiazide-type diuretics, ACE inhibitors, ARBs, β-blockers, and CCBs have each shown benefit in patients with type 1 and 2 diabetes. It should be emphasized that a discussion of which agent is optimal as initial monotherapy is usually fruitless because the majority of diabetics will require two or more medications to achieve goal BP. Despite their predilection for causing hyperglycemia, thiazide-type diuretics appear to be as effective as amlodipine and lisinopril for preventing CVD events in patients with diabetes.

Based on the results from the Heart Outcomes Prevention Evaluation, ACE inhibitors markedly reduce cardiovascular events in high-risk diabetic patients with or without hypertension. Both ACE inhibitors and ARBs are capable of delaying the deterioration in GFR and progression of proteinuria characteristic of diabetic renal disease. Of note, the detailed study indicated that preservation of renal function (measured by GFR) in type 2 diabetics is similar among patients treated with the ACE inhibitor enalapril or the ARB telmisartan *(11)*.

There is insufficient data to comment on the effect of ARBs on cardiovascular end points in patients with diabetes. This is noteworthy because these agents are frequently used in diabetics to preserve renal function and reduce proteinuria.

The biomedical literature is conflicting with respect to the effect of dihydropyridine CCBs on cardiovascular outcomes. However, several recent randomized controlled trials have established CCBs as an effective pharmacological strategy for managing hypertension in patients with diabetes. In the subgroup of patients with diabetes mellitus in ALLHAT, amlodipine was as effective as chlorthalidone except for the end point of HF, where significantly more cases of HF developed in patients taking amlodipine. Nonetheless, the consensus of JNC 7 is that nondihydropyridine CCBs are a rational adjunctive therapy to thiazide diuretics in patients with hypertension and diabetes.

Although β-blockers are beneficial when applied as part of combination therapy, their role as initial monotherapy is less clear compared with the aforementioned agents. JNC 7 suggests that β_1-selective drugs may be preferable to nonselective β-blockers in light of a more favorable metabolic profile in the case of the former. Following publication of the JNC 7 guidelines, the Glycemic Effects in Diabetes Mellitus: Carvedilol-Metoprolol Comparison in Hypertensives (GEM-INI) study was published *(12)*. GEM-INI compared metoprolol, a β_1-selective agent, to carvedilol, a nonselective α/β-blocker, with respect to metabolic end points and found that carvedilol induced fewer, less pronounced metabolic derangements than metoprolol. However, the clinical significance of these findings is unclear (e.g., hemoglobin A1c was 0.13 points lower in carvedilol-treated patients, $p = 0.004$). In addition to causing blood glucose disturbances, β-blockers mask the epinephrine-mediated symptoms of hypoglycemia and impair glycogenolysis and gluconeogenesis, which blunts the natural response to hypoglycemia. Nevertheless, these problems are manageable and do not represent an absolute contraindication to β-blocker therapy.

Chronic Kidney Disease

Chronic kidney disease (CKD) is defined as a GFR less than 60 mL/min or the presence of albuminuria (>300 mg/d or 200 mg/g creatinine). BP should be treated more aggressively in patients with CKD, a target BP of less than 130/80 mmHg is recommended. This recommendation is based on data from the Modification of Diet in Renal Disease study, in which the rate of progression to end-stage renal disease (ESRD) among patients with proteinuria was slowest in patients with SBP below 130 mmHg. Furthermore, a meta-analysis examining this issue identified the following factors as predictors of positive outcomes in this population: (1) SBP of 110–129 mmHg, (2) albumin excretion ratio less than 1.0 g/d, and (3) treatment with an ACE inhibitor. ACE inhibitors and ARBs have been shown in multiple studies to delay the progression of CKD more effectively than other classes of antihypertensives. JNC 7 recommendations echo the sentiments of the American Society for Nephrology and the National Kidney Foundation, which endorse an ACE inhibitor or ARB in combination with a second antihypertensive, most often a diuretic (loop diuretics will be necessary in patients with more advanced disease, GFR <30 mL/min), to control BP. When there is divergence between the goals of preserving renal function and preventing cardiovascular events, risk stratification should be applied to clinical decision making. For instance, if a clinician is faced with the dilemma of selecting an antihypertensive agent that slows the progression of nephropathy and one that reduces the risk of MI, perhaps in a diabetic with proteinuria and history of MI, it is critical to evaluate the patient's risk; in this case the risk of ESRD vs a recurrent cardiovascular event.

Cerebrovascular Disease

BP control is fundamental to stroke prevention. Current data indicate that the absolute decrease in BP rather than the specific antihypertensive selected is the key for stroke risk reduction. In the Losartan Intervention for End Point Reduction study, losartan was more effective than atenolol for preventing strokes in patients with hypertension and left ventricular hypertrophy (LVH), but this benefit was not observed among African Americans, who respond less effectively to drugs that block the renin–angiotensin system. Furthermore, BP was lower throughout the trial in patients treated with losartan, which explains, in part, the reduction in stroke in this arm of the study. In ALLHAT, chlorthalidone was superior to lisinopril for the prevention of stroke; however, BP was reduced significantly more by chlorthalidone. Hence, the bottom line in stroke risk reduction is BP control, rather than any pleiotropic effect of a given antihypertensive agent.

The management of BP in the setting of acute stroke continues to be debated. In patients with acute ischemic stroke whose SBP exceeds 220 mmHg or DBP is 120–140 mmHg, cautious reduction of BP by 10–15% is suggested as a reasonable course of action. Sodium nitroprusside, administered by intravenous infusion is recommended as a first-line agent. In patients who receive thrombolytics, BP must be monitored cautiously to maintain a SBP below 180 mmHg and a DBP below 105 mmHg to minimize the risk of intracerebral hemorrhage.

OTHER CONSIDERATIONS AND COMORBIDITIES

Race

Hypertension is a multifactorial disease and its prevalence, impact, and responsiveness differ across racial and ethnic groups. Because the pathogenesis differs between these groups, it is reasonable to assume that the response to different treatments will also vary. African Americans respond particularly well to weight reduction and sodium restriction. In clinical trials, the response to monotherapy with β-blockers, ACE inhibitors, or ARBs was less pronounced in African Americans than in their white counterparts, whereas diuretics and CCBs lower BP to a similar extent regardless of race. Combining a thiazide with most other classes of antihypertensive agents appears to enhance the overall efficacy of antihypertensive treatment, such that an ACE inhibitor/hydrochlorothiazide or ARB/hydrochlorothiazide combination in an African American patient may ultimately lower BP as effectively as the same combination in other ethnic groups. Major clinical trials have not enrolled other racial or ethnic groups in sufficient numbers to evaluate the responsiveness of these populations to different therapies.

Metabolic Syndrome

JNC 7 has adopted the National Cholesterol Education Panel Adult Treatment Panel III definition of the metabolic syndrome (Table 9). Lifestyle modification is the bedrock for the clinical management of the metabolic syndrome. The goal of managing overweight and obesity is to attenuate the age-related rate of weight gain. A comprehensive lifestyle adjustment is capable of attenuating risk factors associated with the metabolic syndrome and augmenting BP control (Table 7). These include a decrease in sedentary behavior, increased physical activity, and reduction in caloric intake. The Dietary Approaches to Stop Hypertension (DASH) eating plan is particularly well suited for overweight or obese patients with hypertension. It is essential that patients recognize that weight loss of as little as 5 lb was shown to reduce cardiovascular risk by 40% in the Framingham Heart Study, and a 10% reduction in body weight can modulate disease-specific risk factors. Patients should be prescribed regular physical activity for at least 30 min/d on most days of the week. Such a program can be expected to reduce the risk of cardiovascular events by as much as 50% *(13)*.

Left Ventricular Hypertrophy

LVH is a valuable prognostic indicator because patients with LVH are substantially more likely to experience a cardiovascular event or die. Indeed, the presence of LVH confers a greater risk for mortality than does multivessel coronary disease or depressed LVEF. Regression of LVH has been shown to reduce the rate of cardiovascular events. Most antihypertensives, when given in effective doses, will induce LVH regression, weight loss, and sodium restriction. However, a hierarchy has emerged with respect to the degree in which individual antihypertensives reduce LVH, with ACE inhibitors and ARBs being the most effective, followed by diuretics and CCBs, and finally β-blockers. Two recent studies confirmed that LVH regression is associated with improved outcomes in patients with LVH at baseline, irrespective of the antihypertensive used and the BP achieved *(14,15)*. Thus, BP control, not ancillary drug effects, might be the critical determinant for LVH regression.

Table 9
Criteria Included in the Metabolic Syndrome

Presence of three or more of the following risk factors
constitutes the metabolic syndrome

Abdominal obesity
  Waist circumference >40 in. for males (>102 cm)
  Waist circumference >35 in. for females (>88 cm)
Elevated systolic or diastolic blood pressure
  ≥130 mmHg systolic and/or
  ≥85 mmHg diastolic
Insulin resistance
  Fasting glucose ≥110 mg/dL
Dyslipidemia
  Triglycerides ≥150 mg/dL
  HDL cholesterol <40 mg/dL in males or <50 mg/dL in females

HDL, high-density lipoprotein.

Peripheral Artery Disease

Hypertension is a risk factor for peripheral artery disease (PAD). PAD is independently associated with an increased risk of death from CVD. It is reasonable to assume that the presence of atherosclerosis in one vascular bed signifies the presence of atherosclerotic disease in all vascular beds (i.e., patients with PAD are likely to have CAD and cerebrovascular disease). Antihypertensive medications, including vasodilatory agents, are ineffective for alleviating symptoms of PAD or improving walking distance. β-blockers have the potential to cause vasoconstriction (owing to unopposed α_1-receptor stimulation in the presence of β-receptor blockade) and worsen symptoms in patients with intermittent claudication; nevertheless, β-blockers can be used in PAD, especially if compelling indications are present (e.g., HF). Close follow-up is essential following initiation of an ACE inhibitor or ARB because the presence of PAD increases the likelihood of renal artery stenosis.

Elderly

Elderly patients frequently display isolated systolic hypertension. Antihypertensive therapy based on thiazide-type diuretics or dihydropyridine CCBs, lower the risk of cardiovascular events in elderly patients with hypertension. A benefit has been shown even in patients over the age of 80. Meta-analysis of hypertension trials has revealed that the principal determinant of CVD outcome is BP control. Weight loss and sodium restriction are especially potent lifestyle modifications in the elderly. The same algorithm for selecting antihypertensives in the general population should be implemented in the drug selection process for geriatric populations. However, in general, elderly are more susceptible to the adverse effects of antihypertensive medications, thus warranting close follow-up and cautious dose titration. Clinicians should be cognizant of the potential for orthostatic hypotension in older hypertensive patients manifested as postural unsteadiness, dizziness, or syncope. Periodically, lying and standing BPs are indicated in all hypertensives over the age of 50.

α_1-Receptor blockers may be useful in elderly men with symptoms of urinary outflow obstruction caused by benign prostatic hypertrophy (BPH). Terazosin, doxazosin, and prazosin relax prostatic smooth muscle and bladder neck tone, thereby reducing symptoms of BPH. The ALLHAT trial originally consisted of a doxazosin treatment arm, which was discontinued early because of a marked deviation in cardiovascular risk (especially HF). Hence, although it used to be common place to use the "two-for-one" philosophy as a rationale to administer α_1-receptor blockers in men with BPH, the unfavorable cardiovascular outcomes in ALLHAT have relegated these agents to third-tier therapy, at best. It is certainly still appropriate to use α_1-receptor blockers for BPH treatment, but not as foundation therapy for hypertension.

Resistant Hypertension

Resistant hypertension is used to denote the failure to achieve goal BP in patients who are adhering to full doses of appropriate three-drug regimens, including a diuretic. Table 10 lists potential causes of resistant hypertension. If resistant hypertension is not corrected after these underlying factors have been ruled out, and if a secondary cause of hypertension is absent, consultation with a hypertension specialist is indicated.

Women

Women with hypertension should be treated similar to men. However, several considerations are noteworthy. ACE inhibitors and ARBs are contraindicated in pregnant women or women intending to become pregnant and should be used cautiously in women of childbearing age. Elderly women may benefit from the calcium-sparing effect of thiazide diuretics, which have been shown in some epidemiological studies to reduce the risk for fractures.

Treatment of hypertension in pregnant women is controversial. Women with stage I hypertension can often be managed with lifestyle modifications alone. There is evidence that pharmacological lowering of BP in pregnant women increases the number of small-for-gestational-age infants. Thus, some centers opt for discontinuing or withholding antihypertensives unless absolutely necessary, whereas others use agents shown to be safe in pregnant women (Table 11). Antihypertensives should be utilized in women with pre-existing target organ damage or need for multiple antihypertensive medications prior to pregnancy. It is essential to treat severe chronic hypertension, especially in the first trimester, because high rates of fetal loss and maternal mortality have been reported in this setting. Historically,

Table 10
Potential Causes of Resistant Hypertension

Improper BP measurement
Volume overload
   Excessive sodium intake
   Fluid retention from kidney disease
   Inadequate diuretic therapy
Drug-induced (*see* Table 9)
Inadequate drug dosages
Inappropriate drug combinations
Nonadherence
Associated conditions
   Obesity
   Excessive alcohol intake
Identifiable causes of hypertension (*see* Table 3)
White-coat hypertension

Adapted from ref. *1.*

Table 11
Treatment of Chronic Hypertension in Pregnancy

Antihypertensive class	*Comment*
Methyldopa	Preferred based on long-term follow-up studies supporting safety
β-blockers	Reports of intrauterine growth retardation (atenolol)
	Generally safe
Labetalol	Increasingly preferred to methyldopa because of reduced side effects
Clonidine	Limited data
CCB	Limited data
	No increase in major teratogenicity with exposure
Diuretics	Not first-line agents
	Probably safe
ACE inhibitors	Contraindicated
ARBs	Reported fetal toxicity and death

ACE, angiotensin-converting enzyme; ARBs, angiotensin receptor blockers.
Adapted from ref. *1.*

methyldopa has been the preferred agent; however, labetalol is being used more frequently because of stable uteroplacental blood flow and fetal hemodynamics as well as the absence of long-term adverse effects on the development of children sometimes reported with exposure to methyldopa *in utero.* ACE inhibitors and ARBs are contraindicated resulting from reports of fetal toxicity and death.

All antihypertensives are excreted to some extent in breast milk. For this reason, it may be prudent to withhold antihypertensives in lieu of lifestyle changes in women who are breast-feeding. Methyldopa and hydralazine have been used without complication. Of the β-blockers, propranolol and labetalol are preferred. Diuretics should be avoided because they may reduce milk volume, and ACE inhibitors and ARBs should be avoided to protect the infant from potential renal complications.

Children and Adolescents

Lifestyle interventions should play a primary role in hypertensive children and adolescents. There should be high suspicion for identifiable causes of hypertension; however, the incidence of chronic essential hypertension is increasing in adolescents in concert with higher rates of obesity and inactivity. The recommendations for pharmacological treatment are, for the most part, similar for children and adults, although starting dosages may need to be reduced.

Erectile Dysfunction

Erectile dysfunction (ED) is associated with various antihypertensive agents. ACE inhibitors, ARBs, and CCBs have not been noted to increase the incidence of ED. Physically active, nonobese men who do not smoke have a lower incidence of ED, thus, lifestyle modification is important in reducing the risk for this complication. If ED emerges after initiation of an antihypertensive, that agent should be discontinued and an agent from another class initiated. Phosphodiesterase inhibitors (e.g., sildenafil, tadalafil, and vardenafil) can be prescribed safely in most patients provided the patient is not actively using organic nitrates in any form.

Hypertensive Urgency and Emergency

Hypertensive urgencies and emergencies are both characterized by severe elevations in BP (>180/120 mmHg). Emergencies are complicated by the presence of target organ dysfunction such as encephalopathy, intracerebral hemorrhage, acute MI, acute left ventricular failure with pulmonary edema, unstable angina, dissecting aortic aneurysm, or eclampsia. An immediate response is necessary to lower BP to a safer range. Treatment should include parenteral antihypertensive therapy with continuous monitoring in an intensive care unit. The initial goal is to lower BP by a maximum of 25% in the first hour. Over the next 2–6 h, BP can be lowered to 160/100 mmHg. In clinically stable patients who tolerate this level of BP reduction, further attempts can be made to normalize BP over 24–48 h.

Hypertensive urgencies are not associated with target organ damage, although headache, shortness of breath, epistaxis, or anxiety may occur. Patients can often be managed with oral therapies and observation. Oral short-acting agents such

Table 12
Common Drug-Induced Causes of Hypertension

Medications
  Cortico- and mineralocorticoids (e.g., prednisone)
  Estrogens (oral contraceptives more likely than hormone replacement)
  Nonsteroidal anti-inflammatory drugs, including COX-2 inhibitors
  Sympathomimetics (topical or oral decongestants)
  Pseudoepherdrine and related drugs
  Sibutramine, methylphenidate and other anorectics
  Atomoxetine
  Cyclosporine and tacrolimus
  Erythropoietin
  Ergotamine and other ergot containing preparations
  Antidepressants (especially venlafaxine and duloxetine)
  Combination therapy with clonidine and a β-blocker

Herbal and other natural products
  Nicotine, including withdrawal
  Ma huang, ephedrine
  Bitter orange
  Narcotic withdrawal

Food substances
  Sodium
  Ethanol
  Licorice (with MAO-I)

Illicit substances
  Cocaine and cocaine withdrawal
  Phenylpropanolamine analogues, "herbal ecstasy"
  Anabolic steroids
  Phencyclidine
  Ketamine

COX-2, cyclooxygenase-2; MAO-I, monoamine oxidase inhibitor.

as captopril, labetalol, or clonidine are reasonable options. The patient's maintenance antihypertensive regimen should also be re-evaluated. Patients should not leave the emergency room unless a follow-up visit within the next several days has been confirmed.

Drugs and Other Agents That Affect BP

Prescription and over-the-counter mediations, as well as herbal products, can substantially increase BP and may provoke the use of additional antihypertensive agents or unnecessary testing (Table 12). The following are indicators that a medication-induced cause of hypertension may be present: (1) loss of control of previously controlled hypertension, (2) presence of comorbidities

Table 13
Improving Hypertension Control

Provide empathetic reinforcement
Be aware of an monitor for frequent causes of nonadherence in patients
Organize care delivery systems
Educate patients about treatment
Collaborate with other health care providers
Individualize drug therapy regimens
Promote social support systems

(particularly osteoarthritis that may suggest nonsteroidal anti-inflammatory drug [NSAID] use), (3) biochemical evidence of concomitant drug usage (e.g., elevated sodium, potassium, or creatinine in patients using NSAIDs), and (4) sporadic, labile hypertension (e.g., severe, transient hypertension and chest pain accompanying cocaine abuse). Consumption of modest quantities of alcohol is unlikely to substantially affect BP. Because patients often "underestimate" alcohol consumption, it is wise for clinicians to ask for an abstinence period of several days to a week to ascertain whether alcohol is contributing to "resistant" hypertension.

Optimizing Control of Hypertension

Adherence and follow-up are critical for improving hypertension control. Motivation, communication, and empathy are integral for encouraging adherence in patients. There are multiple factors that must be implemented to optimize control of hypertension (Table 13).

SOURCES

1. The Seventh report of the Joint National Committee on Prevention, Detection, Evaluation, and Treatment of High Blood Pressure. From the National High Blood Pressure Education Program, National Heart, Lung, and Blood Institute. Available at www.nhlbi.nih.org.
2. Chobanian AV, Bakris GL, Black HR, et al. (2003) Seventh report of the Joint National Committee on Prevention, Detection, Evaluation, and Treatment of High Blood Pressure. Hypertension 42:1206–1252.
3. Chobanian AV, Bakris GL, Black HR, et al. (2003) The Seventh Report of the Joint National Committee on Prevention, Detection, Evaluation, and Treatment of High Blood Pressure: the JNC 7 report. JAMA 289:2560–2572.
4. Pepine CJ, Handberg EM, Cooper-DeHoff RM, et al. (2003) A calcium antagonist vs. a non-calcium antagonist hypertension treatment strategy for patients with coronary artery disease. The International Verapamil-Trandolapril Study (INVEST): a randomized controlled trial. JAMA 290:2805–2816.
5. Messerli FH, Kupfer S, Pepine CJ. (2005) J curve in hypertension and coronary artery disease. Am J Cardiol 95:160.
6. Pickering TG, Hall JE, Appel LJ, et al. (2005) Recommendations for blood pressure measurement in humans and experimental animals: Part 1: blood pressure measurement in humans: a statement for professionals from the Subcommittee of Professional and Public

Education of the American Heart Association Council on High Blood Pressure Research. Hypertension 45:142–161.

7. Nissen SE, Tuzcu EM, Libby P, et al. (2004) Effect of antihypertensive agents on cardio-vascular events in patients with coronary disease and normal blood pressure: the CAMELOT study: a randomized controlled trial. JAMA 292:2217–2225.

8. Pepine CJ. (2004) What is the optimal blood pressure and drug therapy for patients with coronary artery disease? JAMA 292:2271–2273.

9. Granger CB, McMurray JJ, Yusuf S, et al. (2003) Effects of candesartan in patients with chronic heart failure and reduced left-ventricular systolic function intolerant to angiotensin-converting-enzyme inhibitors: the CHARM-Alternative trial. Lancet 362:772–776.

10. UK Prospective Diabetes Study Group (1998) Tight blood pressure control and risk of macrovascular and microvascular complications in type 2 diabetes: UKPDS 38. BMJ 317: 703–713.

11. Barnett AH, Bain SC, Bouter P, et al. (2004) Angiotensin-receptor blockade versus converting-enzyme inhibition in type 2 diabetes and nephropathy. N Engl J Med 351:1952–1961.

12. Bakris GL, Fonseca V, Katholi RE, et al. (2004) Metabolic effects of carvedilol vs meto-prolol in patients with type 2 diabetes mellitus and hypertension: a randomized controlled trial. JAMA 292:2227–2236.

13. Gregg EW, Cauley JA, Stone K, et al. (2003) Relationship of changes in physical activity and mortality among older women. JAMA 289:2379–2386.

14. Devereux RB, Wachtell K, Gerdts E, et al. (2004) Prognostic significance of left ventricu-lar mass change during treatment of hypertension. JAMA 292:2350–2356.

15. Okin PM, Devereux RB, Jern S, et al. (2004) Regression of electrocardiographic left ven-tricular hypertrophy during antihypertensive treatment and the prediction of major cardio-vascular events. JAMA 292:2343–2349.

16. Pfeffer MA, McMurray JJ, Velazquez EJ, et al. (2003) Valsartan, captopril, or both in myocar-dial infarction complicated by heart failure, left ventricular dysfunction, or both. N Engl J Med 349:1893-1906.

17. Losartan (Cozaar®) prescribing information. Merck. www.cozaar.com/cozaar/shared/documents/pi_cozaar.pdf Accessed on January 6, 2005.

2

Hyperlipidemia

Andrew Cohen, MD
and Neil S. Skolnik, MD

CONTENTS

INTRODUCTION

Cardiovascular disease (CVD) remains the leading cause of overall mortality in America for both men and women. A major risk factor for CVD is hyperlipidemia, a condition referring to elevated levels of at least one of five families of plasma lipoproteins–chylomicrons, very low-density lipoproteins, intermediate-density lipoproteins, low-density lipoproteins (LDL), and high-density lipoproteins (HDL).

The guidelines for the treatment of hyperlipidemia have been dynamic, starting from initial studies to the more recent and accepted recommendations of the Third Report of the Expert Panel on Detection, Evaluation, and Treatment of High Blood Cholesterol in Adults *(1)*. Additionally, since the findings of Adult Treatment Panel III, five major clinical trials have been recognized and have subsequently enriched the guidelines further. These studies include the Heart Protection Study (HPS), the Prospective Study of Pravastatin in the Elderly at Risk (PROSPER), the Antihypertensive and Lipid-Lowering Treatment to Prevent

From: *Current Clinical Practice: Essential Practice Guidelines in Primary Care*
Edited by: N. S. Skolnik © Humana Press, Totowa, NJ

Heart Attack trial—lipid-lowering trial, the Anglo-Scandinavian Cardiac Outcomes Trial—lipid-lowering arm, and the Pravastatin or Atorvastatin Evaluation and Infection—Thrombolysis in Myocardial Infarction 22 trial (PROVE-IT—TIMI 22) *(2)*.

Screening

Universal screening for hyperlipidemia is recommended for all persons aged 20 or older. Screening should consist of a fasting lipoprotein profile, which includes total cholesterol (TC), LDL-cholesterol, HDL-cholesterol, and triglyceride (TG) levels. Blood work should be obtained every 5 yr, unless otherwise indicated.

If the specimen that is collected is nonfasting, only TC and HDL-cholesterol are valid. If the TC is greater than 200 or the HDL cholesterol is less than 40, then a follow-up fasting lipid profile should be performed. Much of the guidelines revolve around LDL-cholesterol, and therefore a follow-up fasting profile is recommended for formal evaluation.

Table 1
Classification

Total cholesterol (mg/dL)	Category
<200	Desirable
200–239	Borderline high
>240	High

LDL-cholesterol (mg/dL)	Category
<100	Optimal
100–129	Near optimal
130–159	Borderline high
160–189	High
>190	Very high

HDL-cholesterol (mg/dL)	Category
<40	Low, increases cardiac risk
40–60	Normal
>60	High, decreases cardiac risk

RISK CATEGORIES AND TARGET LDL-CHOLESTEROL

The treatment of LDL-cholesterol is not solely based on its value. For instance, a healthy 25-yr-old female with an LDL of 174 should be treated differently than a 75-yr-old male with a history of hypertension and stroke having the same LDL. Thus, in addition to the number, treatment is also guided by cardiac risk factors. These risk factors are as follows:

Major cardiac risk factors that modify LDL goals:

- Age
  - Male >45, female >55
- Family history of premature coronary disease in first-degree relative.
  - Male <55, female <65.
- Cigarette smoking.
- Hypertension.
- Low HDL-cholesterol (<40).

Notes:

- High HDL-cholesterol (>60) counts as a negative risk factor 1.
- Diabetes mellitus counts as an independent coronary heart disease equivalent, not merely a risk factor.

Appropriate LDL-cholesterol levels exist for individual patients based on these cardiac risk factors. In patients without coronary disease, having fewer than two cardiac risk factors confers a low risk. For this group, a goal LDL of less than 160 exists.

Having two or more cardiac risk factors confers a moderate to a moderately high risk. For these patients, as further described later, the Framingham score should be used to distinguish those at higher risk. For both of these risk groups, the goal LDL is below 130. However, for those with a moderately high-risk class, or a 10-yr risk of between 10 and 20% based on Framingham, a stronger emphasis is placed on pharmacotherapy.

In patients with a history of coronary disease, or for those with a coronary heart disease equivalent, which is defined as a 10-yr risk of developing a coronary heart event or recurrent event of more than 20%, a goal LDL of less than 100 has been established.

Coronary heart disease includes:

- Myocardial infarction.
- Unstable angina.
- .Evidence of underlying myocardial ischemia.
- Status-post angioplasty or bypass surgery.

Coronary heart disease equivalents include:

- Peripheral arterial disease.

- Abdominal aortic aneurysm.
- Symptomatic carotid artery disease (transient ischemic attack [TIA]/ cerebrovascular accident [CVA] from carotid origin; >50% carotid occlusion).
- Diabetes mellitus.
- Multiple coronary risk factors that confer a 10-yr risk for disease greater than 20% based on Framingham results.

Since the release of ATP III, an optimal LDL goal of less than 70 has been established for those at very high risk, which includes those with established coronary heart disease plus either:

- Multiple major risk factors, especially diabetes.
- Severe and poorly controlled risk factors, especially active cigarette smoking.
- Multiple risk factors of the metabolic syndrome.
- Acute coronary syndrome (ACS).

TREATMENT OF LDL-CHOLESTEROL

The major options for LDL-lowering therapy include therapeutic lifestyle changes (TLCs) and pharmacotherapy. TLCs remain an essential modality in the clinical management of hyperlipidemia and should be initiated for all patients not at goal LDL. In addition, any person at even moderately high risk who has lifestyle-related risk factors (obesity, physical inactivity, elevated TG, low HDL-cholesterol, or metabolic syndrome) is a candidate for TLC to modify these risk factors, regardless of LDL-cholesterol level.

TLC has the potential to reduce cardiovascular risk through several mechanisms beyond purely lowering LDL. The TLC diet emphasizes dietary restriction of saturated fats (<7% of total calories) and cholesterol (<200 mg daily). In addition, weight reduction and increased physical activity are recommended. Physicians are encouraged to refer patients to registered dieticians or other qualified nutritionists.

After 6 wk of TLC, LDL-cholesterol should be remeasured. If the goal has not been achieved, other options should be considered to further lower LDL, such as adding plant stanol/sterols (2 g/d) and viscous soluble fiber (10–25 g/d).

Pharmacotherapy provides the other option in the treatment of elevated LDL-cholesterol. This option should be considered for all patients who have not achieved target levels after TLC implementation.

When LDL-lowering drug therapy is initiated, the intensity of therapy should be aimed at achieving at least a 30–40% reduction in LDL. In patients without coronary disease or the equivalent, recommendations for consideration of drug therapy are again based on the number of cardiac risk factors. For patients with fewer than two risk factors, whose goal LDL is less than 160, drug therapy should be considered when LDL is 190 or higher. Clinical judgment is recommended when LDL is between 160 and 189. Calculation of 10-yr coronary risk is not useful in this group.

For those with two or more risk factors, the Framingham Coronary Risk Assessment Score has been developed to identify individuals at a higher risk, in which consideration should be given to more intensive treatment. The ATP III stratification system uses Framingham calculations to divide persons into those with 10-yr risks for coronary disease of more than 20%, between 10 and 20%, and less than 10%. Scoring calculators can be found in this chapter, on the Internet (at www.nhlbi.nih.gov/guidelines/cholesterol), and for PDAs.

For all patients with two or more risk factors, target LDL-cholesterol is less than 130, as described earlier. For those with a 10-yr risk of less than 10% based on Framingham, drug therapy should be considered when LDL is 160 or more. However, for those with a 10-yr risk of 10–20%, consideration should be given for earlier pharmacotherapy, when LDL is 130 or more. Clinical judgment is reserved for those individuals with LDL levels between 100 and 129; an LDL goal of less than 100 is an option based on the available clinical trial evidence.

In patients with established coronary disease, or risk equivalents, including a 10-yr risk of more than 20%, therapy is favored when LDL is 100 or more. Clinical judgment is recommended for patients whose baseline LDL is less than 100 prior to treatment. Optimal LDL goal for those at very high risk is less than 70. This recommendation evolved from the findings of the PROVE-IT and HPS trials. The PROVE-IT trial evaluated intensive LDL lowering in patients with ACS with high-dose atorvastatin (80 mg/d) against standard-dose pravastatin (40 mg/d). Whereas pravastatin 40 mg lowered median LDL from 106 to 95, atorvastatin 80 mg lowered the median to 62 and was associated with a statistically significant reduction in major cardiovascular events in only 2 yr. The HPS trial found that in a population of high-risk patients with coronary disease, other occlusive arterial disease, or diabetes, with a baseline LDL of less than 116, even in the subgroup with LDL less than 100, there was significant risk reduction with statin therapy. Thus, LDL-cholesterol of 70 seems preferable for very high-risk patients compared with an LDL of 100. In the past, there has been some concern regarding the potential dangers of lowering LDL-cholesterol to very low levels. Early epidemiological studies suggested that very low serum cholesterol levels are associated with an increase in total mortality, largely because of cerebral hemorrhage. This has not been supported in recent clinical trials with statin therapy. No significant side effects from LDL lowering have been formally identified to date. The decision to achieve very low LDL levels in very high-risk patients should be based on clear evidence of benefit with current lack of evidence of harm.

Statins (HMG-CoA reductase inhibitors) are the drugs of choice for elevated LDL, not only for their LDL-reduction capability but also for their anti-inflammatory properties and because of the strength of clinical trial evidence

Table 2
ATP III LDL-Cholesterol Goals and Cutpoints for TLC and Drug Therapy
in Different Risk Categories and Proposed Modifications Based on Recent Clinical
Trial Evidence *(3)*

Risk category	LDL goal	Initiate TLC	Consider drug therapy
High risk: CHD or CHD risk equivalent (10 yr risk >20%)	100 mg/dL (optional goal <70 mg/dL)	≤100 mg/dL	≥100 mg/dL (consider if <100 mg/dL)
Moderately high risk: 2 + risk factors (10 yr risk 10–20%)	<130 mg/dL (optional LDL goal <100 mg/dL)	≥130 mg/dL	≥130 mg/dL (consider drug therapy if 100–129 mg/dL)
Moderate risk: 2 + risk factors (10 yr risk <10%)	<130 mg/dL	≥130 mg/dL	≥160 mg/dL
Lower risk: 0–1 risk factors	<160 mg/dL	≥160 mg/dL	≥190 mg/dL (optional if 160–189 mg/dL)

CHD, Coronary heart disease.

supporting their use. When statin therapy is introduced, the goal should be a reduction in LDL by at least 30–40%. Numerous statins are on the market, each with varying degrees of efficacy.

Table 3
Doses of Statin Required to Obtain a 30–40% LDL-Cholesterol Reduction

Drug	Dose (mg/d)	LDL reduction (%)
Atorvastatin	10	39
Lovastatin	40	31
Pravastatin	40	34
Simvastatin	20–40	35–41
Fluvastatin	40–80	25–35
Rosuvastatin	5–10	39–45

Alternative classes of antihyperlipidemia therapy include nicotinic acid, bile–acid sequestrants, and ezetimibe. These agents should be considered as second-line therapies or, perhaps, first-line therapy for those with intolerance to statins. In addition, some of these agents may be more beneficial should dyslipidemia (depressed HDL, elevated TG) rather than hyperlipidemia exist.

After 6 wk starting pharmacotherapy, LDL should be remeasured. If goal has been achieved, the patient should continue on the present dose. Otherwise, LDL-lowering therapy can be intensified by increasing the dose of the primary medication, or by adding a second medication. If after 12 wk of therapy, LDL levels are not at goal, further intensification should be pursued. Referral to a lipid specialist should be considered if goal LDL is unobtainable.

SPECIAL CONSIDERATIONS

Diabetes

According to ATP III guidelines, patients carrying the diagnosis of diabetes are considered to have an independent coronary heart disease equivalent, not just a risk factor. In the HPS, higher-risk populations of patients with diabetes or other occlusive arterial disease were found to have a risk for coronary events, which was approximately that of nondiabetic patients with established coronary disease. Therefore, for these patients, optimal LDL is less than 100.

However, not all patients with diabetes can be considered to have a 10-yr cardiac risk of more than 20%. For example, an otherwise healthy 20-yr-old male with type 1 diabetes would not be expected to have a significant 10-yr risk. This potentially lower-risk patient was not studied in the HPS; however, and so no formal data have been collected. A potential option remains to use clinical judgment about whether to initiate LDL-lowering therapy if this patient's baseline LDL is below 130. Of note, maximal TLC therapy is clearly indicated.

In the HPS, patients with both diabetes and coronary disease had a very high risk for recurrent coronary disease. This category of patient benefited greatly from statin therapy and thus the data suggests initiation of a statin regardless of baseline LDL levels. For this very high-risk class, optimal LDL is less than 70.

Metabolic Syndrome

The metabolic syndrome, a disease characterized by increased insulin resistance and therefore increased risk for coronary heart disease, is defined by meeting at least three of the following five criteria:

1. Abdominal obesity (males >40 in., females >35 in.).
2. Elevated TG (>150 mg/dL).
3. Depressed HDL (males <40 mg/dL, females <50 mg/dL).
4. Blood pressure above 130/85 mmHg.
5. Impaired fasting glucose (>110 mg/dL).

Treatment of the metabolic syndrome involves TLC therapy (weight reduction and increased physical activity) in an effort to manage the disorder (abdominal obesity, hypertension, depressed HDL), but also to gain control of LDL-cholesterol.

Low HDL-Cholesterol

Low HDL-cholesterol is a strong independent risk factor for heart disease. ATP III specifies low HDL-cholesterol as being a level below 40 mg/dL, a change from the level of 35 mg/dL that was described in ATP II. ATP III does no specify a goal for appropriate elevation of HDL because there is currently no sufficient evidence to define the degree to which HDL should be raised by treatment and available drugs have not been studied sufficiently to make recommendations regarding their use for raising HDL-cholesterol. Reduction of LDL-cholesterol remains the main goal of treatment. Low HDL modifies the risk category, which is assigned to determine goal LDL level.

For all persons with depressed HDL levels, the primary target of therapy remains LDL. After the LDL goal has been attained, emphasis should shift to weight reduction and increased physical activity.

If TGs are between 200 and 499, goal should be to achieve non-HDL goal cholesterol, which is set at 30 mg/dL more than LDL-cholesterol goals. If TGs are less than 200, meaning that the dyslipidemia is solely isolated to low HDL, drugs for HDL raising can be considered. These drugs include nicotinic acid or fibrates. Pharmacotherapy for isolated low HDL is mostly reserved for persons with coronary disease or risk equivalents.

Elevated Serum Triglycerides

Elevated serum TGs are also considered an independent risk factor for coronary disease.

Table 5
Classification of Triglycerides

Serum triglycerides (mg/dL)	Category
<150	Normal
150–199	Borderline high
200–499	High
>500	Very high

Remember that the primary treatment of elevated TGs is to reach LDL goal. Any borderline TGs should be addressed through TLC therapy (weight reduction, increased physical activity). After goal LDL is reached, a secondary goal for non-HDL-cholesterol of 30 mg/dL higher than that of the LDL-cholesterol should be set. Note that non-HDL-cholesterol is the TC–HDL.

For those with high TGs, non-HDL-cholesterol becomes a secondary target for therapy. Weight reduction and increased physical activity should be implemented. Pharmacotherapy can be considered in high-risk persons to achieve the non-HDL-cholesterol goal. This can be achieved by intensifying therapy with an LDL-lowering drug, or by adding nicotinic acid or a fibrate.

The immediate goal of therapy for the patient with very high TGs is to prevent acute pancreatitis through TG lowering. This is usually done through a TG-lowering agent (fibrate or nicotinic acid) in addition to weight reduction, increased physical activity, and a very low-fat diet (15% of total caloric intake). Only after TG levels have fallen to below 500 should LDL lowering be targeted to reduce cardiac risk.

OLDER AND YOUNGER ADULTS

Most cardiovascular events occur in individuals older than 65 yr of age. Elevated LDL-cholesterol and low HDL-cholesterol are predictive for the development of coronary disease in the elderly as well as in the young. ATP III states that older persons should not be denied the benefits of LDL-lowering therapy accorded to other age groups. This recommendation has additional support through both the HPS and the PROSPER trials, which demonstrated that intensive lipid-lowering management for elderly patients with established coronary disease yields similar outcomes as that achieved in younger populations.

Older patients, in general, are at higher risk of developing coronary disease than are younger patients. Quantitative risk assessment in elderly patients without established coronary disease is not as reliable as it is in younger patients. Clinical judgment is therefore recommended when deciding on lipid-lowering therapy. A host of factors must be weighed for these patients, including efficacy, safety, and tolerability. Of note, both the PROSPER and Anglo-Scandinavian Cardiac Outcomes Trial support the efficacy of statin therapy in older, high-risk persons without established CVD.

For all younger adults (males age 20–35, females age 20–45), TLC should be instituted and emphasized when LDL levels surpass 130. Particular attention should be given to young males who smoke and have a high LDL (160–189), as they may be candidates for earlier intervention with LDL-lowering drugs. When young adults have very high LDL levels (>190), pharmacotherapy should be considered, as in other adults.

ADDITIONAL STUDIES SINCE GUIDELINE PUBLICATION

Subsequent to the publication of the 2004 update to ATP III, two trials have been published that futher support intensive treatment of LDL-cholesterol. The Collaborative Atorvastatin in Diabetes Study (CARDS) looked at middle-aged patients with type 2 diabetes without pre-existing cardiovascular disease and at least one other cardiovascular risk factor and mean baseline LDL of 117 (4). Results of CARDS showed that in this group of patients with diabetes and a low LDL-cholesterol, treatment with atorvastatin 10 mg, led to a decrease in first cardiovascular events including MI and stoke. This study, along with the results of the HPS led the American Diabetes Association *(5)* to recommend that all patients older than 40 yr old with diabetes and with a TC over 135 mg/dL be treated with a statin to reduce LDL-cholesterol by 30–40%.

The Treating to New Targets study looked at patients with cardiovascular disease who where already on a statin, and randomized patients to atorvastatin 10 mg vs atorvastatin 80 mg. During the wash-in period, when all patients received atorvastin 10 mg, the mean LDL-cholesterol level was 98 mg/dL. Over the 4.9 yr of the study, there was a relative decrease in cardiovascular events of of 22% (absolute decrease –2.2%) in the group of patients randomized to atorvastatin 80 mg.

In summary, these two studies, both published since the most recent update to ATP III, lend further support to the recommendations of ATP III to pursue aggressive lipid lowering with a target goal consideration of an LDL-cholesterol of less than 70 mg/dL.

SOURCES

1. Detection, Evaluation, and Treatment of High Blood Cholesterol in Adults (ATP III)—NIH publication number 01-3670, May 2001.
2. LaRosa JC, et al. (2005) Intensive lipid lowering with Atorvastatin in patients with stable coronary disease. N Engl J Med 352:1425–1435.
3. Grundy SM (2004) Implications of recent clinical trials for the National Cholesterol Education Program Adult Treatment Panel (III). Circulation 110:227.
4. Colhoun HM, et al. (2004) Collaborative Atorvastatin diabetes study (CARDS). Lancet 364:685–696.
5. Standards of Medical Care in Diabetes American Diabetes Association (2005) Diabetes Care 28:S4–S36.

APPENDIX

Framingham Coronary Risk Assessment Male Based on LDL-Cholesterol

Step 1			Step 2			Step 3		
Age		*Points*	*LDL-cholesterol*		*Points*	*HDL-cholesterol*		*Points*
30–34		–1	<100		–3	<35		2
35–39		0	100–129		0	35–44		1
40–44		1	130–159		0	44–49		0
45–49		2	160–189		1	50–59		0
50–54		3	>190		2	>60		–1
55–59		4						
60–64		5						
65–69		6						
70–74		7						

Step 4

	Blood pressure				
Systolic		*Diastolic*			
	<80	80–84	85–89	90–99	>100
<120	0 pts	–	–	–	–
120–129	–	0 pts	–	–	–
130–139	–	–	1 pts	–	–
140–159	–	–	–	2 pts	–
>160	–	–	–	–	3 pts

When systolic and diastolic measures provide different point scores, use the higher number.

Step 5		Step 6		Step 7
Diabetes	*Points*	*Smoker*	*Points*	Add up all of the points
No	0	No	0	
Yes	2	Yes	2	

Step 8		Step 8 *(Continued)*	
Coronary heart disease risk		*Point total*	*10-Yr risk (%)*
Point total	*10-Yr risk (%)*	5	9
≤–3	1	6	11
–2	2	7	14
–1	2	8	18
0	3	9	22
1	4	10	27
2	4	11	33
3	6	12	40
4	7	13	47
		≥14	≥56

(Continued)

Framingham Coronary Risk Assessment Male Based on Total Cholesterol

Step 1			Step 2			Step 3	
Age	Points		Total cholesterol	Points		HDL-cholesterol	Points
30–34	–1		<160	–3		<35	2
35–39	0		160–199	0		35–44	1
40–44	1		200–239	1		44–49	0
45–49	2		240–279	2		50–59	0
50–54	3		>280	3		>60	–2
55–59	4						
60–64	5						
65–69	6						
70–74	7						

Step 4

	Blood pressure				
Systolic	Diastolic				
	<80	80–84	85–89	90–99	>100
<120	0 pts	–	–	–	–
120–129	–	0 pts	–	–	–
130–139	–	–	1 pts	–	–
140–159	–	–	–	2 pts	–
>160	–	–	–	–	3 pts

When systolic and diastolic measures provide different point scores, use the higher number.

Step 5			Step 6			Step 7
Diabetes	Points		Smoker	Points		Add up all of the points
No	0		No	0		
Yes	2		Yes	2		

Step 8

Coronary heart disease risk		Step 8 (Continued)	
Point total	10-Yr risk (%)	Point total	10-Yr risk (%)
≤ –1	2	6	10
0	3	7	13
1	3	8	16
2	4	9	20
3	5	10	25
4	7	11	31
5	8	12	37
		13	45
		≥14	≥53

(Continued)

Framingham Coronary Risk Assessment Female Based on LDL-Cholesterol

Step 1		Step 2		Step 3	
Age	Points	LDL-cholesterol	Points	HDL-cholesterol	Points
30–34	–9	<100	–2	<35	5
35–39	–4	100–129	0	35–44	2
40–44	0	130–159	0	44–49	1
45–49	3	160–189	2	50–59	0
50–54	6	>190	2	>60	–2
55–59	7				
60–64	8				
65–69	8				
70–74	8				

Step 4

	Blood pressure				
Systolic	Diastolic				
	<80	80–84	85–89	90–99	>100
<120	–3 pts	–	–	–	–
120–129	–	0 pts	–	–	–
130–139	–	–	0 pts	–	–
140–159	–	–	–	2 pts	–
>160	–	–	–	–	3 pts

When systolic and diastolic measures provide different point scores, use the higher number.

Step 5		Step 6		Step 7
Diabetes	Points	Smoker	Points	Add up all of the points
No	0	No	0	
Yes	4	Yes	2	

Step 8

Coronary heart disease risk	
Point total	10-Yr risk (%)
≤–2	1
–1	2
0	2
1	2
2	3
3	3
4	4
5	5
6	6

(Continued)

Step 8 (Continued)

Point total	10-Yr risk (%)
7	7
8	8
9	9
10	11
11	13
12	15
13	17
14	20
15	24
16	27
≥17	≥32

Framingham Coronary Risk Assessment Female Based on Total Cholesterol

Step 1		Step 2		Step 3	
Age	Points	Total cholesterol	Points	HDL-cholesterol	Points
30–34	–9	<160	–2	<35	5
35–39	–4	160–199	0	35–44	2
40–44	0	200–239	1	45–49	1
45–49	3	240–279	1	50–59	0
50–54	6	>280	3	>60	–3
55–59	7				
60–64	8				
65–69	8				
70–74	8				

Step 4

Blood pressure					
Systolic	Diastolic				
	<80	80–84	85–89	90–99	>100
<120	–3 pts	–	–	–	–
120–129	–	0 pts	–	–	–
130–139	–	–	0 pts	–	–
140–159	–	–	–	2 pts	–
>160	–	–	–	–	3 pts

When systolic and diastolic measures provide different point scores, use the higher number.

Step 5		Step 6		Step 7
Diabetes	Points	Smoker	Points	Add up all of the points
No	0	No	0	
Yes	4	Yes	2	

Step 8

Coronary heart disease risk		Step 8 (Continued)	
Point total	10-Yr risk (%)	Point total	10-Yr risk (%)
≤ –2	1	7	6
–1	2	8	7
0	2	9	8
1	2	10	10
2	3	11	11
3	3	12	13
4	4	13	15
5	4	14	18
6	5	15	20
(Continued)		16	24
		≥17	≥ 27

3

Management of Newly Diagnosed Atrial Fibrillation

A Clinical Practice Guideline From the American Academy of Family Physicians and the American College of Physicians

Jaya Udayasankar, MD and Doron Schneider, MD

Contents

INTRODUCTION

Atrial fibrillation (AF) is a common cardiac arrhythmia. The prevalence of AF increases progressively with age, ranging from about 1% for those under 60 yr

From: *Current Clinical Practice: Essential Practice Guidelines in Primary Care*
Edited by: N. S. Skolnik © Humana Press, Totowa, NJ

of age and increases to more than 8% for those over 80 yr of age. AF is more common in males, with the age-adjusted incidence for women being about half that of men. AF can occur in both the normal heart and the structurally abnormal heart. The cardiac conditions most commonly associated with AF are rheumatic mitral valve disease, ischemic heart disease, congestive cardiomyopathy, and hypertension. Other causes include hyperthyroidism, hypoxic conditions, and alcohol intoxication. The most widely accepted theory in the pathogenesis of AF is believed to be multiple re-entry wavelet mechanism. Patients with AF may be asymptomatic or have symptoms such as palpitations, light-headedness, shortness of breath, and poor exercise tolerance. Some symptoms are related to reduction of cardiac output. Patients with AF are at increased risk for systemic thromboembolism. The absolute risk for stroke is dependent on comorbidities and can range from 1 to 15% per year. The goals in the treatment of AF are to reduce the risk of stroke or other systemic embolus, control the symptoms of palpitations, and improve exercise tolerance.

The American College of Cardiology (ACC)/American Heart Association (AHA)/European Society of Cardiology Task Force on Clinical Guidelines for the Management of classified AF into four types: first detected episode, paroxysmal (terminates spontaneously), persistent (electrical or pharmacological termination necessary), and permanent (resistant to electrical or pharmacological conversion or accepted by the physician). The ACC/AHA has recommended using the term "first detected atrial fibrillation" depending on when it was first clinically detected, either by the first onset of symptoms or electrocardiographic evidence of AF. For instances in which the patient is not able to recall symptoms at the onset of the arrhythmia, there can be uncertainty about the duration of the episode and about previous undetected episodes (1).

Guideline

This guideline reflects recommendations on the management strategy for adults with first-detected AF. These recommendations do not apply to patients with class 4 heart failure already taking antiarrhythmic medication, postoperative or postmyocardial infarction AF, or AF in patients with valvular heart disease. The main objective of this guideline is to provide evidence-based guidelines for the practicing internist or family physician for the management of newly detected AF in the adult patient.

A joint American Academy of Family Physicians/American College of Physicians panel (using the Guyatt Approach to Grading Recommendations; *see* Table 1) made recommendations in the following areas: rate vs rhythm control, stroke prevention and anticoagulation, electrical cardioversion vs pharmacological cardioversion, and the role of transesophageal echocardiography (TEE) in guiding therapy and maintenance therapy.

Table 1
Guyatt Approach to Grading Recommendations

Grade	Clarity of risk/benefit	Strength of supporting evidence	Strength of recommendation/ implication
1A	Clear	Randomized trials without important limitation	Strong; applies to most patients in most circumstances
1B	Clear	Randomized trials without important limitation	Strong; likely to apply to most patients
1C	Clear	No randomized controlled trial pertaining to this patient but results from randomized controlled trial including different patients, extrapolated to the patient, under consideration. Overwhelming evidence from observational studies	Strong; can apply to most patients in most circumstances
1C+	Clear	Observational studies	Intermediate; may change when stronger evidence becomes available
2A	Unclear	Randomized trials without important limitations	Intermediate; best action may differ depending on social, patient's value, or circumstances
2B	Unclear	Randomized trials without important limitations	Weak; alternative; approaches may be better for some patients under some circumstances
2C	Unclear	Observational studies	Very weak; other alternatives may be reasonable

RATE CONTROL VS RHYTHM CONTROL

An initial question faced by practitioners is the choice of maintaining rate or attempting to re-establish normal rhythm. This decision must weigh morbidity and mortality data as well as quality-of-life data that are now available from recent clinical trials.

The Atrial Fibrillation Follow-Up Investigation of Rhythm Management Trial (AFFIRM) compared rhythm vs rate control. More than 4000 patients with AF who were at least 65 yr of age or who had risk factors for stroke or death, such as diabetes, coronary artery disease (CAD), hypertension, poor ventricular function, or previous stroke were studied for a mean of 3.5 yr. Anticoagulation was recommended in both arms (although discontinuation was permitted in the cardioversion arm after 4 wk of antiarrhythmic therapy). Physicians were allowed to select pharmacological or nonpharmacological therapies to achieve sinus rhythm. The prevalence of the sinus rhythm in the rhythm-control group was 82, 73, and 63% at 1, 3, and 5 yr, whereas sinus rhythm in the rate-control group was 34.6% at 5 yr. Overall mortality, the Primary End Point of the AFFIRM trial was not different between the two groups. A higher risk of death as noted in the rhythm-control group for patients with CAD, congestive heart failure (CHF), and in the elderly. Although stroke rates did not differ between the two groups, 70% of all strokes occurred in patients who had stopped receiving anticoagulation or who had subtherapeutic international normalized ratio (INR <2). More hospitalizations were reported in the rhythm-control group ($p < 0.001$).

A smaller study conducted in Europe called the Rate Control vs Electrical Cardioversion study, randomly assigned 522 patients to either aggressive rhythm control or rate control. About 64% patients were men, 49% had hypertension, and 27% had CAD. Eligibility criteria consisted of persistent AF lasting less than 1 yr and failure of at least one previous electrical cardioversion. There was no difference between the two groups in the primary end point, which was a composite of cardiovascular mortality, heart failure, thromboembolic complications, bleeding, pacemaker implantation, and severe side effects of antiarrhythmic drugs. In *post hoc* analysis, rate control was superior for patients with hypertension and women.

Another small study, the Pharmacological Intervention in Atrial Fibrillation trial randomly assigned 252 patients aged between 18 and 75 yr with new-onset or permanent symptomatic AF to rate control with diltiazem or conversion to sinus rhythm and its maintenance with amiodarone. The primary end point was symptomatic improvement. The study outcomes were similar in both groups including symptom relief and quality-of-life measures. Hospital admissions were more frequent in the rhythm-control group.

In the Strategies of Treatment of Atrial Fibrillation trial, patients were randomly assigned into two groups: those with short-term anticoagulation after attempted conversion with antiarrhythmic therapy to prevent AF recurrence or a rate-control group with long-term anticoagulation. After 19.6 mo, the annual incidence of the primary end points of death, stroke, transient ischemic attacks, and thromboembolism was similar in the two groups. Only 40% of patients in the rhythm-control group were in sinus rhythm at the end of 1 yr, despite aggressive attempts. In the rhythm-control group, all the thromboembolic end points occurred in patients while they were in AF. It also highlights the fact that a substantial number of patients cannot maintain sinus rhythm despite aggressive conversion methods.

All the trials consistently showed no improvement in mortality or morbidity by aggressively controlling rhythm as opposed to rate control. Moreover, patients randomly assigned to aggressive rhythm control with brief anticoagulation post-cardioversion consistently have more hospitalizations, adverse drug events, and frequently do not maintain sinus rhythm. The population studied in the earlier trials did have sufficient representation in certain subgroups of patients, such as younger patients with healthy hearts, therefore, it is not certain whether these groups may benefit from more aggressive rhythm or rate control.

Recommendation 1

For the majority of patients with AF, rate control with chronic anticoagulation is the preferred treatment modality. Rhythm control has not been shown to be superior to rate control with anticoagulation in reducing morbidity and mortality and may be inferior to rate control in certain patient subgroups. Rhythm control is appropriate when based on other considerations, such as patients' preference, symptom, and exercise tolerance (grade 2A).

PREVENTION OF SYSTEMIC EMBOLIZATION: ROLE OF ANTICOAGULATION IN ATRIAL FIBRILLATION

Meta-analysis of the primary prevention studies reported on the pooled efficacy (prevention of stroke and peripheral embolism) and safety (major and minor bleeding events) of warfarin vs placebo, aspirin vs placebo, and warfarin vs aspirin.

Warfarin is more efficacious than placebo for primary stroke prevention (odds ratio [OR] 0.3 [95% confidence interval {CI}, 0.19–0.48]). There is a concurrent increase in warfarin-related risk of major bleeding (OR, 1.90 [CI, 0.89–4]).

Aspirin performs better than placebo in the prevention of primary stroke (OR, 0.68 [CI 0.46–1.02]), with an inconclusive difference for bleeding risk (OR, 0.82 [CI, 0.37–1.78]). Warfarin has been found to be more efficacious than aspirin for stroke prevention (OR, 0.66 [CI, 0.45–0.99]), with inconclusive evidence for difference in major bleeding (OR, 1.6 [CI, 0.75–3.44]).

Adjusted-dose warfarin is more superior for stroke prevention than low-dose warfarin (OR, 0.52 [CI, 0.25–1.08]) or low-dose warfarin combined with aspirin (OR, 0.44 [CI, 0.14–1.39]) but it increased major bleeding (OR, 1.4 [CI, 0.72–2.7]).

Two trials of secondary prevention evaluated warfarin or aspirin. In one trial, it was found that among the warfarin-eligible patients, warfarin was more efficacious for stroke prevention (OR, 0.38 [CI, 0.22–0.66]) but led to more episodes of major bleeding (OR, 4.1 [CI, 1.2–14]; $p = 0.029$) than did placebo.

The absolute reduction in stroke rate with warfarin as opposed to aspirin was greater in older than in younger patients (15/1000 person-years vs 5.5/1000 person-years, respectively). The evidence suggests that aspirin may be useful for persons with a low risk for stroke. Regarding the use of other antithrombotic agents, there is insufficient evidence in the literature. There is insufficient evidence for the use of low-molecular-weight, low-dose warfarin, or newer antiplatelet agents. Depending on the individual's risk for stroke and bleeding, evidence is sufficient to support the use of warfarin or aspirin. Aspirin may be useful for patients with AF who are at low risk for stroke.

When anticoagulation is appropriate, continuation is generally recommended regardless of return to normal sinus.

Recommendation 2

Patients with AF should receive chronic anticoagulation with adjusted-dose warfarin (INR 2:3), unless they are at low risk of stroke or have a specific contraindication for warfarin (thrombocytopenia, recent surgery or trauma, alcoholism) (grade 1A).

Clinical prediction rules for estimating stroke risk based on existing literature have been designed and validated. One such tool called CHADS2 uses the conventional risk factors for stroke, including "C" for CHF (active within the past 100 d or documented by echocardiography); "H" for hypertension (systolic or diastolic); "A" for old age (at least 75 yr); "D" for diabetes mellitus, "S" for history of stroke or transient ischemic attack. Each risk factor is assigned one point except stroke or transient ischemic attack, which is assigned two points. Risk of stroke is stratified by total score and reflected in the Table 2.

EFFICACY OF DIFFERENT AGENTS IN THE CONTROL OF VENTRICULAR RATE IN ATRIAL FIBRILLATION

The most commonly used drugs for rate control are β-blockers, digoxin, and calcium channel blockers. Evidence-based reports assessing 17 different agents from 48 trials were reviewed. Main outcome measures consist of mean heart rate at rest, maximum heart rate with exercise, and distance or time walked on the exercise test. Comparisons of digoxin with placebo were inconsistent, particularly during exercise. Diltiazem and verapamil are more effective than placebo or digoxin in reducing the ventricular rate at rest and during exercise. Although atenolol and metoprolol were found effective in controlling rest and exercise heart rate, results with other β-blockers were less consistent. Studies of combinations found that digoxin plus diltiazem, digoxin plus atenolol, and digoxin plus betaxolol were effective both at rest and with exercise. Combination therapy should only be employed when single-agent regimens have failed. Labetalol

Table 2
Risk for Stroke Stratified by CHADS2 Score

CHADS2 Score	Adjusted stroke rate (95% CI)	CHADS2 Risk level
0	1.9 (1.2–3)	Low
1	2.8 (2–3.8)	Low
2	4 (3.1–5.1)	Moderate
3	5.9 (4.6–7.3)	Moderate
4	8.5 (6.3–11.1)	High
5	12.5 (8.2–17.5)	High
6	18.2 (10.5–27.4)	High

combined with digoxin was effective only with exertion. Side-effect profile should be considered when selecting agents for rate control.

Recommendation 3

For patients with AF, the following drugs are recommended for their demonstrated efficacy in rate control during exercise and rest: atenolol, metoprolol, diltiazem, and verapamil. Digoxin is only effective for rate control at rest and could be used as a second-line agent for rate control in AF (grade 1B).

ACUTE CONVERSION TO SINUS RHYTHM: EFFICACY OF ELECTRICAL VS PHARMACOLOGICAL CARDIOVERSION

In studies, rates of spontaneous conversion to sinus rhythm have ranged from 0 to 76%. In many active pharmacological conversion trials, the rate of maintenance of sinus rhythm is often less than 50%. The contributing characteristics for the wide variation in the rate of spontaneous conversion and reversion may be resulting from age, enlarged left atrial size, ischemic heart disease, hypertension, valvular disease, and differing durations of AF. However, it is still unclear as to which patient characteristic would be the most reliable predictor for spontaneous conversion to sinus rhythm or reversion to AF.

Electrical Conversion

The efficacy of cardioversion of AF with modern biphasic external defibrillators is consistently about 80–85%. Percutaneous catheter-based cardioversion efficacy is about 90%. Risk of a thromboembolic event is equal in both electrical and pharmacological conversion. Patient preference should drive decision making around the modality of cardioversion. Of all antiarrythmics, only pretreatment with ibutilide provides added efficacy but carries a higher risk for inducing ventricular arrhythmia.

Pharmacological Conversion

In meta-analysis of 54 randomized trials, drugs with strong evidence for efficacy for acute conversion were ibutilide, flecainide, dofetilide, propafenone, and amiodarone. Quinidine demonstrated moderate evidence for efficacy. Evidence for the efficacy of sotalol and disopyramide was insufficient. Small sample size, limited follow-up period, and variable duration of AF limit the quality of the reviewed studies.

Induction of *torsades de pointes* through prolongation of the QT interval is the most important side effect of antiarrhythmic therapy. Risk is greatest in the first 24–72 h of treatment. Meaningful comparison of risk between agents is limited by heterogeneity of reporting in reviewed studies. No reports of ventricular arrhythmia were seen with amiodarone and procainamide. Rates were about 2% for flecainide, propafenone, and sotalol. Rates of up to 9% for ibutilide, 12% for quinidine and dofetilide have been reported. Consideration of the risk of *torsades de pointes* is important when deciding where to start therapy (inpatient or outpatient setting).

There is no reliable way to predict which patients are at risk for arrhythmia. Adverse outcomes from arrhythmias related to acute cardioversion are more common with pharmacological conversion than with electrical cardioversion.

Recommendation 4

For those patients who choose to undergo acute cardioversion to achieve sinus rhythm in AF, both direct-current cardioversion (grade 1C+) and pharmacological conversion (grade 2A) are appropriate options.

No head-to-head trials are available to demonstrate superiority of either modality of cardioversion. Long-term effectiveness in maintaining sinus rhythm is moderate to low for both methods.

THE ROLE OF ECHOCARDIOGRAPHY IN THE ACUTE CONVERSION OF ATRIAL FIBRILLATION

Role of Transesophageal Echocardiography

Risk of thromboembolism during cardioversion is related to intra-atrial clot burden slow return of mechanical contraction. TEE, because of high sensitivity and specificity, is an excellent modality to risk-stratify patients by ruling out pre-existing clot.

The Assessment of Cardioversion Using Transesophageal Echocardiography trial randomized patients with AF of more than 48 h duration to either TEE and anticoagulation 4 wk postcardioversion against 3 wk precardioversion anticoagulation followed by 4 wk postcardioversion anticoagulation. Rates of stroke, transient ischemic attack, or peripheral embolism did not differ between groups. The TEE-guided approach was more cost effective. Rates of maintenance of sinus rhythm at 8 wk were similar in both groups. The rates for major and minor bleeding were higher in the conventional group.

Role of Measurement of Left Atrial Size

An inverse relationship between left atrial size and the success rate for cardioversion exists. Although this qualitative relationship exists, evidence-based recommendation to support the routine measurement of the left atrial size for predicting success cannot be made. However, transesophageal echocardiography can still be useful in evaluating left ventricular function or hypertrophy.

Recommendation 5

For those patients with new-onset AF, the conventional approach would be delayed cardioversion with 4 wk of anticoagulation pre- and postconversion. However, if TEE does not reveal intracardiac thrombus, short-term precardioversion anticoagulation followed by early acute cardioversion with postcardioversion anticoagulation is an appropriate strategy for those patients who elect early cardioversion (grade 2A).

EFFICACY FOR EACH ANTIARRHYTHMIC AGENT FOR THE MAINTENANCE OF NORMAL SINUS RHYTHM AFTER SUCCESSFUL CARDIOVERSION

Maintenance Therapy

Amiodarone, disopyramide, propafenone, and sotalol all been have found efficacious in the maintenance of sinus rhythm. Moderate evidence exists for flecainide, quinidine, and azimilide. Comparison trials show amiodarone to be more efficacious than propafenone and sotalol.

Torsades de points and other ventricular arrhythmias are the most significant antiarrhythmic side effect. However, only 18 out of 35 clinical trials of maintenance therapy reported incidence of ventricular arrhythmia. No ventricular arrhythmia were reported with amiodarone or disopyramide, but it was reported in 0–3% of patients treated with propafenone, 0–5% of those treated with sotalol, and 0–12% of those treated with quinidine. Cessation or dose changes were reported in 50–60% of patients treated with quinidine or disopyramide and 10–25% of patients treated with propafenone, flecainide, amiodarone, or sotalol.

Recommendation 6

Most patients with AF, who were successfully converted to sinus rhythm, should not be placed on rhythm maintenance therapy because the risks outweigh the benefits. However, should AF reoccur in some patients whose quality of life is compromised by the AF, the recommended medications for rhythm maintenance are amiodarone, disopyramide, propafenone, and sotalol. The choice of the agent depends on the risk of side effects based on individual patient characteristics (grade 2A).

Amiodarone, despite more noncardiac side effects than other agents, is considered safer in patients with CHF and left ventricular hypertrophy. Sotalol and amiodarone should be considered in patients with CAD. Flecainide is contraindicated in patients with CAD. For carefully selected patients whose quality of life is substantially compromised by AF, the benefits of maintenance therapy may offset the risks.

SOURCES

1. Annals of Internal Medicine, 16 December, 2003, Volume 139 Issue 12.

4 Antithrombotic Therapy for Venous Thromboembolic Disease

George P. N. Samraj, MD

INTRODUCTION

The following recommendations summarize the anticoagulation guidelines from the seventh American College of Chest Physicians (ACCP) conference on antithrombotic and thrombolytic therapy and employ an evidence grading scale (summarized in Table 5), at the end of the chapter *(1)*.

DEEP VEIN THROMBOSIS

Acute DVT Initial Treatment Options

Acute deep vein thrombosis (DVT) of the leg is treated with anticoagulation therapy to prevent extension of the existing thrombus, prevent recurrence (early and late) of DVT, and prevent pulmonary embolism (PE). In patients in whom DVT suspicion is high, treatment should be instituted pending diagnostic confirmation. The treatment options are subcutaneous low-molecular-weight heparins (LMWH) or unfractionated heparin (UFH), which may be administered subcutaneously or intravenously. The guidelines state that LMWH is the preferred agent of choice. A vitamin K antagonist (VKA; warfarin is the only currently

From: *Current Clinical Practice: Essential Practice Guidelines in Primary Care*
Edited by: N. S. Skolnik © Humana Press, Totowa, NJ

available VKA) should be started on day 1 of treatment. The usual initial starting dose of warfarin is 5–10 mg per day. The heparin may be discontinued once a stable target international normalized ratio (INR) greater than 2 is achieved with warfarin, usually after 5–7 d.

LMWH

LMWH is the treatment of choice for initial management of DVT. LMWH is administered subcutaneously once or twice a day, except in cancer patients, in whom twice-a-day therapy preferred. The outcome of in-patient (grade 1A) therapy is similar to outpatient therapy (grade 1C) for DVT and PE, and for DVT out-patient therapy is recommended if possible. LMWH and UFH generally share similar favorable outcomes. In patients with severe renal failure, intravenous UFH is preferred because LMWH is not effectively cleared (grade 2C). All LMWH are similar in safety and efficacy. Routine monitoring of INR while using LMWH is not necessary, but in unusual circumstances (e.g., renal failure), antifactor Xa-level monitoring is recommended (grade 1A).

UFH

UFH is started with 5000 U intravenous bolus followed by an activated partial thromboplastin time (aPTT)-adjusted infusion (about 30,000 U/24 h) or 80 mg/kg bolus followed by continuous infusion (8 U/kg/h). Anti-Xa-U level measurement is recommended in heparin-resistant patients (i.e., persons receiving high-dose UFH with a nontherapeutic aPTT) because of the unpredictable nature of aPTT in these patients.

Other/Additional Treatment Options

Routine use of intravenous (grade 1A) or catheter-directed thrombolytic therapy or venous thrombectomy (grade 1C) is not recommended in DVT. In the exceptional case of massive ileo-femoral DVT with risk of limb gangrene, catheter-directed thrombolytic therapy (urokinase, tissue plasminogen activator [tPA]), or venous thrombectomy is preferred (grade 2C). Routine use of vena caval filter with anticoagulation is not recommended (grade 1A) except in patients with recurrent DVT or those who cannot tolerate anticoagulation therapy (grade 2C). Use of anti-inflammatory agents (e.g., nonsteroidol anti-inflammatory drugs) as primary treatment for DVT is not recommended (grade 2B), in contrast to superficial thrombophlebitis (ST) (*see* below). Presently, no recommendations are available for the use of new antithrombotic agents (Fondaparinux, Ximelagatran) in the initial treatment of DVT. Ambulation as tolerated, rather than bed rest, is recommended for patents with DVT (grade 1B) as described in Table 1.

Table 1
Treatment of VTE (General Approach)

Condition	Treatment	Duration	Recommendation
High clinical suspicion of DVT	Start anticoagulants while pending confirmation of diagnosis	–	Grade 1C
Acute DVT of leg first episode	Initial treatment with LMWH or UFH for at least 5 d. Start VKA on the first day with target INR 2.5 (2–3) and discontinue heparin when stable INR of >2 achieved	See Table 2	Grade 1A
Postphlebitic syndrome	Elastic compression stocking	Long duration (~2 yr)	Grade 1A
Nonmassive PE (objectively confirmed)	Initial treatment with LMWH or UFH for at least 5 d. Start VKA on the first day with target INR 2.5 (2–3) and discontinue heparin when stable INR of >2 achieved	See Table 3	Grade 1A

VTE, venous thromboembolic disease; DVT, deep vein thrombosis; PE, pulmonary embolism; LMWH, low-molecular-weight heparin; UFH, unfractionated heparin; VKA, vitamin K antagonist; INR, international normalized ratio.

Acute DVT: Long-Term Treatment Options

Standard long-term therapy for DVT targets an INR goal of 2.5 (range 2–3). Higher intensity therapy (INR 3–4) has been associated with greater bleeding risk, without superior preventative outcomes; lower intensity therapy (INR 1.5–1.9) does not provide comparable risk reduction compared with an INR of 2–3. Follow-up with ultrasound or plasma D-dimer test may be performed to evaluate the presence or absence of thrombi (grade 2C), with patients who have thrombus present on follow-up with ultrasound having a higher probability of recurrent DVT.

Patients with DVT require long-term anticoagulation (VKA is preferred) to reduce the frequency of recurrence, thrombus extension, or other thromboembolic events. Short-duration VKA therapy (4–6 wk) or long-duration UFH therapy is not recommended because both are associated with increased thromboembolic complications. When VKA is contraindicated, either LMWH or UFH may be used. The former is generally preferred because of ease of administration. VKA is contraindicated in pregnancy; therefore, UFH or LMWH should be used. In cancer-associated DVT, long-term LMWH treatment (3–6 mo) provides more

Table 2
Duration of Treatment: DVT (Proximal or Calf Vein)[a]

Subgroups	Treatment	Duration	INR	Evidence
DVT–first-episode	Secondary to a transient risk factor	VKA[b]	3 mo	INR (2–3) target 2.5	Grade 1A
	With concurrent cancer	LMWH followed by VKA	3–6 mo indefinitely or until cancer resolved	INR (2–3) target 2.5	Grade 1A Grade 1C
	Idiopathic DVT	VKA	At least 6–12 mo or indefinite (consider)	INR (2–3) target 2.5	Grade 1A Grade 2A
	With a prothrombotic genotype[c]	VKA	12 mo or indefinitely	INR (2–3) target 2.5	Grade 1C+ Grade 2C
Recurrent DVT		VKA	Indefinite	INR (2–3) target 2.5	Grade 2A

[a]INR (2–3) target 2.5.
[b]VKA: when contraindicated use heparin or other agents (LMWH, idraparinux, and ximelagatran).
[c]Patients with a known deficiency (antithrombin III, protein C, protein S) or with a prothrombotic gene mutations (factor V Leiden, prothrombin 20210A), with some known antibodies (e.g., antiphospholipid antibodies) or elevated levels of coagulation factor VIII, homocystine.

favorable reductions in recurrent VTE than VKA (grade 1A) and is the treatment of choice. (*See* Table 2 for duration of treatment recommendations.)

POSTPHLEBITIC SYNDROME

As many as 20–50% of DVT patients develop a symptom complex known as Postphlebitic syndrome (PTS; undocumented DVT may also be followed by PTS). Chronic venous insufficiency may be a primary manifestation of undocumented DVT, presenting as PTS. To reduce PTS, after DVT, use of an elastic compression stocking (ankle pressure of 30–40 mmHg) for 2 yr is recommended (grade 1A). To treat mild edema resulting from PTS, elastic compression stocking (grade 2C) is suggested. For patients with severe edema resulting from PTS, an intermittent pneumatic compression device (40 mmHg) is recommended (grade 2A). Data supporting medical therapy for PTS with LMWH, UFH, and other agents is insufficient to confirm efficacy. Some reports, including a meta-analysis, indicate that oral rutosides like horse chestnut seed (i.e., *O*-β-hydroxyethyl rutoside) are useful in the treatment of mild-to-moderate PTS, reducing calf and ankle sizes in 4–8 wk of therapy (grade 2B).

PULMONARY EMBOLISM

Initial Treatment of Acute PE

The treatments for DVT or PE are the same. Most treated patients with DVT or PE do well: mortality is less than 1.4% for treated PE, and fourfold lower for treated DVT without PE.

For nonmassive acute PE, initiate treatment with LMWH subcutaneously (preferred, except for severe renal failure patients who should receive intravenous UFH [grade 2C]) or UFH infusion after the bolus dose (grade 1A) for at least 5 d (grade 1C). VKA is commenced on the first day of anticoagulation therapy. For patients with high clinical suspicion of PE, anticoagulant therapy should be initiated while awaiting diagnostic confirmation (grade 1A). Routine monitoring of LMWH with antifactor Xa is not recommended (grade 1A). If UFH is used, dose adjustment is done by monitoring aPTT prolongation. Patients with unstable aPTT or those who require large doses of UFH are advised to monitor and adjust the dose of heparin based on anti-Xa-level measurement (grade 1B), the therapeutic goal is a plasma heparin level 0.3–0.7 IU/mL anti-Xa activity by amidolytic assay (grade 1C+).

Other/Additional Treatment Options

Because of complications such as cerebral hemorrhage in as many as 2% of patients, systemic thrombolytic therapy with tPA or other agents are recommended only in selected groups of patients with PE (grade 1A). In hemodynamically unstable patients with massive PE, systemic administration of thrombolytic agents is recommended (grade 2B), rather than catheter-assisted infusion (grade 1C). Short-duration thrombolytic regimens are preferred to long duration (grade 2C). Heparin may be concurrently administered with tPA or reteplase, but is contraindicated with streptokinase and urokinase. There is controversy about the benefit of tPA administration for stable patients with echocardiographically demonstrated right ventricle dysfunction.

In most patients, because of high mortality (5–25%, mean = 10%), mechanical removal of clot through catheter or pulmonary embolectomy is contraindicated (grade 1C). In some critically ill patients with PE, because of lack of sufficient time to administer the thrombolytics, mechanical removal (catheter extraction or fragmentation) or pulmonary embolectomy of the clot is recommended as the initial treatment (grade 2C). Vena caval interruption (filter) is indicated only when anticoagulation is contraindicated. In the case of recurrent PE, vena caval interruption procedure may be added as an adjunct therapy to standard anticoagulation (grade 2C).

LONG-TERM THERAPY FOR PE

Long-term anticoagulation therapy is similar to DVT. (*See* Table 3 for details.)

Table 3
Long-Term Therapy for PE[a]

Subgroups	Treatment	Duration	INR	Evidence	
First-episode PE-hemodynamically stable	Secondary to a transient risk factor	VKA	3 mo	INR (2–3) target 2.5	Grade 1A
Gradegrade 1A	With concurrent cancer	LMWH and VKA	3–6 mo followed by indefinitely or cancer resolved	target 2.5	Grade 1C
	Idiopathic PE	VKA	6–12 mo or consider indefinite therapy	INR (2–3) target 2.5	Grade 1A / Grade 2A
	With antiphospholipid syndrome or have more than two prothrombotic genotype[b] conditions	VKA	12 mo or consider indefinite antithrombotic therapy	INR (2–3) target 2.5	Grade 1C+ / Grade 2C
First-episode PE	Critically ill patient	Systemic thrombolytic therapy	Short duration	–	Grade 2B
	Critically ill patient with lack of time to administer thrombolytics	Catheter extraction (or fragmentation) or pulmonary embolectomy	Initial treatment	–	Grade 2C
Recurrent PE	Recurrent PE	VKA	Indefinite	INR (2–3) target 2.5	Grade 2A
	With chronic thromboembolic pulmonary hypertension	a. Venocaval filter, b. pulmonary thromboendarterectomy, and c. VKA	Indefinite target 2.5	INR (2–3)	Grade 2C / Grade 1C

[a]INR (2–3) target 2.5.
VKA-Vitamin K Antagonist, when contraindicated use heparin or other agents (LMWH, idraparinux, ximelagatran).
[b]Patients with a known deficiency (antithrombin III, protein C, protein S) or with a prothrombotic gene mutations (factor V Leiden, prothrombin 20210A), with some known antibodies (e.g., antiphospholipid antibodies) or elevated levels of coagulation factor VIII, homocysteine.

Table 4
Upper Extremity DVT

Condition	Treatment	Duration		Evidence
Acute care	General	LMWH—(sc) or UFH³—(i.v.)	Short-term	Grade 1C
	Low risk for bleeding	May consider i.v. thrombolytic therapy	Short course	Grade 2C
Anticoagulation	Failure of embolectomy or antithrombolytics	Surgical or catheter extraction	–	Grade
	Contraindication to anticoagulants	SVC filter	–	Grade 2C
Long-term therapy		VKA (similar to DVT-lower leg)	*See* Table 2	Grade 2C
Prevention/reduction of complications (pain and swelling)		Elastic bandage	Long duration	–

SUPERFICIAL THROMBOPHLEBITIS

ST presents as a red, tender swollen area along a course of a vein, often with palpable cords. ST is commonly associated with intravenous lines and in the lower leg and is associated with venous varicosities and valvular incompetencies. Topical diclofenac gel (grade 1B) or oral diclofenac (grade 2B) is recommended for ST secondary to an intravenous line. For patients with spontaneous ST, an intermediate dose of LMWH or UFH (10,000—12,000 U subcutaneously twice a day) for at least 4 wk is recommended (grade 2B).

UPPER EXTREMITY DVT

Upper extremity DVT (UE-DVT) has a multifactorial etiology. It can be associated with central vein line placement, presence of external compression (e.g., tumor, altered body positioning) or idiopathic. UE-DVT presents with pain, edema of the arms, or presence of engorged collateral circulation; without resolution, it may lead to chronic edema of the arms or PE. Common sites for thrombotic obstruction are subclavian, axillary, or brachial veins.

Acute UE-DVT therapy may be a UFH or LMWH-subcutaneously (grade 1C+) or a short course of intravenous thrombolytic therapy (recommended in selected patients with recent onset of UE-DVT and low risk for bleeding) (grade 2C). Patients who fail anticoagulants or thrombolytic therapy, or those with persistent symptoms, should be considered for surgical embolectomy or

Table 5
Clinical Evidence Ratings

Type of evidence	Study	Implications
Grade 1: Strong recommendation. Benefits do or do not outweigh the risk, burden, or cost	–	–
Grade 1A	RCT	Strongest recommendation
Grade 1B	RCT with limitations	Strong recommendation (most circumstances)
Grade 1C	Observational studies	Intermediate recommendation
Grade 1C+	No RCT. Strong observational studies	Strong recommendation (most patients and circumstances)
Grade 2: Unclear recommendations. Expert opinion, committee suggestions	–	–
Grade 2A	RCT	Intermediate recommendation. Depends on circumstances
Grade 2B	RCT inconsistent results	Weak recommendation
Grade 2C	Observational studies	Very weak recommendation
Grade 2C+	Strong observational studies	Weak recommendation. Changes with circumstances

RCT, randomized clinical trial.
Adapted from ref. 2.

catheter extraction (grade 2C). A superior vena cava filter may be considered as initial treatment in patients with contraindication to anticoagulants (grade 2C). Long-term treatment with VKA is recommended for UE-DVT (grade 2C) (similar to lower leg DVT or PE). Similar to lower extremity DVT, application of elastic compression bandages may provide benefit for those who suffer persistent pain or swelling (grade 2C) (see Tables 4 and 5).

SOURCES

1. Büller HR, Agnelli G, Hull RD, et al. (2004) The Seventh ACCP Conference on Antithrombotic and Thrombolytic Therapy. Chest 126:401S–428S.
2. Guyatt G, Schunemann HJ, Cook D, Jaeschke R, Pauker S (2004) Applying the Grades of Recommendation for Antithrombotic and Thrombolytic Therapy Chest 126:179S–187S.

5

Antithrombotic Therapy for Atrial Fibrillation, Valvular Heart Disease, Management of Elevated INRs, and Perioperative Management

Ann Peff, MD and Doron Schneider, MD

CONTENTS

SUMMARY

This chapter will concisely summarize the following sections of the anticoagulation guidelines (for management of deep vein thrombosis [DVT]/pulmonary embolism [PE], *see* chapter on DVT/PE):

1. Prevention of venous thromboembolism (VTE).
2. Antithrombotic therapy in atrial fibrillation (AF).
3. Antithrombotic therapy in valvular heart disease—native and prosthetic.
4. Management of elevated international normalized ratios (INRs) or bleeding in patients receiving vitamin K antagonists (VKA).
5. Managing anticoagulation therapy in patients requiring invasive procedures *(1)*.

The recommendations from the American College of Chest Physicians (ACCP) employ a grading system originally described in 2001. If experts are very certain that benefits do, or do not, outweigh risks, burdens, and costs, they

From: *Current Clinical Practice: Essential Practice Guidelines in Primary Care*
Edited by: N. S. Skolnik © Humana Press, Totowa, NJ

Table 1
Risk Factors for VTE

Surgery
Trauma (major or lower extremity)
Immobility and paresis
Malignancy (varies by cancer type; especially high among patients with brain tumors,
    adenocarcinoma of the ovary, pancreas, colon, stomach, lung, prostate, and kidney)
Cancer therapy (hormonal, chemotherapy, or radiotherapy)
Previous VTE
Increasing age (low risk, <40; moderate risk, 40–60 yr; high risk, >60)
Pregnancy and the postpartum period
Estrogen-containing oral contraception or HRT
SERMs
Acute medical illness
Heart or respiratory failure
Inflammatory bowel disease
Nephrotic syndrome
Myeloproliferative disorders
Paroxysmal nocturnal hemoglobinuria
Obesity
Smoking
Varicose veins
Central venous catheterization
Inherited or acquired thrombophilia

VTE, venous thromboembolism; HRT, hormone replacement therapy; SERMs, selective
estrogen receptor modules.

will make a strong recommendation (grade 1). If they are less certain of the magnitude of the benefits and the risks, burdens, and costs, and thus of their relative impact, they make a weaker grade 2 recommendation. Consistent results from randomized clinical trial (RCTs) generate grade A recommendations. Observational studies with very strong effects or secure generalizations from RCTs generate grade C+. Inconsistent results from RCTs generate grade B recommendations and observational studies generate grade C recommendations.

PREVENTION OF VENOUS THROMBOEMBOLISM

Most hospitalized patients have one or more risk factors for VTE (Table 1). These risk factors are generally cumulative. Although, high-risk groups for VTE can be identified, it is not possible to predict which individual patients in a given risk group will develop a clinically important thromboembolic event. Although the prevention of fatal PE remains the top priority for prophylaxis programs, it is not the only objective. The prevention of symptomatic DVT and PE are also important objectives because these outcomes are associated with considerable acute morbidity and long-term sequelae. High-quality evidence demonstrated little or no increase in the rates of clinically important bleeding with appropriate prophylactic doses of low-dose unfractionated heparin (LDUH), low-molecular-weight heparin (LMWH) or a VKA. Prophylaxis of DVT/PE has been found to be cost effective.

The recommended approach to DVT/PE prophylaxis involves the routine implementation of group-specific prophylaxis for all patients who belong to each of the major target groups, listed next.

General Recommendations

1. Mechanical methods of prophylaxis (graduated compression stocking [GCS], intermittent pneumatic compression devices [IPC], venous foot pump) should be used primarily in patients who are at high risk of bleeding (grade 1C+) or as an adjunct to anticoagulant-based prophylaxis (grade 2A). No mechanical prophylaxis option has been shown to reduce the risk of death or PE.
2. The use of aspirin alone is not recommended for any patient group (grade 1A).
3. Clinicians should consider the manufacturer's suggested dosing guidelines for each of the antithrombotic agents (grade 1C).
4. Consider renal impairment when deciding on doses of LMWH, fondaparinux, and thrombin inhibitors, particularly in elderly patients and those at high risk for bleeding (grade 1C+).
5. When using anticoagulant prophylaxis, special caution should be exercised in all patients undergoing neuraxial anesthesia or analgesia (grade 1C+).

General Surgery

1. *Low-risk patients* undergoing minor surgery and who are under 40 yr of age with no additional risk factors require no specific prophylaxis other than early mobilization (grade 1C+).
2. *Moderate-risk patients* are those undergoing a nonmajor procedure and are between 40 and 60 yr of age or have additional VTE risk factors, or those patients who are undergoing major operations and are below 40 yr of age with no additional risk factors. Recommendation: prophylaxis with LDUH, 5000 U twice a day or LMWH, less than 3400 U once daily (both grade 1A).
3. *Higher risk patients* are those undergoing nonmajor surgery and are older than 60 yr of age or have additional risk factors and patients older than 40 having major surgery. These patients should receive prophylaxis with LDUH, 5000 U three times a day or LMWH more than 3400 U daily (grade 1A).
4. In high-risk general surgery patients with multiple risk factors, the recommendation is the same as just given, combined with GCS or IPC (grade 1C+).
5. In selected high-risk general surgery patients, including those who have undergone major cancer surgery, it is suggested that LMWH be used post-hospital discharge (grade 2A).

Vascular Surgery

1. If patients have no additional VTE risk factors, routine prophylaxis is not recommended (grade 2B).

2. Patients undergoing major vascular surgical procedures who have additional risk factors, prophylaxis with LDUH, or LMWH is recommended (grade 1C+).

Gynecological Surgery

1. A brief procedure, less than 30 min, for benign disease has no specific prophylaxis other than early mobilization.
2. Patients undergoing laproscopic procedures, in which additional VTE risk factors are present should receive LDUH, LMWH, IPC, or GCS (grade 1C).
3. Prophylaxis should be used in all major gynecological surgery and should be continued until hospital discharge (grade 1C).
4. Major surgery in benign disease, without additional risk factors use LDUH 5000 U bid (grade 1A) or once daily prophylaxis with LMWH less than 3400 U/d (grade 1C+) or IPC started just before surgery and used continuously while the patient is not ambulating (grade 1B).
5. For patients undergoing extensive surgery for cancer, and for patients with additional VTE risk factors LDUH, 5000 U three times a day (grade 1A) or higher doses of LMWH (i.e., >3400 U/d) (grade 1A). IPC alone until hospital discharge (grade 1A) or a combination of LDUH or LMWH and GCS or IPC is an alternative (all grade 1C).
6. For Patients at particularly high risk, including those who have undergone cancer surgery and who are over 60 yr of age or have had a prior VTE, it is recommended that prophylaxis be continued for 2–4 wk after hospital discharge (grade 2C).

Urological Surgery

1. For transurethral or other low-risk procedures, prophylaxis other than early and persistent mobilization is not recommended (grade 1C+).
2. For major, open procedures, LDUH two or three times a day is recommended (grade 1A). Alternatives include IPC and/or GCS (grade 1B) or LMWH (grade 1C+).
3. Mechanical prophylaxis with GCS (grade 1C+) should be used for patients who are actively bleeding or who are at high risk of bleeding.
4. For patients with multiple risk factors, combine GCS and/or IPC with LDUH or LMWH (grade 1C+).

Laparoscopic Surgery

1. Other than aggressive mobilization, no routine prophylaxis is recommended (grade 1A).
2. If additional VTE risk factors exist, use one or more of the following: LDUH, LMWH, IPC, or GCS (grade 1C+).

Orthopedic Surgery

1. Elective hip arthroplasty
   Use one of the following: (all grade 1A)

   a. LMWH at a usual high-risk dose, started 12 h before surgery or 12–24 h after surgery, or 4–6 h after surgery at half the usual high-risk dose and then increasing to the usual high-risk dose the following day.

   b. Fondaparinux, 2.5 mg started 6–8 h after surgery, or

   c. Adjusted-dose VKA started preoperatively or the evening after surgery, with a target INR of 2.5 with range 2–3.

  Extend prophylaxis for 28–35 d (grade 1A).

2. Elective knee arthroplasty:

   a. Use the same protocol for elective intraperitoneal arthroplasty (THR), above (all grade 1A).

   b. Extend prophylaxis for at least 10 d.

   c. The optimal use of IPC is an alternative option to anticoagulation (grade 1B).

3. Knee arthroscopy:

   a. Early mobilization only. However, if the patient is at a higher than usual risk or has a prolonged and complicated procedure, prophylax with LMWH (grade 2B).

4. Hip fracture surgery:

   a. Use fondaparinux (grade 1A), LMWH at the usual high-risk dose (grade 1C+), adjusted-dose VKA with a target INR of 2.5 with range 2–3 (grade 2B) or LDUH (grade 1B). A decision about the timing of initiation of pharmacological prophylaxis should be based on the efficacy-to-bleeding tradeoffs for that particular agent (grade 1A). For LMWH there are only small differences between starting preoperatively or postoperatively, and both options are acceptable (grade 1A). One systematic study found LMWH administered close to the time of surgery (<2 h before, at half the usual high-risk dose or 6–8 h after surgery) reduced the risk of VTE compared with VKA, but this benefit was offset by an increased risk of major bleeding.

   b. Use of aspirin alone is not recommended (grade 1A).

   c. Delayed surgery initiates prophylaxis with either LDUH or LMWH during the time between hospital admission and surgery (grade 1C+).

   d. Extend prophylaxis for 28–35 d after surgery (grade 1A).

   e. If there is a high risk of bleeding making anticoagulation contraindicated, use mechanical prophylaxis (grade 1C+).

5. Isolated lower extremity injury:

   a. Thromboprophylaxis is not routinely recommended.

Elective Spine Surgery

1. If no additional risk factors, routine prophylaxis, apart from early mobilization, is not recommended (grade 1C).

2. Some form of prophylaxis (post-operative LDUH or LMWH alone, perioperative GCS or IPC alone or combined) is recommended if the patient has history

of, or risk factors for, VTE, or an anterior surgical approach (grade 1B). If the patient has multiple risk factors, combine LDUH or LMWWH with GCS or IPC (grade 1C+).

Neurosurgery

1. Use routinely in patients undergoing major neurosurgery (grade 1A).
2. Use IPC with or without GCS (grade 1A) or post-operative LMWH or LDUH for intracranial procedures.
3. In high-risk patients, use LDUH or LMWH in combination with mechanical prophylaxis (grade 2B).

Trauma

1. If the patient has at least one risk factor for VTE, he or she should receive thromboprophylaxis (grade 1A).
2. LMWH should be started as soon as it is considered safe (grade 1A).
3. If LMWH is delayed or contraindicated, IPC or GCS should be used (grade 1B).
4. Duplex ultrasonography screening should be performed in patients who are at high risk for DVT (e.g., the presence of a spinal cord injury, lower extremity or pelvic fracture, major head injury, or an indwelling femoral venous line), and who have received suboptimal prophylaxis or no prophylaxis (grade 1C).
5. Prophylaxis should be continued through in-patient rehabilitation (grade 1C+). After discharge, continue with LMWH or a VKA with target INR of 2.5 in patients with major impaired mobility.

Medical Conditions

Patients admitted with congestive heart failure or severe respiratory diseases, or who are confined to bed and have one or more additional risk factors should receive LDUH (grade 1A) or LMWH (grade 1A). If there is a contraindication to anticoagulation, prophylax with GCS or IPC (grade 1C+).

Cancer Patients

1. Refer to the appropriate surgical procedures described earlier.
2. Cancer patients who are hospitalized and bedridden with a medical illness should receive prophylaxis appropriate for their risk state (grade 1A).
3. LMWH and fixed-dose warfarin should not routinely be used to prevent thrombosis related to long-term central venous catheters in cancer patients (Grades 2B and 1B, respectively).

Critical Care

1. Moderately ill patients in the intensive care unit (post-operatively or medically ill) should receive LDUH or LMWH (grade 1A).

2. Patients at higher risk (major trauma or orthopedic procedures) should receive LMWH (grade 1A).
3. Patients at high risk for bleeding should receive GCS and/or IPC (grade 1C+).

Long-Distance Travel (Flights More Than 6 H)

1. General measures should include avoidance of constrictive clothing around the lower extremities or waist, avoidance of dehydration, and frequent calf muscle stretching.
2. Additional risk factors for VTE present: below-knee GCS providing 15–30 mmHg of pressure at the ankle (grade 2B) or a single dose of LMWH injected prior to departure (grade 2B).

Acute Spinal Cord Injury

1. Prophylaxis should be provided to all spinal cord injury patients (grade 1A).
2. LDUH, GCS, and IPC should not be used in isolation (grade 1A).
3. LMWH should be commenced as soon as hemostasis is achieved. IPC with either LDUH or LMWH is an alternative to LMWH alone.
4. IVC filters should not be used as primary prophylaxis for PE.
5. LMWH with conversion to VKA (INR target 2.5 with range 2–3) should occur during the rehab phase.

Burns

Burn patients with additional VTE risk factors should receive prophylaxis with either LDUH or LMWH starting as soon as possible.

ANTITHROMBOTIC THERAPY IN ATRIAL FIBRILLATION

Background

The risk of cardiovascular accident (CVA) because of atrial flutter (AF) increases with age. Warfarin decreases the risk of CVA because of AF in all age groups. In younger patients, for example, warfarin (at target INR 2–3) decreases the annual stroke risk from 4.5 to 1.4% (relative risk reduction [RRR] 68%, absolute risk reduction [ARR] 3.1%, and number needed to treat [NNT] = 32). Annual major bleeding risk is 1.3% in warfarin group and 1% in controls.

The evidence supporting the superiority of aspirin to placebo is less robust than the evidence for warfarin. There may be a 22% risk reduction with aspirin, but the confidence interval for this risk reduction is large. There is a 36% RRR of all stroke with adjusted-dose oral anticoagulation compared with aspirin. In patients with AF and atherosclerosis who are receiving oral anticoagulation (OAC) for stroke prevention, it is acceptable to add aspirin in doses up to 100 mg/d to OAC (INR, 2–3) for added prevention of ischemic coronary events. This combination is associated with a higher risk of bleeding than treatment with either agent alone.

Atrial Fibrillation and Anticoagulation

- Atrial fibrillation (or paroxysmal AF [PAF]) and any high-risk factor (prior ischemic stroke, transient ischemic attack [TIA], or systemic embolism, age >75 yr, moderately or severely impaired left ventricular systolic function and/or congestive heart failure, history of hypertension, or diabetes mellitus)— long-term warfarin therapy—goal INR 2.5 with range 2–3 (grade 1A).
- Atrial fibrillation (or PAF) and age 65–75 yr, in the absence of other risk factors, antithrombotic therapy is recommended (grade 1A). Either an oral VKA, such as warfarin (target INR 2.5 with range, 2–3), or aspirin, 325/d, are acceptable alternatives in this group of patients who are at intermediate risk of stroke.
- Atrial fibrillation (or PAF), age younger than 65 and no high-risk or moderate-risk factors, aspirin 325 mg daily is recommended (grade 1B). It is recognized that VKA (warfarin) is superior in reducing stroke risk but this benefit may be offset by increased bleeding risk in the low and intermediate CVA risk patient.
- AF: decisions follow the same risk-based recommendations as for AF (grade 2C).
- AF and mitral stenosis—anticoagulation with an oral VKA (warfarin) (target INR 2.5 with range, 2–3) (grade 1C+).
- AF and prosthetic heart valves: anticoagulation with an oral VKA, such as warfarin. The target intensity of anticoagulation may be higher than the usual INR, with a recommended INR 3 with range 2.5–3.5) (grade 1C+). It may be appropriate to add aspirin, depending on the type and position of the prosthesis.
- AF following cardiac surgery: for AF lasting more than 48 h, anticoagulation with an oral VKA, such as warfarin. Target INR is 2.5 with range, 2–3). Anticoagulation should continue for several weeks following reversion to normal sinus rhythm (grade 2C).

Elective Cardioversion of AF or Atrial Flutter

1. If AF is of more than 48 h or of unknown duration and pharmacological or electrical cardioversion is planned, anticoagulate with an oral VKA to target INR 2.5 with range, 2–3, for 3 wk before and 4 wk after elective cardioversion.
2. An alternate strategy for patients with AF of more than 48 h or of unknown duration undergoing cardioversion is anticoagulation with unfractionated intravenous heparin with target partial thromboplastin time of 60 s (range, 50–70 s), or at least 5 d of warfarin with target INR of 2.5 with range, 2–3) with subsequent screening transesophageal echocardiogram (TEE). If thrombus is absent, cardioversion is performed and anticoagulation is continued for 4 wk. Continuation of anticoagulation beyond 4 wk is based on whether the patient has experienced more than one episode of AF and on their risk-factor status. Patients experiencing more than one episode of AF should be considered as having PAF.
3. For patients with AF of known duration less than 48 h, cardioversion can be performed without anticoagulation. However, if no contraindications to anticoagulation are present, begin intravenous heparin (target PTT, 60 s; range, 50–70 s) or LMWH (at full DVT treatment doses) at presentation.
4. For emergency cardioversion in which a TEE-guided approach is not possible, use intravenous unfractionated heparin (target PTT, 60 s; range, 50–70 s)

started as soon as possible, followed by 4 wk of anticoagulation with an oral VKA, such as warfarin (target INR 2.5 with range, 2–3), if normal sinus rhythm persists after cardioversion.

ANTITHROMBOTIC THERAPY IN VALVULAR HEART DISEASE: NATIVE AND PROSTHETIC

Rheumatic Mitral Valve Disease (Mitral Stenosis and/or Mitral Regurgitation)

• History of systemic embolism or presence of PAF or chronic AF—warfarin INR range, 2–3.
• Recurrent systemic embolism, despite adequate warfarin therapy—add aspirin (75–100 mg/d); for patients unable to take aspirin, add dipyridamole (400 mg/d) or clopidogrel.
• Mitral valvuloplasty—anticoagulation with VKA with a target INR of 2.5 with range, 2–3 for 3 wk prior to the procedure and for 4 wk after the procedure.

Mitral Valve Disease in Normal Sinus Rhythm

• Normal sinus rhythm with a left atrial diameter less than 5.5 cm—do not need antithrombotic therapy.
• Normal sinus rhythm; left atrial diameter greater than 5.5 cm—Consider long-term warfarin INR range, 2–3.

Mitral Valve Prolapse

• No systemic embolism, unexplained TIA or AF—antithrombotic therapy should not be given.
• Unexplained TIA—long-term, low-dose aspirin (50–162 mg/d).
• Systemic embolism or recurrent TIA, despite aspirin therapy—long-term VKA therapy (warfarin) (target INR 2.5 with range, 2–3).

Mitral Annular Calcification

Systemic embolism—long-term VKA therapy (warfarin), INR range, 2–3.

Aortic Valve and Aortic Arch Disorders

• OAC is not indicated unless there is another indication for anticoagulation.
• OAC is indicated in patients with mobile aortic atheromas and aortic plaques greater than 4 mm as measured by TEE.

Mechanical Heart Valves

• All patients with mechanical valves need OAC and heparin or LMWH should be given until the INR is within therapeutic range for the next consecutive 2 d.
• St. Jude Medical bileaflet valve in the aortic position—target INR 2.5 (range 2–3).
• Tilting disk valves and bileaflet mechanical valves in the mitral position—target INR—3 (range 2.5–3.5).

- CarboMedics bileaflet valve or Medtronic Hall tilting disk mechanical valves in the aortic position, normal left atrium size, and sinus rhythm—INR 2.5 (range, 2–3).
- Mechanical valves and additional risk factors (AF, myocardial infarction, left atrial enlargement, endocardial damage, and low ejection fraction)—target INR 3 (range 2.5–3.5), combined with low-dose aspirin, 75–100 mg/d.
- Caged ball or caged disk valves—target INR 3 (range, 2.5–3.5) in combination with aspirin, 75–100 mg/d.
- Mechanical prosthetic heart valves with systemic embolism despite a therapeutic INR—aspirin, 75–100 mg/d, in addition to VKA, and maintenance of the INR at target of 3 (range 2.5–3.5).
- Prosthetic heart valve patients in whom VKA must be discontinued—LMWH or aspirin 80–100 mg/d.

Prosthetic Heart Valves: Bioprosthetic Valves

First 3 mo after bioprosthethic valve insertion:

- *Mitral position:* VKA with a target INR of 2.5 (range 2–3) for the first 3 mo after valve insertion.
- *Aortic position:* VKA (warfarin)—target INR of 2.5 (range 2–3) for the first 3 mo after valve insertion or aspirin 80–100 mg/d.
- *Patients who have undergone valve replacement:* It suggests heparin (LMWH unfractionated) until the INR is stable at therapeutic levels for the next consecutive 2 d.
- *Patients with bioprosthetic valves with a history of systemic embolism:* VKA (warfarin) for 3–12 mo.
- *Patients with bioprosthetic valves who have evidence of a left atrial thrombus at surgery:* VKA (warfarin)—target INR of 2.5 (range 2–3).
- *Bioprosthetic valves:* long-term treatment.
- *Bioprosthetic valves with AF:* Long-term treatment with VKA (warfarin)—target INR of 2.5 (range 2–3).
- *Bioprosthetic valves with sinus rhythm (do not have AF):* aspirin, 75–100 mg/d.

Infective Endocarditis and Nonbacterial Thrombotic Endocarditis

- Mechanical prosthetic valve and endocarditis—continuation of long-term VKA (warfarin).
- Nonbacterial thrombotic endocarditis and systemic or pulmonary emboli—full-dose unfractionated intravenous or subcutaneous heparin.
- Disseminated cancer or debilitating disease with aseptic vegetations—full-dose unfractionated heparin.

RECOMMENDATIONS FOR MANAGING ELEVATED INRs

If warfarin therapy is indicated after high doses of vitamin K_1 are given, heparin or LMWH can be used until the effects of vitamin K are reversed and the patient is again responsive to warfarin (Table 2).

Table 2
Recommendations for Managing Elevated INRs or Bleeding
in Patients Receiving Vitamin K Antagonists

INR	Action
INR more than target range but <5, no significant bleeding	Decrease or hold dose, monitor frequently, restart at lower dose when INR therapeutic; if only minimally above target range, a dose reduction may not be required (grade 2C).
INR >5 but <9, no significant bleeding	Hold next one or two doses, monitor more frequently and resume at lower dose when INR is therapeutic. Alternative-omit dose and give vitamin K (<5 mg orally), particularly if at increased risk of bleeding. If more rapid reversal is required, vitamin K (2–4 mg orally) can be given with the expectation that a reduction of the INR will occur in 24 h. If the INR is still high, additional vitamin K (1–2 mg orally) can be given (grade 2C).
INR >9, no significant bleeding	Hold warfarin and give higher dose of vitamin K (5–10 mg orally), the INR should be reduced in 24–48 h. Monitor more frequently and use additional vitamin K if needed. Resume therapy at lower dose when INR therapeutic (grade 2C).
Serious bleeding at any elevation of INR	Hold warfarin and give vitamin K (10 mg by slow IV infusion), supplemented with fresh plasma or prothrombin complex concentrate, depending on urgency of the situation; recombinant factor VIIa may be considered as alternative to prothrombin complex concentrate; vitamin K_1 can be repeated every 12 h (grade 1C).
Life-threatening bleeding	Hold warfarin therapy and give prothrombin complex concentrate supplemented with vitamin K (10 mg by slow i.v. infusion); recombinant factor VIIa may be considered as alternative to prothrombin complex concentrate; repeat if necessary, depending on INR (grade 1C).

RECOMMENDATIONS FOR MANAGING ANTICOAGULATION THERAPY IN PATIENTS REQUIRING INVASIVE PROCEDURES

The management of anticoagulation is dependent on the risk of thromboembolic events in the absence of anticoagulation. The annualized risk of complications is lone atrial fibrillation—1%; average risk for AF—5%; high-risk AF—12%; dual-leaflet (St. Jude) aortic valve prosthesis—10–12%; single-leaflet (Bjork-Shiley) aortic valve prosthesis—23%; dual-leaflet (St. Jude) mitral valve prosthesis 22%; multiple St. Jude prostheses—91%.

Low Risk for Thromboembolism

Stop warfarin about 4 d before surgery and allow the INR to return to near-normal levels; if intervention increases risk for thrombosis then begin low-dose UFH (5000 U subcutaneously) or a prophylactic dose of LMWH, and simultaneously begin warfarin therapy. Alternatively, a low dose of UFH or a prophylactic dose of LMWH also can be used preoperatively.

Intermediate Risk for Thromboembolism

Stop warfarin about 4 d before surgery and allow the INR to reduce; about 2 d preoperatively, give either low-dose heparin (5000 U subcutaneously) or a prophylactic dose of LMWH; postoperatively, give low-dose heparin (or LMWH) and warfarin.

High Risk for Thromboembolism

Discontinue warfarin therapy about 4 d before surgery, and allow the INR to return to normal range; about 2 d preoperatively, as the INR decreases, give full-dose heparin or full-dose LMWH. Heparin can be given subcutaneously on an outpatient basis, and if admitted to the hospital presurgically, as a continuous IV infusion, and discontinued 5 h before surgery; alternatively, continue subcutaneous heparin or LMWH therapy until 12–24 h before surgery. Restart LDUFH (or LMWH) and warfarin therapy postoperatively.

Patients With a Low Risk of Bleeding

Continue warfarin therapy at a lower dose and operate at an INR of 1.3–1.5. The dose of warfarin can be lowered 4 or 5 d before the patient undergoes surgery. Warfarin can be restarted postoperatively and supplemented with a low dose of UFH (5000 U subcutaneously) or a prophylactic dose of LMWH if needed.

Dental Procedures

Anticoagulant therapy is recommended to be continued. Studies have shown no difference in postprocedure bleeding at low or higher levels of INR. In patients, in which there is a need to control local bleeding, may use tranexamic acid mouthwash or epsilon amino caproic acid mouthwash without interrupting anticoagulant therapy.

SOURCES

1. The seventh ACCP Conference on Antithrombotic and Thrombolytic Therapy. Chest (Suppl.). Volume 126/number 3/September, 2004.

6

Prevention of Bacterial Endocarditis

Recommendations by the American Heart Association

Margot Boigon, MD *and* Doron Schneider, MD

CONTENTS

INTRODUCTION

Antimicrobial prophylaxis for bacterial endocarditis in select patients has become the standard of medical care in the United States. This practice exists despite the fact that there are no randomized controlled human studies in patients with underlying structural heart disease that definitely establish that antibiotic prophylaxis provides protection against endocarditis during procedures that induce bacteremia. This chapter is based on the recommendations formulated and published by the American Heart Association (AHA) in 1997 *(1)*. When the AHA published the recommendations, it was expressly stated that the document was meant as a guideline and is "not intended as the standard of care or as a substitute for clinical judgment." The 1997 guidelines represent an update from recommendations published by the AHA in 1990.

The updated version reflected the following changes:

1. It emphasized that most cases of endocarditis are not attributable to an invasive procedure.
2. If endocarditis does develop, cardiac conditions were stratified into high, moderate, and negligible risk categories based on the potential outcome.

From: *Current Clinical Practice: Essential Practice Guidelines in Primary Care*
Edited by: N. S. Skolnik © Humana Press, Totowa, NJ

Table 1

High risk	Prosthetic cardiac valves, including bioprosthetic and homograft valves
	Previous bacterial endocarditis
	Complex cyanotic congenital heart disease (single ventricle states, transposition of the great vessels, tetralogy of Fallot)
	Surgically constructed systemic pulmonary shunts or conduits
Moderate risk	Most other congenital cardiac malformations (other than above and in negligible risk)
	Acquired valvar dysfunction
	Hypertrophic cardiomyopathy
	MVP with valvar regurgitation and/or thickened leaflets
Negligible risk— endocarditis prophylaxis not recommended	Isolated secundum atrial septal defect
	Surgical repair of atrial septal defect, ventricular septal defect, or patent ductus arteriosus (without residual beyond 6 mo)
	Previous CABG
	MVP without valvar regurgitation
	Physiological, functional, or innocent heart murmurs
	Previous Kawasaki disease without valvar dysfunction
	Previous rheumatic fever without valvar dysfunction
	Cardiac pacemakers (epicardial and intravascular) and implanted defibrillators

MVP, mitral valve prolapse; CABG, coronary artery bypass graft.

3. There is clearer specification of procedures that may cause bacteremia and for which prophylaxis is recommended.
4. The algorithm of mitral valve prolapse (MVP) is recommended for the prophylaxis.
5. The initial amoxicillin dose for oral and dental procedures is reduced to 2 g, and a follow-up dose was no longer recommended.
6. For penicillin-allergic patients, clindamycin and other alternatives replaced erythromycin as the drug of choice.
7. Prophylactic regimens for gastrointestinal (GI) and genitourinary (GU) procedures were simplified.

WHICH CARDIAC CONDITIONS SHOULD BE PROPHYLAXED?

The AHA recommends prophylaxis for those patients with a higher risk of developing endocarditis than the general population and for those patients at risk of high morbidity or mortality if endocarditis occurs. This includes patients with conditions classified as high or moderate risk (*see* Table 1).

In the 1997 guidelines, MVP was recognized to represent a spectrum of valvular changes and clinical conditions. When normal valves prolapse with one or more systolic clicks but no murmurs and no Doppler-demonstrated mitral regurgitation, the risk of endocarditis is not increased over the normal population. Antibiotic prophylaxis is not recommended in this scenario. Antibiotic prophylaxis is recommended in MVP associated with audible clicks and murmurs of mitral regurgitation or by Doppler-demonstrated mitral insufficiency. Likewise, myxomatous mitral valve degeneration with regurgitation is an indication for antibiotic prophylaxis.

WHICH PROCEDURES ARE BACTEREMIA-PRODUCING PROCEDURES?

The AHA recommendations define significant bacteremias as those caused by organisms commonly associated with endocarditis and attributable to identifiable procedures. These significant bacteremias result from the following:

Dental and Oral Procedures

The degree of oral inflammation and infection directly influences the magnitude and incidence of bacteremias resulting from dental and oral procedures. The greater the degree of inflammation, the more likely it will result in bacteremia. Optimal oral health through regular professional care and the use of appropriate dental products such as toothbrushes and floss is advised especially for individuals who are at risk of developing bacterial endocarditis.

Endocarditis prophylaxis is recommended for the following procedures in patients with high- and moderate-risk cardiac conditions:

1. Dental extractions.
2. Periodontal procedures including surgery, scaling, and root planing, probing and recall maintenance.
3. Dental implant placement and reimplantation of avulsed teeth.
4. Endodontic (root canal) instrumentation or surgery only beyond the apex.
5. Subgingival placement of antibiotic fibers or strips.
6. Initial placement of orthodontic bands but not brackets.
7. Intraligamentary local anesthetic injections.
8. Prophylactic cleaning of teeth or implants where bleeding is anticipated.

Endocarditis prophylaxis is not recommended in these procedures:

1. Restorative dentistry.
2. Local anesthetic injections.
3. Intracanal endodontic treatment; postplacement and buildup.
4. Placement of rubber dams.
5. Postoperative suture removal.
6. Placement of removable prosthodontic or orthodontic appliances.

7. Taking of oral impressions.
8. Fluoride treatments.
9. Taking of oral radiographs.
10. Orthodontic appliance adjustment.
11. Shedding of primary teeth.

Respiratory, Gastrointestinal, and Genitourinary Tract Procedures

The guidelines recommend endocarditis prophylaxis for the following procedures:

Respiratory tract:

- Prophylaxis recommended for high- and moderate-risk patients.
- Tonsillectomy and/or adenoidectomy.
- Surgical operations that involve respiratory mucosa.
- Bronchoscopy with a rigid bronchoscope.

GI Tract:

- Prophylaxis recommended for high-risk patients; optional for moderate-risk patients.
- Sclerotherapy for esophageal varices.
- Esophageal stricture dilation.
- Endoscopic retrograde cholangiography with biliary obstruction.
- Biliary tract surgery.
- Surgical operations that involve intestinal mucosa.

GU Tract:

- Prophylaxis recommended for high- and moderate-risk patients.
- Prostatic surgery.
- Cystoscopy.
- Urethral dilation.

Endocarditis prophylaxis is not recommended for these procedures:

Respiratory tract:

- Endotracheal intubation.
- Bronchoscopy with a flexible bronchoscope, with or without biopsy.*
- Tympanostomy tube insertion.

GI tract:

- Transesophageal echocardiography (TEE).*
- Endoscopy with or without GI biopsy.*

GU tract:

- Vaginal hysterectomy.*
- Vaginal delivery.*
- Cesarean section.

---

*Prophylaxis is optional for high-risk patients.

In uninfected tissue:

• Urethral catheterization.
• Uterine dilation and curettage.
• Therapeutic abortion.
• Sterilization procedures.
• Insertion or removal of intrauterine devices.

Other procedures in which prophylaxis is not recommended include the following:

• Cardiac catheterization including balloon angioplasty.
• Implanted cardiac pacemakers.
• Implanted defibrillators and coronary stents.
• Incision biopsy of surgically scrubbed skin.
• Circumcision.

WHAT PROPHYLACTIC REGIMENS SHOULD BE USED?

Prophylaxis should be given perioperatively in doses that are high enough to ensure an adequate concentration in the bloodstream during and after the procedure. To avoid antimicrobial resistance, the antibiotics should be initiated shortly before the procedure and not continued for more than 6–8 h after. The guidelines suggest practitioners use their own judgment when determining the choice of antibiotics and the number of doses to be administered in individual cases or in special circumstances. Because endocarditis may occur despite appropriate antibiotic prophylaxis, health care providers should maintain a high index of suspicion for endocarditis when evaluating unexpected clinical signs or symptoms. These might include unexplained fever, night chills, weakness, or arthralgias.

Regimens for Dental, Oral, Respiratory Tract, or Esophageal Procedures

Streptococcus viridans is the most common cause of endocarditis following these procedures (*see* Table 2).

Regimens for GU and Nonesophageal GI Procedures

Enterococcus faecalis is the most common cause of bacterial endocarditis that occurs following GU and GI tract surgery or instrumentation. The guidelines recommend parenteral antibiotics in high-risk patients. In moderate-risk patients, a parenteral or oral regimen is provided. For procedures in which prophylaxis is not routinely recommended, physicians may choose to give antibiotics to high-risk patients (*see* Table 3).

Special Situations

PATIENTS ALREADY ON ANTIBIOTICS

If the patient is taking an antibiotic normally used for endocarditis prophylaxis, the suggestion is to select a drug from a different class rather than increasing the

Table 2

Situation	Agent	Regimen
Standard general prophylaxis	Amoxicillin	Adults: 2 g; children: 50 mg/kg orally 1 h before procedure
Unable to take oral medications	Ampicillin	Adults: 2 g i.m. or i.v.; children: 50 mg/kg i.m. or i.v. within 30 min before procedure
Allergic to penicillin	Clindamycin or Cephalexin or cefadroxil or Azithromycin or clarithromycin	Adults: 600 mg; children: 20 mg/kg orally 1 h before procedure Adults: 2 g; children: 50 mg/kg orally 1 h before procedure Adults: 500 mg; children: 15 mg/kg orally 1 h before procedure
Allergic to penicillin and unable to take oral medications	Clindamycin or cefazolin	Adults: 600 mg; children: 20 mg/kg i.v. 30 min before procedure Adults: 1 g; children: 25 mg/kg i.m. or i.v. within 30 min before procedure

i.m., intramuscularly; i.v., intraveneously.

dose of the current antibiotic. For example, if a patient is taking oral penicillin for the secondary prevention of rheumatic fever, he or she may have relatively resistant *viridans streptococci* in his or her oral cavities. In this situation, the patient should be placed on clindamycin, azithromycin, or clarithromycin.

PROCEDURES INVOLVING INFECTED TISSUES

Incision and drainage or other procedures involving infected tissues may result in bacteremia with the same organism causing the infection. Prophylaxis for endocarditis should be given to individuals at high or moderate risk of endocarditis using a therapy directed at the most likely pathogen causing the primary infection.

PATIENTS WHO RECEIVE ANTICOAGULANTS

Patients on anticoagulants should be prophylaxed with intravenous or oral regimens rather than intramuscular injections.

PATIENTS WHO UNDERGO CARDIAC SURGERY

The guidelines recommend careful preoperative dental evaluation so that dental treatment can be completed before cardiac surgery whenever possible. *Staphylococcus aureus*, coagulase-negative staphylococci, or diptheroids most often causes endocarditis associated with open-heart surgery. Streptococci, Gram-negative bacteria, and fungi are cited as being less common. No single antibiotic

Table 3

Situation	Agent	Regimen
High-risk patients	Ampicillin plus gentamycin	Adults: ampicillin 2 g i.m. or i.v. plus gentamycin 1.5 mg/kg (not to exceed 120 mg) within 30 min of starting the procedure; 6 h later ampicillin 1 g i.m./i.v. or amoxicillin 1 g orally Children: ampicillin 50 mg/kg i.m. or i.v. (not to exceed 2 g) plus gentamycin 1.5 mg/kg within 30 min of starting the procedure; 6 h later, ampicillin 25 mg/kg i.m./i.v. or amoxicillin 25 mg/kg orally
High-risk patients allergic to ampicillin/ amoxicillin	Vancomycin and gentamycin	Adults: vancomycin 1 g i.v. over 1–2 h plus gentamycin 1.5 mg/kg (not to exceed 120 mg) complete injection/infusion within 30 min of starting the procedure; Children: vancomycin 20 mg/kg i.v. over 1–2 h plus gentamycin 1.5 mg/kg, complete injection/infusion within 30 min of starting the procedure
Moderate-risk patients	Amoxicillin or ampicillin	Adults: amoxicillin 2 g orally 1 h before procedure, or ampicillin 2 g i.m./i.v. within 30 min of starting the procedure Children: amoxicillin 50 mg/kg orally 1 h before procedure, or ampicillin 50 mg/kg i.m./i.v. within 30 min of starting the procedure
Moderate-risk patients allergic to ampicillin/ amoxicillin	Vancomycin	Adults: vancomycin 1 g i.v. over 1–2 h complete injection/infusion within 30 min of starting the procedure Children: vancomycin 20 mg/kg i.v. over 1–2 h complete injection/infusion within 30 min of starting the procedure

i.m., intramuscularly; i.v., intravenously.

regimen is effective against all these organisms. Prophylaxis should therefore be aimed primarily against staphylococci. First generation cephalosporins are most often used. Perioperative prophylactic antibiotics are recommended for patients with cardiac conditions that predispose them to endocarditis and for patients having surgery for placement of prosthetic heart valves or prosthetic intravascular or intracardiac materials.

SOURCES

1. JAMA, June 11, 1997:277(22).

II   RESPIRATORY

7

Clinical Guidelines for the Diagnosis and Treatment of Asthma

Michael Gagnon, MD and Neil S. Skolnik, MD

CONTENTS

INTRODUCTION

Asthma is a chronic inflammatory disorder of the airways with episodic airway constriction manifesting as chest tightness, wheezing, and cough, particularly at night and early in the morning. Approximately 14–15 million people in the United States suffer from asthma and it is the most common chronic disease of childhood, with an estimated 4.8 million affected children. Asthma accounts for close to 500,000 hospitalizations each year in the United States and approx 5000 deaths each year.

Airway inflammation is central to asthma and is caused by a multitude of inflammatory mediators in response to environmental triggers. Inflammation is caused by both the direct action of the inflammatory cells and through neurovascular mechanisms resulting in the increased hyper-responsiveness to airway stimuli. Airway inflammation and hyper-responsiveness results in episodic brochoconstriction, airway edema, and mucus plugging. Asthma has

From: *Current Clinical Practice: Essential Practice Guidelines in Primary Care*
Edited by: N. S. Skolnik © Humana Press, Totowa, NJ

been shown to have specific immunohistopathological features such as mast cell activation and inflammatory cell infiltration with collagen deposition below the basement membrane and airway denudation and edema. Microvascular leakage is noted along with airway smooth muscle hypertrophy. Chronic inflammation is now thought to cause airway remodeling and persistent airway obstruction. The National Asthma Education and Prevention Program Expert Panel has set out guidelines for the management of asthma (1,2). The current guidelines for asthma management are divided into the following four components:

1. Initial assessment and diagnosis.
2. Control of factors contributing to asthma severity.
3. Pharmacotherapy.
4. Education for a partnership in asthma care.

COMPONENT 1: INITIAL ASSESSMENT AND DIAGNOSIS

The establishment of a proper diagnosis of asthma is necessary for early intervention that may help prevent irreversible airway remodeling. In order to establish a diagnosis of asthma, there should be episodic wheezing or airflow obstruction that is at least partially reversible either spontaneously or with treatment. The exclusion of other diseases is also required to establish a diagnosis of asthma. Important diagnostic clues in the clinical history include a history of wheezing, increased nocturnal cough in the absence of illness, chest tightness, or difficulty breathing. History may also include increased symptoms associated with exercise, infection, exposure to animal fur, house dust, pollen, changes in weather, and extremes of emotion. Other supporting associations include a positive family history, eczema, or hay fever. On physical examination, the clinician may look for a hyperexpanded chest, hunched shoulders, or chest deformities. Wheezing with forced exhalation is a poor diagnostic sign of airway limitation as it may be absent in mild intermittent disease or between exacerbations. Increased nasal secretions, mucosal swelling, and nasal polyps are also associated with asthma.

Assessment of Severity

Every asthma patient needs to be assessed for severity of disease based on frequency of symptoms and peak flow values (Table 1).

Spirometry

Spirometry is a simple yet useful test to help establish a diagnosis as well as manage asthma. Spirometry measures forced expiratory volume in 1 s (FEV_1) and forced vital capacity as well as the ratio between the two of these. A typical obstructive pattern is one in which the FEV_1 is reduced below 80% with respect to the predicted value for age, height, sex, and race along with a ratio of FEV_1/forced vital capacity below 65%. To establish reversibility of airway disease, a change of 12% or more in FEV_1 and 200 mL after inhalation of a short-acting β_2-agonist is

Table 1
Classification of Asthma Severity

	Symptoms	Nighttime symptoms	Lung function
Severe persistent	Continual symptoms Limited physical activity Frequent exacerbations	Frequent	FEV_1 or PEF <60% predicted PEF variability >30%

Moderate persistent	Daily symptoms
	Daily use of short-
	    acting β_2-agonist
	Exacerbations affect activity
	Exacerbations >2 times/wk
	    may last days
		1 time/wk	FEV_1 or PEF
			>60 to <80%
			predicted
			PEF variability
			>30%

Mild persistent	Symptoms >2 times
	    per wk<1 time/d
	Exacerbations may
	    affect activity
		>2 times/mo	FEV_1 or PEF
			>80% predicted
			PEF variability
			20–30%

Mild intermittent	Symptoms <2 times/wk
	Asymptomatic and
	    normal PEF between
	    exacerbations
	Exacerbations brief (hours
	    to days) intensity
	    may vary
		<2 times/mo	FEV_1 of PEF >80%
			predicted
			PEF variability
			<20%

The presence of one feature of severity is sufficient to place a patient in a category. Patients should be assigned to the most severe grade in which any feature occurs. Asthma is highly variable and an individual category classification may vary over time.

Patients at any level of severity can have mild, moderate, or severe exacerbations.

PEF, peak expiratory flow.

considered relevant. Spirometry should be performed using equipment and techniques that meet the standards of the American Thoracic Society.

Additional Testing

Additional pulmonary function testing is warranted when considering a coexisting diagnosis of chronic obstructive pulmonary disease (COPD), restrictive lung disease, emphysema, or a centrally obstructive lesion. Provocation testing by methacholine, histamine, or exercise must be performed by a trained individual and should not be done if the FEV_1 is less than 65% of predicted. The provocation test is exquisitely sensitive and all but rules out asthma if it is negative. Other testing that may be considered includes chest X-ray, allergy testing, and testing for gastroesophageal reflux disease (GERD).

Differential Diagnosis

The differential diagnosis for asthma is dependent on the age of the patient. In children and infants, wheezing is associated with an acute illness that can happen in both allergic and nonallergic individuals. Allergic individuals will tend to have associated eczema, allergic rhinitis, and food allergies, whereas nonallergic individuals will tend to stop wheezing when their airways become larger in the preschool years. Both groups benefit in the acute phase of an illness with treatment.

Vocal cord dysfunction (VCD) manifests as recurrent breathlessness and wheeze, and therefore, can mimic asthma. VCD is most common in young adults with psychological disorders. Differentiating between VCD and asthma is difficult; however, the presence of a monophonic wheeze loudest over the glottis points toward VCD. Flow volume curves can be helpful in diagnosis and definitive diagnosis can only be achieved with direct visualization of the vocal cords. For a comprehensive differential diagnosis *see* Table 2.

Patient Education

It is important for the physician to establish the patient's concerns regarding their diagnosis of asthma and to educate patients about their disease. Patients should be aware of their triggers and understand that asthma is a chronic inflammatory disorder and although there may be periods without bronchospasm, in many cases anti-inflammatory medication must be taken daily to avoid exacerbations. Patients need to understand the treatment plan for their disease as well as have a written action plan for exacerbations. There is some evidence that those patients with written action plans have overall better control of their asthma than those without.

Referral Guidelines

It is recommended that asthma patients be referred to a specialist in the following situations:

- *Difficulty with diagnosis/assessment:* atypical symptoms and signs, complicating comorbidities, confirmation of environmental, or occupational exposures.
- *Education and specialized testing:* if the patient needs additional education or guidance, problems with avoidance of triggers, or is being considered for immunotherapy.
- Patients with a life-threatening exacerbation or patients with severe persistent asthma requiring step 4 care.
- Patients requiring continuous oral corticosteroids or more than two bursts of oral steroid within 1 yr.
- Patients younger than 3 yr of age requiring step 3 or 4 care and referral should be considered for patients younger than 3 yr who require step 2 care.

Table 2
Differential Diagnosis When Considering Asthma

Infants and children

Upper airway disease
   Allergic rhinitis and sinusitis

Obstruction of large airways
   Foreign body aspiration
   Vocal cord dysfunction
   Vascular ring or laryngeal webs
   Laryngotracheomalacia, tracheal stenosis, and brochostenosis

Obstruction of small airways
   Viral bronchiolitis
   Cysti fibrosis
   Bronchopulmonary dysplasia
   Heart disease

Others
   Recurrent cough not as a result of asthma
   Gastroesophageal reflux disease
   Adults
   Chronic obstructive pulmonary disease
   Congestive heart failure
   Pulmonary embolism
   Laryngeal dysfunction
   Mechanical obstruction (benign or malignant tumor)
   Pulmonary infiltrate with psychological disorders

- A specialist in asthma is generally considered a fellowship trained allergist or pulmonologist; however, can be considered a primary care physician with extra training and experience in asthma treatment.

Periodic Assessment and Monitoring

Frequent assessment and monitoring is key to appropriate asthma management.

Goals of Therapy

The goals of asthma therapy include the prevention of symptoms, including cough and breathlessness, prevention of exacerbations, maintenance of near normal peak flows, and activity levels. Optimal pharmacotherapy should be used and reassessed frequently to keep patients on the appropriate therapy for their disease severity, while minimizing side effects. Families and patients should also be routinely questioned as to their understanding of the disease and their degree of satisfaction with the treatment. Quality of life is important and should be inquired about, including missed school or work, reduction in activity level or sleep disturbances because of asthma.

Areas to Monitor

Nocturnal cough, wheeze, daytime breathlessness, chest tightness, and any morning symptoms not relieved within 15 min of using a short-acting β_2-agonist should be noted. Exacerbations since last visit should be noted as well as any temporally associated precipitants thought to have been associated with the exacerbations.

Physicians should ask about signs of poor control, including nighttime wakening and increased oral steroid or β_2-agonist use. The use of more than one canister of short-acting β_2-agonist per month is also a sign of poor control. Any hospitalizations or acute care visits should be documented. If a patient remains poorly controlled, the physician needs to consider several possibilities including poor inhaler technique, poor compliance with medication use, new or increased environmental exposures, or an alternative diagnosis.

Patients need to know the signs of inadequate control and should have a sick day plan in writing. When questioning patients regarding symptoms, it is generally best to discuss the last 2 or 3 wk at most, because more distant time periods are subject to poor recall. Medications should be reviewed at each visit and inhaler technique should be reviewed often. Peak flows and technique should be reviewed for all patients.

Pulmonary Function Testing

It is recommended that spirometry be used at the time of diagnosis as well as after treatment has been established and symptoms and peak expiratory flow (PEF) times have stabilized, to document "normal" spirometry. Spirometry should then be repeated every 1–2 yr to follow disease progression.

PEF time is a simple quantitative and reproducible measure of airway obstruction. The literature would suggest that using peak flows in asthma management results in better outcomes than using symptom monitoring alone. It is recommended that all patients with moderate-to-severe persistent asthma have a peak flow monitor at home. Patients need to be shown how to use the monitor and how to establish a baseline value for themselves. Peak flow times are a relative measure to a personal best and the percentage of personal best is a good indicator of disease severity. The peak flow machine can be set with color-coordinated markers to show levels of severity for the patient. With each zone, patients should understand what the plan is. For example:

1. *Green zone* >80% of normal, take medications as usual.
2. *Yellow zone* >50%, <80% of normal may indicate asthma is not under good control, take your inhaled β_2-agonist immediately and recheck frequently that day.

3. *Red zone* <50% of normal, may indicate poor control, take β_2-agonist immediately and call physician or go to the emergency room.

Therefore, peak flow monitoring can act as a guide for severity of asthma exacerbations and determine treatment based on a predetermined sick day plan. Peak flow monitoring is used to monitor response to treatment and in those patients who are poor perceivers of airway obstruction, it offers them a quantitative measure of impairment. Peak flows can also assist in determining temporal relationships between exposure to possible precipitants and exacerbations as well as help establish response to a change in therapy. Patients with mild intermittent to mild persistent asthma under adequate control for at least 3 mo should be seen in the office a minimum of every 6 mo. Patients with more severe asthma should be seen more frequently (Fig. 1).

COMPONENT 2: CONTROL OF FACTORS CONTRIBUTING TO ASTHMA SEVERITY

There are many factors that contribute to asthma exacerbations and severity. Inhalant allergens such as house dust mite and animal dander are common exposures that can influence asthma severity, as are occupational exposures to allergens. Nonallergic irritants such as tobacco smoke and environmental pollution also contribute to asthma symptoms. Finally, other associated factors such as allergic rhinitis and sinusitis, GERD, aspirin and nonsteroidal anti-inflammatory drug (NSAID) sensitivity, sulfite intake, β-blocker use, and viral upper respiratory tract infections can all exacerbate asthma. Physicians need to assess each asthma patient's potential for exposure to allergens and give practical advice on how to avoid triggers once they are established. Establishing sensitivity is sometimes difficult and may require skin testing or in vitro testing for IgE antibodies to indoor exposures. Any positive allergy test needs clinical correlation as to the significance for each patient.

Animal Allergens

The house dust mite lives in areas of high humidity such as carpets, pillow cases, mattresses, bed covers, and soft toys. Dehumidifiers that can keep the house at less than 50% humidity are desirable for this reason. It is recommended that mattresses be enclosed in an allergen impermeable cover and pillow cases and blankets are washed at least once a week in water over 130°F. Ideally, there should be no carpet in the bedroom and a minimal number of stuffed toys for children. Pet dander can be a potent irritant as well and it is ideal if the animal can be removed from the household. If this is unacceptable, then there should be no animals in the patient's bedroom and the bedroom door should remain closed. Washing pets weekly can decrease the amount of dander in the air.

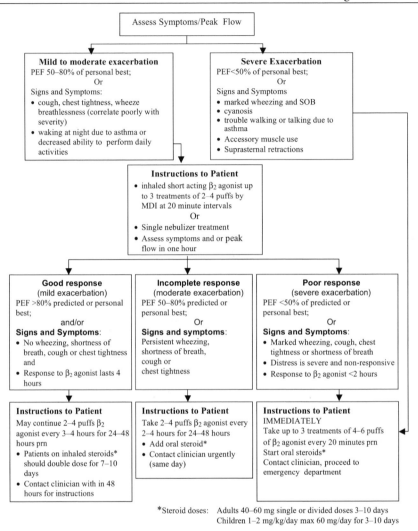

Fig. 1. Management of asthma exacerbation: home treatment.

Seasonal Allergies

Air conditioning in the summer is helpful to reduce exposure to allergens and reduces the humidity in the air. Asthmatics should avoid going outside near midday and the early afternoon when spore counts are highest. The use of medications to control upper airway inflammation can be helpful in reducing lower airway hyper-responsiveness.

Indoor Air

The house should be vacuumed once or twice a week and if patients are vacuuming they should use a mask.

Rhinitis/Sinusitis

Intranasal steroids have been proven to reduce nasal inflammation, obstruction, and discharge, and reduce lower airway hyper-responsiveness. Antihistamines and decongestants have no proven benefits for associated lower airway symptoms. Intranasal cromolyn has also been shown to reduce symptoms in ragweed season; however, less than steroids. When antibiotics are indicated, they should be prescribed for sinusitis as upper airway inflammation contributes to lower airway hyper-responsiveness.

GERD

Any patient with persistent nocturnal asthma despite therapy should be investigated for GERD. Medical or surgical management of GERD may alleviate asthma symptoms.

Aspirin Sensitivity

Many asthmatics are sensitive to aspirin and other NSAIDs and a thorough history should enquire concerning any past reactions. Patients should be informed that subsequent reactions can be severe and even fatal and that acetaminophen and salsalates are much safer alternatives. It is recommended that patients with severe persistent asthma or nasal polyps should be counseled regarding the use of aspirin and NSAIDs and that sensitivity increases with age and severity of asthma.

Sulfites

Sulfites, which are preservatives found in processed potatoes, shrimp, dried fruit, beer, and wine, can cause severe exacerbations.

β-Blockers

Nonselective β-blockers, both topical ophthalmic drops and systemic can cause bronchospasm in asthmatics. Cardioselective β-blockade can sometimes be tolerated.

Infection

Viral infections are the most common precipitant of wheezing in infancy. Many of these children will cease to wheeze as they become preschoolers and their airways enlarge. The annual flu shot is recommended for all asthmatics as the influenza virus is capable of precipitating life-threatening exacerbations.

COMPONENT 3: PHARMACOTHERAPY

Asthma morbidity and mortality is largely associated with underdiagnosis or under/inappropriate therapy. There are clear guidelines for stepwise therapy in all categories of asthma (*see* Tables 3 and 4). During exacerbations, the initial exacerbation is treated aggressively with step-up therapy and once stable then

Table 3
Stepwise Approach to Management of Asthma in Adults and Children Older Than 5 yr of Age

Classify severity: clinical features before treatment or adequate control	Symptoms/day PEF or FEV1 Symptoms/night PEF variability	Medications required to maintain adequate long-term control
Step 4: Severe persistent	Continual <60% Frequent >30%	Preferred treatment: high-dose inhaled corticosteroid and long-acting β_2-agonist. And if needed: corticosteroid tablets or syrup (2 mg/kg/d do not exceed 60 mg/d). Make repeat attempts to reduce systemic corticosteroid and maintain with high-dose inhaled steroid
Step 3: Moderate persistent	Daily >60 to <80% >1 d/wk >30%	Preferred treatment: low- to medium-dose inhaled corticosteroid and long-acting β_2-agonist Alternative treatment (listed alphabetically). Increased inhaled corticosteroid within the medium-dose range; or low- to medium-dose inhaled steroid and either a leukotriene modulator or theophylline If needed (particularly patients with recurrent severe exacerbations). Preferred treatment: increased inhaled corticosteroid within medium-dose range and long-acting β_2-agonist Alternative treatment (listed alphabetically) Increased inhaled corticosteroid within the medium dose range and add either a leukotriene modulator or theophylline

Step 2: Mild persistent	>2 times/wk but <1 times/d >80% >2 nights/mo 20–30%	Preferred treatment: low-dose inhaled corticosteroid: Alternative treatments (listed alphabetically) cromolyn, leukotriene modifier, nedocromil OR sustained-release theophylline to serum concentrations 5–15 mg/mL
Step 1: Mild intermittent	<2 d/wk >80% <2 nights/mo <20%	No daily medications needed: severe exacerbations may occur separated by long periods of normal lung function and no symptoms. A course of systemic corticosteroids is recommended
Quick relief		Short-acting bronchodilator: two to four puffs of short-acting β_2-agonist as needed for symptoms
All patients		Intensity of treatment dependent on severity: up to three treatments at 20 min intervals or one nebulizer treatment. Systemic steroid may be needed. Use of short-acting β_2-agonist >2 times a week in intermittent asthma or increased use in persistent asthma may indicate poor control and need for addition of (increase of) long-term control medication

Table 4
Stepwise Approach to Management of Asthma in Infants and Young Children (5 yr of Age and Younger)

Classify severity: clinical features before treatment or adequate control	Symptoms/day Symptoms/night	Medications required to maintain adequate long-term control
Step 4: Severe persistent	Continual frequent	Preferred treatment: high-dose inhaled corticosteroid and long-acting β_2-agonist And if needed: corticosteroid tablets or syrup (2 mg/kg/d do not exceed 60 mg/d) Make repeat attempts to reduce systemic corticosteroid and maintain with high-dose inhaled steroid
Step 3: Moderate persistent	Daily >1 d/wk	Preferred treatment: low-dose inhaled corticosteroid and long-acting β_2-agonist; or medium-dose inhaled corticosteroid Alternative treatment: low-dose inhaled steroid and either a leukotriene modulator or theophylline if needed (particularly patients with recurrent severe exacerbations) Preferred treatment: medium-dose inhaled corticosteroid and long-acting β_2-agonist Alternative treatment (listed alphabetically) Medium-dose range and add either a leukotriene modulator or theophylline

Step 2: Mild persistent	>2 times/wk but <1 time/d >2 nights/mo	Preferred treatment: low-dose inhaled corticosteroid via nebulizer or MDI with holding chamber with or without face mask Alternative treatments (listed alphabetically) Cromolyn (nebulizer preferred or MDI with holding chamber) or Leukotriene receptor antagonist
Step 1: Mild intermittent	<2 d/wk <2 nights/mo	No daily medications needed: severe exacerbations may occur separated by long periods of normal lung function and no symptoms. A course of systemic corticosteroids is recommended
Quick relief All patients		Bronchodialator as needed for symptoms Preferred treatment: short-acting β_2-agonist by nebulizer or face mask with holding chamber Alternative treatment: oral β_2-agonist. With viral upper respiratory infections; give short-acting β_2-agonist every 4 h for 24 h (longer with physician input) not more than once every 6 wk Consider systemic corticosteroid if patient has severe exacerbation or history of severe exacerbation

93

step-down therapy back to more appropriate long-term therapy can be instituted. There are two general categories of medication in the treatment of asthma—quick-relief medication and long-term control medication.

Long-Term Control Medications

Anti-inflammatory medications, long-acting bronchodilators, and leukotriene modifiers have all been shown to reduce airway inflammatory markers in airway tissue as well as airway secretions and reduce the intensity of airway hyper-responsiveness.

INHALED STEROIDS

Corticosteroids have long been the mainstay of asthma management and still remain the most effective long-term therapy. Inhaled daily corticosteroids have been shown to reduce daily symptoms, increase peak flows, reduce exacerbations, reduce airway hyper-responsiveness, and prevent airway remodeling. The anti-inflammatory effects of inhaled steroids have been noted both in clinical trials and through analysis of airway histology. Prior to increasing the dose of inhaled corticosteroid it is currently recommended for patients 5 yr of age and older that a long-acting β_2-agonist be added to attempt to gain better control of symptoms.

CROMOLYN SODIUM AND NEDOCROMIL

These medications have distinct but similar anti-inflammatory actions, including blockade of chloride channels and the ability to modulate mast cell mediator release and eosinophil recruitment. Both medications inhibit the early and late asthmatic response to allergen challenge and exercise induced bronchospasm. Nedocromil has been shown to be more effective than cromolyn at reducing exercise induced bronchospasm; however, they both reduce symptoms, increase morning peak flows, and reduce short-acting β_2-agonist usage. Clinical trials have shown them to be equally efficacious. Both are available in a metered dose inhaler and require four times a day dosing, although there is some evidence that nedocromil may be effective at twice-daily dosing. The clinical response to these is much less predictable than steroids, however the safety profile is excellent.

LONG-ACTING β_2-AGONISTS

These medications have the same mechanism of action as the quick relief β_2-agonists, however, they can last up to 12 h. Stimulation of β_2 receptors in the lung causes an increase in cAMP production that antagonizes bronchoconstriction. These medications are not of use in acute exacerbations but rather as adjunctive therapy to anti-inflammatory control. Long-acting β_2-agonists are especially helpful with nocturnal symptoms and exercise-induced bronchospasm and should be added to low-dose inhaled steroid prior to increasing the steroid dose.

(*Note.* since guideline issued: FDA issued a statement [http://www.fda.gov/cder/drug/InfoSheets/HCP/salmeterolHCP.htm, accessed 12/13/05], based on data from a large placebo-controlled US [SMART—Salmeterol Multicenter Asthma Research Trial]. This study compared the safety of salmeterol or placebo added to usual asthma therapy and showed an increase in asthma-related deaths in patients receiving salmeterol [13 deaths out of 13,176 patients treated for 28 wk on salmeterol vs 3 deaths out of 13,179 patients on placebo]. Therefore, long-acting β-agonists should not be used alone in the treatment of asthma).

METHYLXANTHINES

Theophylline as a sustained-release preparation may be used as an alternative medication for long-term prevention; however, it is not the preferred medication as it has a small therapeutic window and its serum level must be monitored. It is thought to have mild anti-inflammatory effects at low doses.

LEUKOTRIENE MODIFIERS

Leukotrienes are biochemical inflammatory mediators released from mast cells, eosinophils, and basophils that cause airway smooth muscle to contract, increase vascular permeability, increase mucus secretions, and attract further inflammatory cells. Zilueton is a 5-lipoxogenase inhibitor, whereas zafirlukast and montelukast are both leukotriene receptor antagonists. The have all been shown to improve lung function and reduce the use of short-acting β_2-agonists. They can function as alternative monotherapy in mild persistent asthma or in combination with an inhaled steroid in moderate persistent therapy, also as alternative therapy.

Quick-Relief Medications

Quick-relief medications are designed to relieve acute asthma symptoms such as bronchospasm, cough, chest tightness, and wheeze. These medications include both β_2-agonists and anticholinergic medications. Oral steroids may be comprised in this category as well, although they may take several hours to begin taking effect. They are effective in acute exacerbations at preventing progression, speeding recovery, and preventing early relapses.

β_2-AGONISTS

Short-acting β_2-agonists are the main type of quick-relief medicine used in acute asthma. These medications act on β_2-receptors to antagonize bronchospasm and relax airway smooth muscle causing prompt increase in airflow.

ANTICHOLINERGIC MEDICATION

Ipratroprium bromide is an inhaled anticholinergic medication used to antagonize the cholinergic regulation of airway smooth muscle tone. It is not frequently used in asthma; however, may be helpful in some patients with concomitant COPD.

SYSTEMIC CORTICOSTEROIDS

Oral corticosteroids provide relief of airway inflammation in moderate-to-severe asthmatic exacerbations. Their onset is generally within 4 h and they have been shown to reverse inflammation, prevent progression of exacerbations, speed recovery, and reduce relapse rates. Short-term, they can be used from 3 to 10 d until the patient consistently achieves more than 80% of his or her normal peak flow. Patients receiving more than 5 d of oral steroid may require a taper prior to discontinuing the course.

Safety

INHALED CORTICOSTEROIDS

There is a small but increased risk of adverse events associated with the use of inhaled corticosteroids. Adverse reactions include oral candidiasis, dysphonia, reflex cough, and bronchospasm as well as dose-dependent linear growth delay and osteoporosis.

Oral thrush can be avoided by advising patients to rinse their mouths with water (swish and spit) after administration of steroid. Dysphonia is reported with vocal stress and increased doses of inhaled steroid. Vocal rest, use of a spacer, and if required a short-term reduction in steroid dose, generally alleviates the problem. Reflex cough and bronchospasm can also be alleviated by the use of a spacer device. There is no evidence that use of a short-acting β_2-agonist prior to steroid use increases the amount of medication that reaches the lungs.

Severe asthma itself can cause linear growth delay. The evidence for linear growth retardation with inhaled corticosteroid use seems to be largely dose-dependent. Most long-term studies on low-to-moderate doses of inhaled steroid have found no reduction in ultimate adult height, only transient reductions in growth rates. Physicians should, however, always use the lowest effective dose of inhaled steroid to manage symptoms of asthma and to monitor the growth of children with asthma carefully. In severe asthma, the use of inhaled corticosteroids show significantly less adverse effects on linear growth than the use of systemic steroids.

The risk of inhaled corticosteroids effecting bone metabolism and causing osteoporosis seems to be limited. There is some evidence that suggests a reduction in bone mineral content in asthma patients taking inhaled corticosteroid. Elderly female patients may be more at risk for these effects resuting from concurrent osteoporosis and previous oral corticosteroid use. If inhaled corticosteroids are used in this group, it is reasonable to recommend supplementation of calcium and vitamin D.

SHORT-ACTING β_2-AGONISTS

The increased use of short-acting β_2-agonist medication should alert the clinician that there may be poor overall control and the patient may require increased anti-inflammatory medication use. The scheduled use of short-acting β_2-agonists is not recommended as it has not shown any proven benefit over as-needed therapy and the later can act as a barometer for control.

Special Treatment Groups

INFANTS AND PRESCHOOLERS

As in other groups, these children should follow the stepwise therapy outlined in Table 4. Children requiring treatment of symptoms more than twice a week should be given a trial of a long-term anti-inflammatory medication (nedocromil, cromolyn, or inhaled corticosteroid). Frequent office visits for symptom monitoring in the first month are required. Once the child is under adequate control for 3 mo, step-down therapy can be considered. In this age group cromolyn, nedocromil, and leukotriene receptor antagonists are often tried prior to initiation of steroids. If the therapy does not seem to be working, a change in therapy or an alternative diagnosis must be considered. Oral corticosteroids may be required for moderate to severe exacerbations or for those patients with a history of severe exacerbations associated with viral upper respiratory infections. Consider that medications must be given via a device that is age appropriate and that doses received may vary considerably owing to poor technique.

CHILDREN AGED 2 OR LESS

Nebulized therapy is preferred for the use of high-dose, short-acting β_2-agonists or nedocromil. A metered dose inhaler (MDI) with a spacer device and face mask can be used for inhaled corticosteroid; however, appropriate sizing is required as well as review of technique prior to leaving the office.

CHILDREN 3–5 YR

Children of this age should be able to use an MDI with spacer effectively; however, some may still require the use of a face mask with the device or nebulizer treatments if the desired effect of the medication is not achieved.

SPACER DEVICES

There are a large variety of shapes and sizes of spacer devices. Spacers are designed to hold aerosolized medication so dispensing the medication and inhalation do not have to be perfectly coordinated to achieve adequate delivery to the lungs.

SCHOOL-AGED CHILDREN

Stepwise management is required for this age group and it may be appropriate to try nedocromil, cromolyn, or leukotriene receptor antagonists as an anti-inflammatory because of their efficacy and their safety profile. Children with moderate or severe persistent asthma will often require inhaled corticosteroid. Adverse effects of inhaled corticosteroids including concerns with linear bone growth are discussed elsewhere in the text. Physicians should attempt to step-down therapy to the lowest dose of inhaled corticosteroid required to reduce side effects.

OLDER ADULTS

It is recommended that older adults taking inhaled corticosteroid be given calcium and vitamin D supplementation to combat the possibility of increased risk of osteoporosis. Oral steroids are more likely to cause confusion and agitation in the elderly and irregularities in glucose metabolism.

EXERCISE-INDUCED ASTHMA

A history of cough, shortness of breath, chest tightness, and wheezing with onset during exercise and peaking shortly after ceasing exercise is consistent with exercise-induced asthma. Most patients do not need to limit their activity but should abide by the recommended control measures. Control measures include two to four puffs of a short-acting β_2-agonist 5–60 min before exercise, which can be helpful for up to 3 h. An alternative is to use a long-acting β_2-agonist within 30 min of exercise, which will continue to have effects for up to 12 h. Many patients with exercise-induced asthma benefit from a short warm-up period prior to vigorous activity. Children at school should have teachers who are informed of their condition and have a written action plan for an acute asthma attack.

PATIENTS UNDERGOING SURGERY

Asthma patients undergoing surgery should be evaluated as to their control over the last 6 mo. When possible, therapy should be initiated in order to improve these patients to predicted peak flow values. These therapies include the use of oral corticosteroids. Any patient having received oral steroids for more than 14 d in the previous 6 mo requires stress-dose steroids during surgery. Patients should be given 100 mg of hydrocortisone intravenously every 8 h during the procedure and quickly taper in the first day following surgery.

PREGNANT PATIENTS

Most pregnant patients can have their asthma regimen unchanged throughout pregnancy without risk of harm to the fetus. There is evidence to suggest that poorly controlled asthma is associated with low birthweight infants and increased risk of prematurity. Many antibiotics cannot be used in acute exacerbations and α-adrenergic agonists (other than pseudoephedrine) are not safe during pregnancy.

COMPONENT 4: EDUCATION FOR A PARTNERSHIP IN ASTHMA CARE

Physicians need to arm patients and their families with the tools required to take the appropriate actions to control their asthma. Patients should have frequent visits to their primary care physician and at each visit medication compliance must be checked. Peak flows should be monitored.

In order to increase compliance in asthma patients, the plan must be tailored to their needs and their lifestyle. Goals of therapy must be discussed with the patient. Written instructions can be helpful with compliance as well as a written agreement between the physician and the patient regarding the long-term management plan of the patient's asthma. Physicians need to follow-up either with frequent office visits or telephone calls to reinforce the treatment plan. The physician should find out when the easiest time to take medications is for the patient and attempt to tailor therapy to fit the patient's and his or her family's or schedule. Action plans for exacerbations frequently and ask them to repeat them to you. As many helpful family members as possible should be recruited to learn and understand the long-term treatment plan as well as the plan for exacerbations.

Like any chronic disease, the best management of asthma will be in partnership with an educated and motivated patient. The patient should be involved in all aspects of his or her care and should be empowered to make educated decisions according to his or her symptoms. Exacerbations can be a time to educate and allow patients to further understand their disease.

SOURCES

1. Expert Panel Report 2. *Guidelines for the Diagnosis and Management of Asthma,* National Asthma Education and Prevention Program, Clinical Practice Guidelines, National Institutes of Health; No. 97-4051 July 1997.
2. Expert Panel Report: *Guidelines for the Diagnosis and Management of Asthma,* Update on Selected Topics 2002. National Asthma Education and Prevention Program, National Institutes of Health; No. 02-5074 June 2003.

III INFECTIOUS DISEASE

8

Community-Acquired Pneumonia and Health Care-Associated Pneumonia Clinical Guidelines

John Russell, MD

CONTENTS

OVERVIEW AND EPIDEMIOLOGY
CHEST RADIOGRAPHY
OTHER DIAGNOSTIC TESTING
SITE OF TREATMENT DECISION
PORT SEVERITY INDEX
DISCHARGE CRITERIA
SPECIFIC PATHOGENS
EMPIRIC THERAPY
SPECIFIC ANTIBACTERIAL AGENTS
SPECIAL POPULATIONS AND CIRCUMSTANCES
UPDATE ON PERFORMANCE INDICATORS
PREVENTION
SOURCES

The Infectious Disease Society of America (IDSA) produced clinical guidelines on the care of community-acquired pneumonia (CAP) in immunocompetent adults in 2000 and 2003 *(1,2)*. Throughout the guidelines, a grading system is used to categorize the strength of evidence behind various recommendations *(3)*, as listed in Table 1.

OVERVIEW AND EPIDEMIOLOGY

In the United States, pneumonia is a major cause of mortality and the sixth leading cause of death. The most common cause of death being from infectious

From: *Current Clinical Practice: Essential Practice Guidelines in Primary Care*
Edited by: N. S. Skolnik © Humana Press, Totowa, NJ

Table 1
IDSA-US Public Health Service Grading of Recommendations

Category, grade	Interpretation
Strength of recommendation	
A	Good evidence to support a recommendation for use
B	Moderate evidence
C	Poor evidence
D	Moderate evidence to support recommendation against its use
E	Good evidence to support a recommendation against use
Quality of evidence	
I	>1 Randomized, controlled trial
II	>1 Well-designed trial without randomization; might be cohort, case-controlled studies
III	Evidence from opinions of authorities or expert committees

disease. William Osler referred to pneumonia as "the old man's friend" and "captain of the men of death." These spoke to the high lethality the disease had at the turn of the 20th century. Still, pneumonia is the cause of great morbidity and mortality, despite advances in antibacterial therapies. Overall, there are 2–3 million cases of pneumonia in the United States and approx 500,000 hospitalizations. Mortality rates range from less than 1% in those treated as out-patients to up to 30% in hospitalized patients. Overall, the incidence of pneumonia is higher during the winter.

CAP is defined as an acute infectious process of the lower respirator tract in a patient living outside of a nursing care facility or not hospitalized in the previous 2 wk. Patients should have evidence of pneumonia on a chest radiograph by way of an infiltrate or finding on physical examination consistent with pneumonia. These findings might include diminished breath sounds or localized rales. Because physical examination findings are neither sensitive nor specific, it is recommended that patients receive further testing by way of chest radiographs (A–II).

CHEST RADIOGRAPHY

Chest radiography is indicated for all patients with suspected pneumonia (A–II). The radiograph is essential for establishing a diagnosis and distinguishing pneumonia from acute bronchitis. Physical examination is neither sensitive nor specific in establishing the diagnosis of pneumonia. There may be times when one is unable to obtain a chest radiograph because of limited resources but, because of the lack of clinical accuracy of the physical examination, this practice should be discouraged. The incidence of false-negative chest radiographs can be up to 30% in *Pneumocystis carinii* pneumonia, but this is not true in the case of immunocompetent adults.

OTHER DIAGNOSTIC TESTING

For the ambulatory patient who is to be treated as an outpatient, recommendations do not favor a search for an etiological agent but, rather empiric therapy. The clinician may decide to perform an air-dried, pretreatment, deep cough sputum sample that may have some utility (C–III). Patients who are being hospitalized or evaluated for possible hospitalization should have the following testing, that includes a complete blood count, electrolyte and blood urea nitrogen (BUN) measurement, liver functions, and oxygen saturation (B–II). Patients between 15 and 54 yr of age should be considered for HIV testing with proper consent (B–II).

Patients who are being hospitalized for pneumonia should have been tested or searched for an etiology of the pneumonia. Patients should have two pretreatment blood cultures obtained (A–II) as well as Gram stain and culture of the expectorated sputum (B–II). The sputum should be obtained before antibiotic therapy (B–II). Induced sputum should be reserved only for evaluation of *Mycobacterium tuberculosis* and *P. carinii* (A–I).

SITE OF TREATMENT DECISION

The decision regarding place of treatment is an important step in the management of CAP. In the United States, 75% of the 1 million pneumonia admissions come through emergency care units. The IDSA recommends that the decision on place of treatment is based on three steps: (1) safety and ability for patient to be treated at home, (2) clinical judgment, and (3) calculation of the pneumonia outcomes research team (PORT) severity index (PSI) with home therapy for PSI risk classes I–III (A–II). Use of the PSI scoring system is currently recommended by the IDSA, Canadian Thoracic Society, Canadian Infectious Disease Society, and the American College of Chest Physicians. Multiple studies have shown that patients in low PSI risk classes can be safely managed as outpatients.

PORT SEVERITY INDEX

Patients are classified into one of five risk classes with class I having the lowest risk and class V the highest. Initially, patients are screened for low-risk status based on age less than 50, comorbid illness (cancer, congestive heart failure, renal disease, liver disease, and cerebrovascular disease), vital signs, and mental status. Patients not assigned to class I are further evaluated by a point system based on age, comorbid illnesses listed previously, physical examination findings, presence of abnormal oxygenation, elevated BUN, acidosis on arterial blood gas, hyponatremia (<130 mmol/L), hyperglycemia (>250 mg/dL), anemia (hematocrit <30%), and presence of pleural effusion. The patient's sex and residence in a nursing facility also are part of the scoring system. Patients in classes I–III have an overall low mortality and can be treated safely at home unless there are preventing social factors.

DISCHARGE CRITERIA

Hospitalized patients can be safely changed to oral antibiotics when the patient, with a functioning gastrointestinal (GI) tract, is improving clinically, able to take oral medications, and hemodynamically stable (A–I). For a patient to be safely discharged from the hospital the following criteria are needed. The patient can have not more than one of the following characteristics in the 24 h before discharge: temperature over 37.8°C; pulse over 100/min; respiratory rate greater than 24 breaths/min; systolic blood pressure less than 90 mmHg, oxygen saturation below 90%, and ability to take oral medications (B–I). The physician should be aware of any of these characteristics that are abnormal at baseline.

SPECIFIC PATHOGENS

Streptococcus pneumoniae

A new method of testing is a pneumococcal urine antigen assay. It is a immunochromatographic membrane test that detects pneumococcal cell wall polysaccharide. It should yield results in approx 15 min. It can be used in conjunction with Gram stain and culture of sputum for diagnosis. Potentially, the urine antigen assay will provide accuracy similar to Gram stain in a more timely manner (B–II). The testing has been found to have a sensitivity in the 50–80% range, with a specificity of approx 90%.

Chlamydophilia pneumoniae

C. pneumoniae is a common respiratory pathogen. There is no clear "gold standard" for the diagnosis. The IDSA CAP Committee recommends testing methods that include serology, culture, polymerase chain reaction (PCR), and tissue diagnostics or immunochemistry. Acceptable ways to obtain the diagnosis for C. pneumonia pulmonary infections are the demonstration of a fourfold increase in IgG or a individual IgM titer of more than 1:16 via a microimmunofluorescence assay, isolation of a tissue culture, or a PCR assay of respiratory secretions (B–II). In patient-care settings, acute and convalescent titers may not be practical and the clinician should use the more timely PCR or IgM testing.

Legionella *Spp*

Legionella is implicated in 0.5–6% of CAP cases. Risk factors for *Legionella* are exposure, increasing age, smoking, and compromised cell-mediated immunity. Epidemiological risk factors include travel outside of home, exposure to spas, changes in domestic plumbing, and comorbid illnesses including renal failure, liver failure, diabetes, and malignancy. Overall mortality rates are 5–25%. A large percentage of hospitalized patients require ICU admission. Testing for *Legionella* is appropriate for any hospitalized patient with an enigmatic pneumonia (C–II). These patients are most likely critically ill, part of an epidemic, or nonresponders to β-lactam therapy (A–III). Testing should be performed via urine antigen assay and culture of respiratory secretions using selective media (A–II). The urine test is a rapid assay that detects 80–95% of CAP cases. In the setting of epidemiological evidence of disease, treatment should be administered despite negative testing (B–III). The preferred treatment of hospitalized patients is azithromycin or a fluoroquinolone (B–II). For out-patients, treatment options include erythromycin, azithromycin, clarithromycin, doxycycline, or a fluoroquinolone (A–II). Treatment should begin as rapidly as possible (A–II).

Viral Pneumonia

Respiratory viruses are a common cause of CAP. They are seen most commonly in the elderly, patients with chronic obstructive pulmonary disease or other comorbidities. The incidence of viral infections in CAP ranges from 4 to 39% in studies. Three-quarters of the viral infections are one of three viruses: respiratory syncytial virus (RSV), influenza, and parainfluenza viruses. There can be secondary bacterial infection in 26–77% of hospitalized adult patients with viral pneumonias. The most common pathogen seen is *S. pneumoniae* but, earlier studies found *Staphylococcus aureus* in 25% of cases. Empiric treatment of bacterial superinfection should provide activity against *S. pneumoniae*, *S. aureus*, and *Hemophilus influenzae*. Antibiotics choices should include amoxicillin-clavulanate, cefpodoxime, cefprozil, cefuroxime, or a respiratory quinolone (B–III).

RSV antigen detection tests are readily available but are insensitive for detecting disease in adults and are not generally recommended (C–III). The rapid detection test for influenza is recommended for both epidemiological and treatment purposes (C–II). Tests that can distinguish between influenza A and B are recommended (C–III). Treatment within 48 h of the onset of symptoms with antivirals targeted against influenza is recommended. Influenza A and B can be treated with oseltamivir or zanamivir, whereas amantadine and rimantadine only treat influenza A (B–I). Patients with symptoms of uncomplicated influenza for more than 48 h should not be treated with medications (D–I). The drugs can be used to reduce viral shedding in patients hospitalized with CAP (C–III).

Table 2
Outpatient Empiric Therapy of CAP

Outpatient characteristics	
Previously healthy	
No recent antibiotics	Erythromycin or doxycycline
Recent antibiotics	Levofloxacin, moxifloxacin, gemifloxacin or gatifloxacin alone, or azithromycin, clarithromycin plus high-dose amoxicillin, or azithromycin, clarithromycin plus high-dose amoxicillin-clavulanate
Comorbid illnesses	
No recent antibiotics	Azithromycin, clarithromycin, or levofloxacin, moxifloxacin, gemifloxacin, or gatifloxacin
Recent antibiotics	Levofloxacin, moxifloxacin, gemifloxacin, or gatifloxacin or azithromycin, clarithromycin plus a β-lactam
Suspected aspiration	Amoxicillin-clavulanate or clindamycin
Nursing home	Levofloxacin, moxifloxacin, gemifloxacin, or gatifloxacin, or azithromycin, clarithromycin plus amoxicillin-clavulanate
Influenza with bacterial superinfection	A β-lactam or levofloxacin, moxifloxacin, gemifloxacin, or gatifloxacin

Patients with pneumonia caused by *varicella zoster* virus should be treated by parenteral acyclovir (A–II). Other viral pneumonias caused by RSV, parainfluenza virus, adenovirus, metapneumovirus, Hantavirus, and the severe acute respiratory syndrome agent have no effective treatment (D–I).

EMPIRIC THERAPY

In the most diligent of CAP studies, an etiological agent is only found in 40–60% of cases. Clinicians need to treat patients empirically based on certain historical data until a specific pathogen can be found. Treatment can then be tailored to the specific pathogen. For empiric treatment of outpatients, please refer to Table 2 and for empiric treatment of hospitalized patients refer to Tables 3 and 4.

SPECIFIC ANTIBACTERIAL AGENTS

Macrolides

Macrolides are active against most common pathogens that cause CAP. Data from clinical trials has shown good results against strains with resistance

Table 3
In-Patient Empiric Therapy of CAP

In-patient characteristics	
Medical ward	
No recent antibiotics	Levofloxacin, moxifloxacin, gemifloxacin (orally only) or gatifloxacin or azithromycin, clarithromycin plus a β-lactam
Recent antibiotics	Azithromycin, clarithromycin plus a β-lactam levofloxacin, moxifloxacin, gemifloxacin (orally only) or gatifloxacin
Intensive care	
Pseudomonas infection is not an issue	A β-lactam plus azithromycin, clarithromycin or levofloxacin, moxifloxacin, gemifloxacin (orally only) or gatifloxacin
Pseudomonas infection is not an issue but patient has a β-lactam allergy	Levofloxacin, moxifloxacin, gemifloxacin (orally only) or gatifloxacin ± clindamycin
Pseudomonas infection is an issue	Piperacillin, piperacillin-tazobactam, imipenem, meropenem, or cefepime + ciprofloxacin or Piperacillin, piperacillin-tazobactam, imipenem, meropenem, or cefepime + aminoglycoside + respiratory fluoroquinolone or macrolide
Pseudomonas infection is an issue but patient has a β-lactam allergy	Aztreonam plus levofloxacin or, aztreonam plus moxifloxacin or gatifloxacin ± aminogylocoside
Nursing home	Same as medical ward or ICU[a]

[a]*See also* section at end of chapter on health care-associated pneumonia.

Table 4
Initial Empiric Antibiotic Therapy for HAP, VAP, and HCAP in Patients With Late-Onset Disease or Risk Factors for Multidrug-Resistant Pathogens (All Disease Severity)

Antipseudomonal cephalosporin (cefipime, ceftazidime)
or
Antipseudomonal carbepenem (imipenem or meropenem)
or
β-Lactam/β-lactamase inhibitor (piperacillin-tazobactam)
plus
Antipseudomonal fluoropunolone (ciprofloxacin or levofloxacin)
or
Aminoglycoside (amikacin, gentamicin, or tobramycin)
plus
Linezolid or vancomycin

HAP, hospital-acquired pneumonia; VAP, ventilator-associated pneumonia; HCAP, health care-associated pneumonia.

in vitro. The extended spectrum macrolides, azithromycin, and clarithromycin, can each be given once daily. Drawbacks are related to resistance and tolerability. Macrolide resistance can occur in 20–30% cases of *S. pneumonia*. Resistance can develop during therapy. The resistance occurs more often than in fluoroquinolones or β-lactams. Overall, erythromycin is less well tolerated resulting from GI side effects. Erythromycin is also less effective against *H. influenzae*.

Ketolides

Ketolides are semisynthetic derivatives of macrolides. They were designed to be effective against macrolide-resistant Gram-positive cocci. Telithromycin is a ketolide that may be an alternative to macrolides in CAP. Telithromycin is a once-daily, well-tolerated antibiotic. It is active against *S. pneumoniae*, including macrolide-resistant strains, *H. influenzae*, *Moraxella catarrhalis*, as well as *Legionella*, *Mycoplasma*, and *Chlamydophylia* species.

Amoxicillin

Amoxicillin is the preferred drug of choice for oral treatment of susceptible strains of *S. pneumoniae*. At doses of 3–4 g daily, it covers 90–95% of strains of pneumococccus. The drawback to using amoxicillin as a treatment is that there is no coverage of atypical pathogens. It is also problematic that very high doses are required for coverage of *S. pneumoniae*.

Amoxicillin–Clavulanate

Compared with amoxicillin, the combination has better coverage against anaerobes, *H. influenzae*, and methicillin-sensitive *S. aureus*. Like amoxicillin, it has no activity against atypical pathogens. It is more expensive than amoxicillin and GI symptoms are common.

Cephalosporins

Oral cephalosporins are active against 75–85% of *S. pneumoniae* and almost all species of *H. influenzae*. Ceftriaxone and cefotaxime are injectable medications that cover 90–95% of *S. pneumoniae* and *H. influenzae* and methicillin-sensitive *S. aureus*. Neither the oral or injectable forms of cephalosporins are active against atypical agents.

Doxycycline

Doxycycline is active against 90–95% of strains of *S. pneumoniae*, as well as *H. influenzae* and atypical pathogens. It is also active against many agents used in bioterrorism. Despite being an affordable and well-tolerated medication, it is rarely used for CAP in clinical practice.

Fluoroquinolones

As a class, the fluoroquinolones are active against a broad spectrum of agents that cause CAP. This includes more than 98% of strains of *S. pneumoniae* in the United States. Despite its wide spectrum of activity, there are fears of increasing resistance to these medications. They can be given once daily and are very well tolerated. Overall, they are far more expensive than erythromycin and doxycycline.

Clindamycin

Clindamycin is active against 90% of strains of *S. pneumoniae* but not *H. influenzae* and atypical pathogens. It also has very good activity for anaerobic infections. It is favored for toxic shock owing to pneumonia associated with group A *streptococci*. Clindamycin can cause high rates of diarrhea and *Clostridium difficile* colitis.

SPECIAL POPULATIONS AND CIRCUMSTANCES

Pneumonia in Elderly Persons

With 60,000 annual deaths, pneumonia is the sixth leading cause of death in senior citizens. Elderly persons who live in extended-care facilities are at increased risk of morbidity and mortality from pneumonia. The most common pathogen is *S. pneumoniae* CAP, which is also the most common pathogen in younger patients. The elderly, especially those with comorbidities or those living in extended-care facilities, are more likely to have Gram-negative bacteria and *S. aureus* as etiological agents than their younger counterparts. Risk factors in addition age that put seniors at increased risk are institutionalization, difficulty swallowing, inability to take oral medications, lung disease, heart disease, immunosuppression, alcoholism, and male sex.

When elderly patients present with pneumonia, they are likely to have fewer symptoms than younger adults. The fewer number of symptoms are mostly related to a decrease in the febrile response to illness (chills, sweats). Prevention of pneumonia through vaccination against pneumococcus and influenza should be part of the primary care management of senior citizens. Antimicrobial choice for elderly patients with CAP is the same as for all adults with CAP (B–III). For nursing home patients with pneumonia that is severe enough to require hospitalization (health care-associated pneumonia [HCAP], please *see* updated guidelines for hospital-acquired pneumonia [HAP] in the last section of this chapter).

SARS

SARS is a termed first used in 2002 to describe a pneumonia outbreak that began in southern China. As of July 2003, there had been more than 8000 cases in 28 nations worldwide. Most of the cases were seen in people with close contact with infected patients. The transmission rate was relatively high. The transmission was felt to be via respiratory droplets. Health care workers must be vigilant in recognizing SARS because of important issues regarding transmissibility to close contacts including health care workers and close personal contacts (A–III). Health care workers should use standard infection control precautions as well as contact and respiratory precautions (A–I), which would include hand washing; wearing of gowns, goggles, gloves, fit-tested respirators; which and negative pressure rooms.

The infectious agent is a novel coronavirus. The signs and symptoms in patients are temperature over 38°C and more than one of the constellation of cough, dyspnea, and hypoxia in the setting of possible exposure to a person with SARS or a region with community transmission of SARS. Diagnostic criteria include clinical and epidemiological features and also diagnostic studies (A–I). Recommendations for virological studies include culture for SARS coronavirus, detection of antibody during the acute phase of illness, or detection of SARS coronavirus RNA by second PCR assay.

In most cases, the illness resolves spontaneously in 1–2 wk. In 20% of patients, symptoms over 2–3 wk will progress to a more severe respiratory illness. Overall, 10–15% of cases have died of progressive respiratory failure. Mortality rates have been highest in the elderly or in those with heart or lung disease. At this point, the major therapeutic intervention is supportive care (B–III).

Pneumonia in the Context of Bioterrorism

With the ability to disseminate some infectious agents via an aerosolized route, bioterrorism attacks might presents as pneumonia. The agents with the greatest risk of severe respiratory illness are *Bacillus anthracis, Franciella tularensis,* and *Yersinia pestis.* A case of inhaled anthrax would always indicate bioterrorism, whereas pneumonic tularemia or pneumonic plague may or may not be caused by bioterrorism. Clinicians should know the clues to bioterrorism and the mechanism of alerting public health officials in cases of suspected bioterrorism (A–III).

In 2001, there were 11 cases of inhalation anthrax from contaminated mail in the United States. Diagnostic features that might distinguish inhalational anthrax from CAP include a widened mediastinum on chest X-ray, hyperdense mediastinal lymph nodes on chest computed tomography (CT) scan, and a bloody pleural effusion. Blood cultures were positive eight of eight untreated patients in 2001. The blood cultures were positive on the first day. Mortality rates are in the 45–80% rate. The incubation period was approx 4 d. The work-up of inhalation anthrax should include a blood culture (A–I) and a chest CT scan (A–I). The most important therapeutic interventions are antibiotic therapy and draining of pleural effusions. Antibiotic treatment should be prolonged resulting from the potential persistence of spores in animal models. Prophylaxis can be achieved with prolonged courses (60–100 d) of doxycycline or ciprofloxacin.

F. tularensis causes less than 200 infections a year in the United States. An aerosolized attack with *F. tularensis* is referred to as a "typhoidal" or "pneumonic" tularemia. After an incubation period of 3–5 d, the patient might present nonspecific symptoms of fever, dry cough, malaise, and pleuritic chest pain. The chest X-ray should show a pneumonia with mediastinal adenopathy. Cultures of blood, pharynx, and sputum should be obtained and evaluated in a biocontainment level-3 laboratory owing to safety concerns (A–I).

Standard treatment is streptomycin but gentamicin is an acceptable alternative. Tetracycline and chloramphenicol have also been used, but with higher failure rates. Ciprofloxacin is not approved for tularemia but has had clinical success in human and animal studies. Treatment should last 2 wk. Mortality rate has been found in studies to be 1.4%.

Y. pestis is an ideal biological weapon because of its high mortality without treatment and can be transmitted from person to person. Patients might present with high fevers, chills, headache, cough, bloody sputum, leukocytosis, and bilateral pneumonia on chest radiograph. Patients can decompensate quickly to septic shock and death. Patients lack the swollen, tender lymph node, or bubo that is characteristic of bubonic plague.

Patients should have blood culture, sputum culture, and Gram stain (A–I). The Gram stain shows safety pin-shaped Gram-negative coccobacilli. Health care workers should use respiratory precautions until the patient has undergone 48 h of therapy. Antibiotic treatment would be streptomycin or gentamicin for 10 d. Patients with face-to-face contact or suspected exposure should receive 7 d of prophylaxis with tetracycline or fluoroquinolone.

UPDATE ON PERFORMANCE INDICATORS

Previous IDSA guidelines recommended starting antibiotics within 8 h of admission. A more recent medicare analysis of pneumonia hospitalizations found that earlier treatment with antibiotics improved outcomes. Patients who received antibiotics within 4 h of arrival at the hospital had a mean length of stay that was 0.4 d shorter than patients who received their antibiotics later. Earlier initiation of antibiotics had a greater impact than antibiotic choice. These factors have led to a change in the IDSA guidelines. Patients hospitalized with CAP should have antibiotics initiated within 4 h of registration at the hospital. Patients being hospitalized for pneumonia should have blood cultures performed prior to initializing antibiotic therapy (B–III).

Patients should also have assessment of oxygenation by pulse oximetry or arterial blood gas measurement within 8 h of admission (A–III). There should also be a documented infiltrate on chest X-ray or other imaging study in all patients except those with decreased immune function that might not be able to mount an inflammatory response (A–I).

In intensive care patients with severe enigmatic pneumonia, a target of at least 50% of patients should receive some type of testing for *Legionella* by either urine antigen testing or culture (A–III). Smoking has a long and heralded connection with respiratory diseases. Smoking is the biggest risk factor for pneumococcal bacteremia in immunocompetentent, nonelderly adults. Smoking cessation should be a goal for persons who smoke and are hospitalized with CAP (B–II).

PREVENTION

Influenza

All persons over the age of 50 or younger patients with risk factors for pneumonia should receive a yearly inactivated influenza vaccine each fall (A–I). Household contacts, aged 5–49 yr, of patients at risk for influenza may receive the nasally administered live, attenuated influenza vaccine (C–I). The live attenuated vaccine should not be used in those with asthma or immunodeficiency. The influenza vaccine should be offered to at-risk patients on hospital discharge, or outpatient encounters in the late fall or early winter (C–III). All health care workers, in any setting, should receive annual influenza vaccine (A–I).

Pneumococcal Vaccine

Pneumococcal polysaccharide vaccine is indicated for all persons aged 65 yr or older and selected high-risk patients (B–II). High-risk patients include those with diabetes, cardiovascular disease, lung disease, alcohol abuse, liver disease, cerebrospinal fluid leaks, HIV, renal failure, sickle cell disease, nephrotic syndrome, hematological malignancies, or those on long-term immunosuppressive medications. Patients should receive a repeat vaccination in 5 yr if they received their first dose before the age of 65 yr. Vaccination can occur on hospital discharge or during outpatient therapy (C–III).

Management of Adults With Hospital-Acquired, Ventilator-Associated, and Health Care-Associated Pneumonias

Additional guidelines on the management of adults with HAP, ventilator-associated pneumonia, and HCAP, were issued jointly by the American Thoracic Society and the IDSA in 2005. The guidelines acknowledge that they emphasize (VAP) because there is far less clear evidence on HAP in nonintubated patients and for HCAPs. HAP is defined as pneumonia that occurs 48 h or more after hospital admission. HCAP is defined as including any patient who was hospitalized in an acute care hospital for 2 or more days within 90 d of the development of the current pneumonia; any patient residing in a nursing home or long-term care facility; any patient who has received recent intravenous antibiotic therapy, chemotherapy, or wound care (in the last 30 d);

Table 5
Doses of Recommended Antibiotics for HAP, VAP, and HCAP in Patients With Late-Onset Disease or Risk Factors for Multidrug-Resistant Pathogens (All Disease Severity)

Antibiotic	Dosage[a]
Antipseudomal cephalosporin	
Cefepime	1–2 g every 8–12 h
Ceftazidime	2 g every 8 h
Carbepenems	
Imipenem	500 mg every 6 h or 1 g every 8 h
Meropenem	1 g every 8 h
β-Lactam/β-lactamase inhibitor	
Piperacillin-tazobactam	4.5 g every 6 h
Aminoglycosides	
Gentamicin	7 mg/kg/d[b]
Tobramycin	7 mg/kg/d[b]
Amikacin	20 mg/kg/d[b]
Antipseudomonal qunolones	
Levofloxacin	759 mg every d
Ciprofloxacin	400 mg every 8 h
Vancomycin	15 mg/kg every 12 h[c]
Linezolid	600 mg every 12 h

[a]Doses are based on normal renal and hepatic function.
[b]Trough levels for gentamicin and tobramycin should be less than 1 mg/mL, and for amikacin less than 4–5 mg/mL.
[c]Trough levels for vancomycin should be 15–20 mg/mL.

or who has attended a hemodialysis unit. These guidelines, were created because of the increasing prevalence of multidrug-resistant (MDR) bacterial pathogens.

HCAP in elderly patients in long-term care facilities have pathogens that are similar to those of patients with HAP and VAP. The guidelines quote two studies of patients in nursing homes with severe pneumonias. One of the studies looked specifically at patients who failed to respond to initial antibiotics over 72 h and found a high level of resistant pathogens. Common organisms that cause HCAP include aerobic Gram-negative bacilli (*Pseudomonas aeruginosa*, *Klebsiella pneumoniae*, and *Acinetobacter*), Gram-positive cocci (*S. aureus* [often methicillin resistant *S. aureus*], *S. pneumoniae, and H. influenzae* cause early-onset HAP, but are uncommon in late-onset infection) (*see* Tables 5 and 6).

The guidelines discuss that work-up of patients with VAP should include a lower respiratory tract sample for culture and that absence of organisms is strong evidence that a pneumonia does not exist and that absence of MDR organisms shows that there is a low likelihood of MDR organisms causing the pneumonia. The benefit and the negative predictive value of an expectorated

Table 6
Initial Empiric Antibiotic Therapy for HAP or VAP, in Patients With Early-Onset Disease and No Known Risk Factors for Multidrug-Resistant Pathogens (All Disease Severity)

Cefriaxone
or
Levofloxacin, moxifloxacin, or ciprofloxacin
or
Ampicillin/sulbactam
or
Ertapenem

Note: This is not HCAP, which by definition has risk factors for MDR bacteria.

sputum sample in patients who are not intubated (i.e., HCAP) is not clear. The management strategy for VAP, HAP, and HCAP recommended is as follows:

1. Obtain lower respiratory tract sample for culture and microscopy.
2. Begin empiric antibiotics.
3. On days 2 and 3, check cultures and assess clinical response:
   a. If there is clinical improvement over 48–72 h:
      i. If cultures are positive, "de-escalate antibiotics" and treat selected patients for 7–8 d.
      ii. If cultures are negative, consider stopping antibiotics (decision to stop antibiotics should be influenced by the way the sample was collected and the estimated accuracy of the sample.
   b. If there is no clinical improvement over 46–72 h:
      i. If cultures are positive, adjust antibiotic therapy and reassess diagnosis, and look for complications.
      ii. If cultures are negative, look for other pathogens and reassess diagnosis, and look for complications.

The choice of antibiotics is influenced by the likelihood of MDR pathogens. The guidelines suggest that for HAP, VAP, or HCAP, which occurs as late-onset (>5 d after admission) disease or which have risk factors for MDR pathogens (essentially all HCAP as defined earlier), patients should receive broad spectrum antibiotics to cover for MDR organisms. Combination antibiotic therapy is recommended for this group, as listed in Table 1. The guidelines note that no data exist to document the superiority of combination antibiotic therapy when compared with monotherapy, but combination therapy increases the chances of selecting at least one effective antibiotic during initial treatment. In selecting antibiotics for patients who have recently received antibiotics, it is preferable to select an antibiotic from a different class than the antibiotic the patient was just on. If the patient's regimen includes an aminoglycoside, the aminoglycoside can be stopped after 5–7 d if the patient is responding. Duration of treatment can be as short as 7 d in patients with a good clinical response who do not have a documented infection with *P. aeruginosa*. Clinical improvement usually takes 48–72 h and so therapy should not be changed in that time period unless there is clinical decline. In patients who respond to treatment, therapy can be narrowed on the basis of cultures.

SOURCES

1. Update of Practice Guidelines for the Management of Community-Acquired Pneumonia in Immunocompetent Adults (2003) Clin Inf Dis 37:1405–1433.
2. Practice Guidelines for the Management of Community-Acquired Pneumonia in Adults (2000) Clin Inf Dis 31:347–382.
3. Guidelines for the Management of Adults with Hospital-acquired, Ventilator-associated, and Healthcare-associated Pneumonia (2005) Am J Respir Crit Care Med 171:388–416.

9

Diagnosis and Management of Otitis Media

Joint Guidelines From the American Academy of Pediatrics and American Academy of Family Physicians

Richard Neill, MD

CONTENTS

INTRODUCTION

Acute otitis media (AOM) is one of the most common reasons for sick child visits in the United States. Controversy over its diagnosis and appropriate management has led the American Academy of Pediatrics and American Academy of Family Physicians to author evidence-based clinical practice guidelines. These guidelines are used for the healthy children aged 2 mo to 12 yr. The guidelines do not apply to children with underlying conditions that alter the nature of middle ear disease. Underlying conditions include anatomic abnormalities such as cleft palate and genetic conditions such as Down syndrome, immunodeficiencies, and the presence of cochlear implants.

The guidelines categorize its recommendations according to the strength of evidence supporting the recommendation. Four levels of recommendations

From: *Current Clinical Practice: Essential Practice Guidelines in Primary Care*
Edited by: N. S. Skolnik © Humana Press, Totowa, NJ

119

included are the strong recommendation, recommendation, option, and no recommendation. There are six key recommendations included in the guidelines:

1. *Recommendation:* To diagnose AOM, the clinician should confirm a history of
   acute onset, identify signs of middle ear effusion, and evaluate for the presence
   of signs and symptoms of middle ear inflammation (MEI).
2. *Strong recommendation:* The management of AOM should include an assessment of pain. If pain is present, the clinician should recommend treatment to
   reduce pain *(1)*.
3a. *Option:* Observation without use of antibacterial agents in a child with uncom-
    plicated AOM is an option for selected children based on diagnostic certainty,
    age, illness severity, and assurance of follow-up.
3b. *Recommendation:* If a decision is made to treat with an antibacterial agent, the
    clinician should prescribe amoxicillin for most children. Option: When amox-
    icillin is used, the dose should be 80–90 mg/kg/d.
4. *Recommendation:* If the patient fails to respond to the initial management
   option within 48–72 h, the clinician must reassess the patient to confirm AOM
   and exclude other causes of illness. If AOM is confirmed in the patient initially
   managed with observation, the clinician should begin antibacterial therapy. If
   the patient was initially managed with an antibacterial agent, the clinician
   should change the antibacterial agent.
5. *Recommendation:* Clinicians should encourage the prevention of AOM
   through reduction of risk factors.
6. *No recommendation:* There is insufficient evidence to make a recommendation
   regarding the use of complementary and alternative medicines (CAMs) for AOM.

DIAGNOSIS

The guidelines provide a common definition of AOM comprised of three
required elements: abrupt onset of symptoms, presence of a middle ear effusion
(MEE), and signs or symptoms of MEI (*see* Table 1). Even with clear criteria
for diagnosis, application of the criteria in real life presents many challenges.
For adequate examination, it is often difficult to clear the external canal of ceru-
men. Even when visible, documenting MEE can be a challenge.

The biggest diagnostic challenge is differentiating AOM from otitis media
with effusion, a similar condition defined by the presence of fluid in the middle
ear cavity without signs or symptoms of acute middle ear infection.

A diagnosis of AOM requires all of the following:

1. A history of recent, usually abrupt, onset of signs, and symptoms of MEI.
2. The presence of middle ear effusion that is indicated by any of the following:
   a. Bulging of the tympanic membrane.
   b. Limited or absent mobility of the tympanic membrane.
   c. Air–fluid level behind the tympanic membrane.
   d. Otorrhea.

Table 1
Diagnosis of Acute Otitis Media

A diagnosis of acute otitis media requires all of the following:
1. A history of recent, usually abrupt, onset of signs and symptoms of middle-ear inflammation

and

2. The presence of middle ear effusion that is indicated by any of the following:
   a. Bulging of the tympanic membrane
   b. Limited or absent mobility of the tympanic membrane
   c. Air-fluid level behind the tympanic membrane
   d. Otorrhea

and

3. Signs or symtoms of middle-ear inflammation as indicated by:
   a. Distinct erythema of the tympanic membrane or
   b. Distinct otalgia (discomfort clearly referable to the ear[s] that results in interface with or precludes normal activity or sleep)

3. Signs or symptoms of MEI as indicated by:
   a. Distinct erythema of the tympanic membrane or
   b. Distinct otalgia (discomfort clearly referable to the ears that results in interference with or precludes normal activity or sleep).

MANAGEMENT OF PAIN

All patients should have an assessment of pain, including adequate treatment, especially within the first 24–48 h of onset. Oral ibuprofen and acetaminophen are the mainstays of treatment, although topical agents such as benzocaine may offer a brief incremental benefit in children more than 5 yr old. Home remedies such as external heat or cold, distraction, or oil may have limited effectiveness. Tympanostomy may be used when the potential benefit outweighs the risk of the procedure.

TREATMENT OPTIONS

Clinicians have two initial treatment options based on the child's age (i.e., the certainty of the diagnosis and severity of illness). Uncertain diagnosis means less than three diagnostic criteria met from among history, MEE and MEI, whereas severe illness is defined as fever of at least 39°C or moderate to severe otalgia.

Initial observation is appropriate for children 2 yr or older with nonsevere illness without regard to diagnostic certainty. Children 6 mo or older and nonsevere illness might be observed only if the diagnosis is uncertain. Antibiotics should be used in all children 6 mo old and older and in those ages from 6 mo to 2 yr with a certain diagnosis.

In all instances in which observation is chosen, it should be reserved only for children in whom follow-up can be ensured. A parent or adult should be identified who will reliably observe the child, recognize signs of serious illness, and should be able to provide prompt access to medical care, if improvement does not occur.

If antibiotic therapy is chosen, high-dose amoxicillin (80–90 mg/kg/d divided into two or three doses) is the preferred agent for patients with non-severe illness. Patients with severe illness should receive amoxicillin–clavulanate. Penicillin-allergic patients should receive a second-generation cephalosporin (if no type I allergy) or macrolide (if a type I penicillin allergy). Penicillin-allergic children with severe illness should receive ceftriaxone.

TREATMENT FAILURE

A clear plan for follow-up should be negotiated with the adult caregiver at the initial visit. Improvement in fever, irritability, eating, and sleeping patterns should be expected in the first 48–72 h. If no improvement occurs, either another disease is present or the therapy is inadequate and re-evaluation of the child is warranted.

Children who have failed initial observation should be offered antibiotic therapy as if they are diagnosed initially (amoxicillin for nonsevere illness and amoxicillin–clavulanate for severe illness). Initial amoxicillin failure should be treated with amoxicillin–clavulanate, whereas, initial amoxicillin–clavulanate failure should be treated with ceftriaxone.

Failure of antibiotic treatment in penicillin-allergic children should include ceftriaxone or clindamycin. Failure in penicillin-allergic children with severe illness should be treated with clindamycin preferentially.

Secondary antibiotic therapy failure warrants consideration of tympanocentesis for bacterial identification.

RISK FACTOR REDUCTION

Whenever possible, parents should be encouraged to modify or eliminate known risk factors that cause otitis media. Although the magnitude of effect varies among the interventions, encouragement of breast-feeding, reducing child care attendance, avoiding supine bottle feeding, reducing or eliminating pacifier use in the second 6 mo of life, eliminating exposure to passive tobacco smoke, and age-appropriate immunization have all been shown to reduce episodes of AOM.

COMPLEMENTARY MEDICINE APPROACHES TO AOM

The panel found insufficient evidence to make a recommendation regarding the use of CAM for AOM. Treatments studied include homeopathy, acupuncture, and nutritional supplements, although none of them showed convincing evidence of benefit. Clinicians should remain aware of parents' health beliefs and encourage discussion of treatments with an eye toward potential benefits or risks.

SOURCES

1. Diagnosis and Management of Acute Otitis Media. Subcommittee on Management of Acute Otitis Media, American Academy of Pediatrics and American Academy of Family Physicians. Pediatrics 2004, 113(5):1451–1465.

10

Appropriate Antibiotic Use for Treatment of Nonspecific Upper Respiratory Infections, Rhinosinusitis, and Acute Bronchitis in Adults

Tina H. Degnan, MD
and Neil S. Skolnik, MD

Contents

BACKGROUND

Acute sinusitis, bronchitis, pharyngitis, and nonspecific upper respiratory tract infections (URIs) account for the majority of antibiotics prescribed by primary care physicians in the United States. The emergence of antibiotic-resistant bacteria in the community setting is now an issue for individual patients as well as society at large, and it is the responsibility of all clinicians to limit antibiotic treatment to those patients who are most likely to benefit from it. The vast majority of acute respiratory infections are caused by viruses. Antibiotic treatment of patients with these infections selects for resistant nasopharyngeal bacteria, acutely increasing the spread of resistant pathogens through secretions and predisposing the treated patient to more serious bacterial infections in the future. The guidelines summarized in this chapter were designed by a panel of physicians representing family medicine, internal medicine, emergency medicine, and infectious diseases to provide a practical

From: *Current Clinical Practice: Essential Practice Guidelines in Primary Care*
Edited by: N. S. Skolnik © Humana Press, Totowa, NJ

125

approach to the appropriate diagnosis and treatment of previously healthy adults with nonspecific URI, acute sinusitis, or acute bronchitis in the ambulatory care setting. Recommendations for the diagnosis and treatment of pharyngitis are provided in a separate chapter.

NONSPECIFIC URI

The diagnosis of nonspecific URI should be applied to a patient with an acute infection involving sinus, pharyngeal, and upper airway symptoms without a prominent symptom with which to make a more specific diagnosis of sinusitis, pharyngitis, or bronchitis. Antibiotics are ineffective in treating nonspecific URIs because most often, a virus is the causative agent. Mild cases are most frequently caused by rhinoviruses. Patients with more severe symptoms, especially when accompanied by myalgia and fatigue, are likely to be infected with influenza or parainfluenza viruses. Other sources of URI symptoms include adenovirus and respiratory syncytial virus (RSV).

Multiple studies have failed to show a benefit for antibiotic treatment in adults with URI. Purulent secretions and prevention of complications are two common justifications for antibiotic treatment of URI. The clinical finding of purulent sputum or rhinorrhea in a patient with URI symptoms is not a reliable indicator of bacterial infection and should not be used to justify treatment of the URI with antibiotics. Bacterial complication of a viral URI is rare, and antibiotics have not been shown to prevent complications such as pneumonia or hasten the resolution of URI in previously healthy adults. On the contrary, unnecessary antibiotic use predisposes patients to carriage of antibiotic-resistant *Streptococcus pneumoniae* and to invasive infection with this bacterium in the future.

RHINOSINUSITIS

Acute rhinosinusitis (acute sinusitis) is a common primary care diagnosis and physicians prescribe an antibiotic to 85–98% of patients with this illness. Although primary care physicians tend to think of rhinosinusitis as an acute bacterial infection, the majority of cases are caused by a virus. The lack of straightforward diagnostic criteria or available testing with which to distinguish a bacterial sinusitis that might benefit from antibiotic therapy from a viral infection has led to the clinical overdiagnosis of bacterial sinus infections and the overprescription of antibiotics.

Symptom duration is one criterion that has been used to diagnose acute bacterial sinusitis. By definition, acute rhinosinusitis symptoms last less than 4 wk, but patients and physicians begin to suspect bacterial rather than viral infection when symptoms last longer than a few days. Studies of rhinovirus infection describe duration of symptoms from 1 to 33 d, with an average illness lasting about 7–10 d. An estimated 0.2–2% of viral URIs are complicated by sinus ostia obstruction leading to bacterial infection. Although studies have shown that few patients with symptoms lasting less than 7 d will have bacterial infections, the small percentage of bacterial compared with viral sinus infections and the underestimation of the duration of viral symptoms suggest that the majority of illnesses lasting longer than 7 d are caused by viruses and will not benefit from antibiotic treatment.

The gold standard method for diagnosis of bacterial sinusitis is sinus puncture, with *S. pneumoniae* and *Haemophilus influenzae* being the most commonly isolated organisms. This invasive test is clearly impractical for routine use in the primary care office. Sinus radiography is another test that has limited value for routine diagnosis of bacterial infection. Just as the symptoms of viral and bacterial rhinosinusitis overlap, so do the radiographic changes they produce. Most patients with viral sinusitis will have abnormal sinus radiographs, and determination of the degree of mucosal thickening and sinus obstruction becomes a judgment call with predictive value similar to that of clinical findings alone.

A further similarity of viral and bacterial rhinosinusitis is that all infections with mild to moderate symptoms are likely to resolve with symptomatic treatment alone. Therefore, rather than assigning treatment based on the difficult distinction of acute viral vs bacterial rhinosinusitis, antibiotic treatment should be prescribed for those patients with severe symptoms regardless of duration or patients with moderate symptoms that persist beyond 7 d. Patients who experience severe symptoms of purulent nasal discharge *accompanied by* maxillary tooth or facial pain, especially when unilateral, unilateral sinus tenderness, and worsening of symptoms after initial improvement should be treated with narrow-spectrum antibiotics such as amoxicillin, doxycycline, or trimethoprim–sulfamethoxazole in addition to the symptomatic treatments recommended for all patients with acute rhinosinusitis. Patients with mild symptoms or moderate symptoms persisting for less than 7 d should be treated with appropriate doses of analgesics, antipyretics, and decongestants and educated about their diagnosis and the chosen treatment strategy.

Recently published, updated guidelines from the American Academy of Allergy, Asthma and Immunology support the use of narrow-spectrum antibiotic therapy, specifically amoxicillin, as the first choice in the treatment of uncomplicated sinusitis in children and adults. Depending on the local prevalence of β-lactamase-producing strains of bacteria, it might be reasonable to add potassium clavulanate, in the form of amoxicillin-potassium clavulanate, which is usually effective against β-lactamase-producing *H. influenzae, M. catarrhalis, S. aureus,* and anaerobic bacteria. These guidelines indicate that in certain areas there are high rates of resistance to sulfamethoxazole-trimethoprim present in *S. pneumoniae, H. influenzae,* and *M. catarrhalis,* so that sulfamethoxazole-trimethoprim would not be an ideal first choice.

ACUTE BRONCHITIS

Acute bronchitis is a clinical diagnosis defined as an acute respiratory infection in which cough is a predominant symptom. Cough may be dry or productive of sputum but by definition lasts less than 3 wk. Cough illness lasting longer than 3 wk should be categorized as chronic or persistent cough illness and evaluated as such. Assessment of patients with chronic cough often begins with chest radiography and is beyond the scope of this chapter. As with the URI and sinusitis guidelines, the recommendations for acute bronchitis summarized here apply only to healthy adults without underlying lung disease.

The majority (70%) of previously healthy adults presenting to the primary care office with a chief complaint of cough will have acute bronchitis associated with URI. The next most common diagnoses are asthma (6%) and pneumonia (5%). Previously undiagnosed asthma in a patient with acute cough is an important consideration, but it is difficult to distinguish asthma from transient bronchial hyperresponsiveness and abnormal spirometry associated with uncomplicated acute bronchitis. Pneumonia is potentially the most serious diagnosis associated with acute cough illness and can be fairly accurately distinguished from acute bronchitis based on clinical examination findings. Therefore, the primary objective of the office visit for acute cough should be to exclude a diagnosis of pneumonia.

Non-elderly adult patients with normal vital signs (heart rate ≤100, respiratory rate ≤24, and oral temperature ≤38°C) and chest examination (absence of signs of focal consolidation such as asymmetric breath sounds, rales, egophony, or fremitus) are unlikely to have pneumonia. A patient with cough for less than 3 wk, whose clinical examination is not suspicious for pneumonia may be considered to have acute bronchitis, which is likely because of infection with a respiratory virus. Chest radiography or other diagnostic tests are rarely warranted in a previously healthy adult in whom pneumonia has been excluded based on clinical presentation.

Acute bronchitis is caused by both upper and lower respiratory tract viruses. Lower respiratory tract viruses such as influenza A and B, parainfluenza 3, and RSV are the most common causes of acute bronchitis, but upper tract viruses such as coronavirus, adenovirus, and rhinovirus may also cause acute cough illness. *Bordetella pertussis, Mycoplasma pneumoniae,* and *Chlamydia pneumoniae* (strain TWAR) are the only nonviral causes of uncomplicated acute bronchitis in previously healthy adults, accounting for 5–10% of cases. Gram stain and culture of sputum does not reliably identify these agents and, therefore, it is not recommended for evaluation of acute bronchitis in adults without underlying lung disease.

Randomized controlled trials have shown that antibiotic treatment of acute bronchitis in previously healthy adults is not beneficial. The two uncommon exceptions to this rule include cases of bacterial superinfection as evidenced by infiltrate on chest X-ray and cases of suspected pertussis. Because previously immunized adults often do not present with the characteristic whooping cough of pertussis, it is difficult to distinguish this disease in this patient population from other causes of acute bronchitis. It is recommended that antibiotic treatment for pertussis should be limited to those adults with a high probability of exposure to the disease, such as during documented outbreaks. Treatment is largely beneficial as it decreases shedding of the organism. As pertussis is rarely suspected prior to 7–10 d of illness it is too late to speed resolution of symptoms.

Influenza infection is one other circumstance in which antimicrobial treatment of acute bronchitis may be warranted. Influenza viruses are the most common causes of uncomplicated acute bronchitis. It has been shown that during documented influenza outbreaks, clinical judgment can be as accurate as rapid diagnostic tests, which have a sensitivity of 63–81%. However, judgment must also be used in weighing the high cost of the newer neuraminidase inhibitors, which are active against both influenza A and B, against their rather limited benefit of 1 d of less illness in addition to the requirement that they be taken within 48 h of symptom onset and may contribute to the emergence of resistant viral strains.

In summary, a previously healthy adult patient with acute cough illness without signs of pneumonia or exposure to pertussis will not benefit from antibiotic treatment. Chest radiography should be limited to those cases in which pneumonia is suspected or cough has persisted for more than 3 wk in the absence of other known causes. Some patients with acute bronchitis will expect antibiotic treatment for uncomplicated acute bronchitis based on past experience. When antibiotic treatment is not warranted, all patients will benefit from the explanation that they have acute bronchitis, a self-limiting viral infection that may be thought of as a "chest cold," and discussion about why antibiotics are not being prescribed. Patients should be prepared for the possibility that cough could last an average of 10–14 d. Analgesics, antipyretics, antitussives, β-agonist inhalers, and vaporizers should be offered, with the explanation that they will not shorten the course of illness but will provide symptomatic relief.

SOURCES

1. Principles of Appropriate Antibiotic Use for Treatment of Acute Respiratory Tract Infections in Adults: background, Specific Aims, and Methods (2001) Ann Inter Med 134:479–486.
2. Principles of Appropriate Antibiotic Use for Treatment of Nonspecific Respiratory Tract Infections in Adults (2001) Ann Intern Med 134:487–489.
3. Principles of Appropriate Antibiotic Use for Acute Sinusitis in Adults (2001) Ann Intern Med 134:495–497.
4. Principles of Appropriate Antibiotic Use for Treatment of Acute Bronchitis in Adults (2001) Ann Intern Med 134:518–520.
5. Slavin RG. The diagnosis and management of sinusitis: a practice parameter update. J Allergy Clin Immunol 2005;116:S13–47.

11

Group A Streptococcal Pharyngitis
The Infectious Disease Society of America

Mario Napoletano, MD

CONTENTS

INTRODUCTION
DIFFERENTIAL DIAGNOSIS
MANAGEMENT OF GROUP A STREPTOCOCCAL PHARYNGITIS
TREATMENT REGIMENS
RECURRENT STREPTOCOCCAL INFECTIONS
SOURCES

INTRODUCTION

Group A streptococcal pharyngitis is defined as an acute infection of the oropharynx and sometimes the nasopharynx by *Streptococcus pyogenes*. The purpose of this guideline is to provide recommendations for the accurate diagnosis and optimal treatment of Group A streptococcal pharyngitis in children and adults. Following these recommendations should result in fewer cases of acute rheumatic fever, fewer cases of suppurative complications (e.g., peritonsillar abcesses, cervical lymphadenitis, and mastoiditis), a more rapid return to usual activities, and a decrease in infectivity. This decrease in infectivity will result in a reduced transmission of Group A β-hemolytic streptococci among family members and close contacts of the patient. Another important benefit to the widespread use of this guideline will be the minimization of inappropriate antibiotic therapy use.

Acute pharyngitis accounts for about 2% of all outpatient visits in the United States. Of these visits, only about 10% are actually infected by Group A β-hemolytic streptococci. Accurate diagnosis of the etiology of this presenting complaint is critical because of the small number of cases that actually do

From: *Current Clinical Practice: Essential Practice Guidelines in Primary Care*
Edited by: N. S. Skolnik © Humana Press, Totowa, NJ

require antibiotic therapy. Despite these statistics, most patients presenting with acute pharyngitis receive presumptive antibiotic therapy. One large retrospective study revealed that 73% of adults presenting to their primary care doctors with acute pharyngitis were prescribed with antibiotics; 68% of which were broad spectrum, expensive, and not recommended in established guidelines. This vast potential for inappropriate antibiotic use represents a significant contribution to growing antimicrobial resistance.

DIFFERENTIAL DIAGNOSIS

Most cases of acute pharyngitis are of viral etiology. These possible viral agents include adenovirus, influenza, parainfluenza, rhinovirus, and respiratory syncytial virus. Less common viral agents include coxsackievirus, echoviruses, herpes simplex virus, Epstein–Barr virus, cytomegalovirus, rubella, and measles.

The most common cause of bacterial pharyngitis is Group A β-hemolytic streptococci. This bacterium is also the only common cause of pharyngitis for which antibiotic therapy is definitely indicated with the exception of two very rare pathogens: *Corynebacterium diphtheriae* and *Neisseria gonorrhoeae*. For most patients presenting with acute pharyngitis, the clinical decision to be made is whether the infection is caused by a virus or Group A β-hemolytic streptococci. Other less common causes of bacterial pharyngitis normally have other historical or physical exam findings associated with them. These include Groups C and G streptococci, which can cause tonsillitis with a scarlatiniform rash. Mixed anaerobes may cause Vincent's angina. *N. gonorrhoeae* may cause a pharyngitis and tonsillitis in sexually active patients. *C. diphtheriae* can cause a pseudomembranous pharyngitis. *Arcanobacterium haemolyticum* can also cause a pharyngitis with a scaratiniform rash. *Yersinia enterocolitica* can cause enterocolitis along with pharyngitis.

Clinical Diagnosis

Group A β-hemolytic streptococcal pharyngitis has specific clinical features and epidemiological characteristics. Typically, it is a disease of children aged 5–15. It also typically occurs in winter and early spring in temperate climates. Patients with Group A β-hemolytic streptococcus typically present with sudden onset of a sore throat, severe pain during swallowing, and fever. At times, children may present with headache, nausea, vomiting, and abdominal pain.

Objectively, patients present with tonsillopharyngeal erythema, sometimes with exudates, and enlarged, tender anterior cervical lymph nodes. Other clinical findings can include an erythematous, swollen uvula, petechia on the palate, excoriated nares, and a scarlatiniform rash. It is important to keep in mind that none of these findings are specific for Group A β-hemolytic streptococcal pharyngitis. The absence of fever or the presence of conjunctivitis, cough, hoarseness, coryza, anterior stomatitis, discrete ulcerative lesions, viral exanthema, or diarrhea strongly suggests a viral etiology. In many cases, the signs and symptoms of streptococcal pharyngitis overlap with those of nonstreptococcal pharyngitis too much to make a diagnosis based on clinical criteria alone. Microbiological testing is often necessary to establish a definitive diagnosis.

Microbiological Testing

Certainly the application of either throat culture or rapid antigen detection testing (RADT) is necessary to properly diagnose many presenting cases of acute pharyngitis. Accurate diagnosis on clinical presentation alone is simply not possible even by the most experienced clinicians. However, testing is normally not necessary for patients presenting with acute pharyngitis of clearly viral etiology. Selective application of diagnostic microbiological tests will increase the percentage of positive test results for patients who are truly infected with Group A β-hemolytic streptococcus and helps to avoid regular antibiotic therapy for those who are in a transient carrier state. The application of any clinical algorithm for the diagnosis and treatment of acute pharyngitis that does not incorporate microbiological testing is not recommended. These algorithms result in an unacceptably large number of patients receiving inappropriate antibiotic therapy.

Throat Culture

Culture of a throat swab on sheep-blood agar remains the standard for documenting the presence of Group A streptococci in the upper respiratory tract. It is also the standard for confirming the clinical diagnosis of an acute streptococcal pharyngitis. With proper technique throat culture yields a sensitivity of 90–95% for detecting Group A β-hemolytic streptococci. The method in which the throat culture is obtained is crucial in order to maintain this level of sensitivity. The swab should be of both tonsils or tonsillar fossae and the posterior pharyngeal wall. Other areas of the mouth and pharynx should never be touched with the swab. False-negative results may be obtained if the patient has been taking antibiotics either shortly before or at the time of obtaining the throat swab. Another factor that can affect the sensitivity of throat culture is the length of incubation. A culture should be incubated at 35°C–37°C for 18–24 h before reading. An additional 24 h of incubation will yield a considerable number of positive throat culture results that would not have otherwise been identified. Therefore, although initial therapeutic decisions can be made based on culture results after 24 h of incubation, the throat culture should be examined again after 48 h before it is read as negative.

The most widely used method of differentiating Group A streptococci from other β-hemolytic streptococci on a culture plate is the bacitracin disk test. More than 95% of Group A streptococci demonstrate a zone of inhibition around the bacitracin disk, whereas 83–97% of non-Group A streptococci do not demonstrate this zone of inhibition. Another method of establishing specificity of a throat culture involves the identification of streptococcal serogroups by detection of group-specific cell wall carbohydrate antigen in isolated bacterial colonies. These tests are highly specific and most commonly used in clinical microbiology laboratories.

Rapid Antigen Detection Testing

RADT has been developed for the immediate detection of Group A β-hemolytic streptococci from throat swabs. Because RADT does not require 24–48 h to yield results, patients are treated earlier, return to work or school earlier, and reduce the risk of spreading of Group A β-hemolytic streptococci. The majority of RADTs currently available have an excellent specificity of more than 95%. False-positive test results are unusual and so therapeutic decisions can be made based on a positive test result. Unfortunately, the older RADTs use either latex agglutination methods or enzyme immunoassay techniques, which yield a sensitivity of 80–90% when compared with throat culture. This relatively high rate of false-negative results for RADTs led to the prior recommendation that any negative RADT should be followed up with a confirmatory throat culture. However, the newest RADTs, which involve optical immunoassay and DNA probes, offer sensitivity that rivals that of throat cultures. There is conflicting data involving the optical immunoassay RADT and other commercially available RADTs, as well as the lack of studies directly comparing the different commercially available RADTs.

It is recommended that physicians confirm that the RADT being used in their own particular office has a sensitivity and specificity comparable with that of throat culture, especially if RADTs are being used in the evaluation of children and adolescents. If the practice-specific RADT evaluation is not available, then negative RADTs in children and adolescents should be followed by a confirmatory throat culture. However, a negative RADT in an adult is sufficient evidence to support withholding antibiotic therapy. The physician should also realize that some of the RADTs require proper certification of the physician's laboratory under the Clinical Laboratory Improvement Act of 1988.

ASO Titers

Antistreptococcal antibody titers are of no value in the detection of acute streptococcal pharyngitis because they reflect past immunological events. They are useful for the confirmation of previous streptococcal infections in patients suspected of having acute rheumatic fever or poststreptococcal acute glomerulonephritis. They are also helpful epidemiologically in distinguishing patients with acute infection from those who are carriers.

No microbiological test is able to differentiate between acutely infected patients and asymptomatic carriers of Group A β-hemolytic streptococci, who happen to have a viral pharyngitis. These tests do allow physicians to withhold antibiotic therapy for the majority of patients who present with a sore throat and negative culture or RADT results. This is extremely significant because nationally 70% of patients presenting to their primary care doctor with a sore throat receive antibiotics.

MANAGEMENT OF GROUP A STREPTOCOCCAL PHARYNGITIS

Antimicrobial therapy is indicated in patients with symptomatic pharyngitis if the presence of Group A β-hemolytic streptococci is confirmed by throat culture or RADT. If there is a high index of suspicion for this specific infection, antimicrobial therapy can be initiated, whereas the results of a throat culture are pending as long as the antibiotic is discontinued, if the culture results are negative. Group A streptococcal pharyngitis is usually a self-limited disease. Even without the use of antibiotics, symptoms commonly go away spontaneously within 3 or 4 d of onset. Antimicrobial therapy can be safely postponed for up to 9 d after the appearance of symptoms and still safely prevent acute rheumatic fever. These facts offer the physician flexibility in initiating antibiotic therapy during the evaluation of a patient with presumed Group A streptococcal pharyngitis.

Numerous antibiotics have been examined in clinical trials and have been shown to eradicate Group A streptococci from the upper respiratory tract. However, the only antibiotic that has been examined in controlled studies and has been shown to prevent an acute attack of rheumatic fever is intramuscular repository penicillin therapy. These studies were performed with procaine penicillin G in oil containing aluminum monostearate, which has since been supplanted with benzathine penicillin G. It is because of this that none of the recommended antibiotic regiments are rated A–I. There are data indicating that benzathine penicillin G is effective in the prevention of acute rheumatic fever after Group A streptococcal pharyngitis. Other antibiotics can effectively clear Group A streptococci from the upper respiratory tract. It is assumed that eradication is equivalent to primary prevention of rheumatic fever.

TREATMENT REGIMENS

Standard

- Penicillin V: children: 250 mg bid or tid po × 10 d; adults: 250 mg tid or qid po × 10 d OR 500 mg bid × po 10 d.
- Amoxicillin can be used in place of penicillin.
- First- and second-generation cephalosporins also are effective.
- Benzathine Pen G: Children: 600,000 U intramuscular once, Adults: 1,200,000 U intramuscular once.

For Penicillin-Allergic Patients

- Erythromycin (dose varies with formulation).
- Note: Sulfonamides and tetracyclines are not recommended for streptococcus Group A because of resistance.

RECURRENT STREPTOCOCCAL INFECTIONS

It is recommended that patients with recurrent Group A streptococcal pharyngitis receive a throat culture. If the throat culture is positive for streptococcal, explanations include carrier state with intercurrent viral illnesses, noncompliance with the antibiotics prescribed, and newly acquired infection from a close contact. Treatment failures for Group A streptococcal pharyngitis are rare. When "Ping-Pong" effect with multiple family members passing streptococcal on to each other is suspected, all family members can be cultured and those with positive tests can be treated at the same time. There is no evidence that pets spread streptococcal (1).

For patients with multiple episodes of streptococcal for more than 6–24 mo, tonsillectomy may decrease recurrences (NEJM 1984;310:674). For patients who are having multiple recurrent episodes of culture-positive streptococcal pharyngitis, treatment to eradicate streptococcal from the pharynx has been effective using clindamycin, amoxicillin/clavulanate, or benzathine Penicillin G.

SOURCES

1. Infectious Disease Society of America's Practice Guidelines for the Diagnosis and Management of Group A Streptococcal Pharyngitis (2002) Clin Infect Dis 35:113–125.

12 Prevention of Perinatal Group B Streptococcal Disease

Ross Albert, MD, PhD, *Neil S. Skolnik,* MD, *and Richard Neill,* MD

CONTENTS

INTRODUCTION

The 2002 *Prevention of Perinatal Group B Streptococcal Disease* guidelines from the Center for Disease Control (CDC) represents a revision of a prior set of guidelines represented by the CDC in 1996. Group B streptococcus (GBS) remains a leading cause of serious neonatal infection despite the significant efforts in the disease prevention through the 1990s, including recommendations presented by the CDC, the American College of Obstetricians and Gynecologists (ACOG), and by the American Academy of Pediatrics (AAP). The updated 2002 guidelines were based on clinical evidence and expert opinions gathered since the 1996 recommendations *(1)*. Significant changes in the newer guidelines included a recommendation for universal prenatal screening for GBS;

From: *Current Clinical Practice: Essential Practice Guidelines in Primary Care*
Edited by: N. S. Skolnik © Humana Press, Totowa, NJ

detailed instructions on specimen collection, processing and testing; updated prophylaxis regimens for penicillin-allergic women; recommendations against routine antipartum antibiotic prophylaxis for GBS-colonized women undergoing planned cesarean deliveries prior to the onset of labor or the rupture of membranes; a suggested algorithm for management of threatened preterm delivery; and an updated algorithm for the management of newborns exposed to intrapartum antibiotics.

BACKGROUND

In the 1970s, GBS emerged as the primary cause of neonatal death in the United States. Common presentations of GBS infection are pneumonia and sepsis, with less common presentations including meningitis, osteomyelitis, and septic arthritis. GBS infections have been classified as early or late onset. Early-onset infections occur in the first week of life. These infections make up the majority of neonatal GBS infections. Late-onset infections occur in infants after the first week of life, typically until 3 mo of age. The primary risk factor for neonatal GBS infection is maternal GBS colonization. Other risk factors for infection include gestational age less than 37 wk, greater than 12 h of membrane rupture, intra-amniotic infection, previous delivery of an infant with invasive GBS disease, young maternal age, black race, hispanic ethnicity, and low maternal levels of anticapsular antibody.

Early studies in the 1980s showed that administration of antibiotics during labor could prevent invasive GBS disease in the first week of life. The first official statements regarding the use of intrapartum antibiotics from the ACOG and by the AAP were set forth in the early 1990s. The incidence of neonatal invasive GBS disease decreased significantly following these initial recommendations. They supported the use of antibiotics in the intrapartum period; however, neither of the guidelines suggested using only screening based or only risk factor-based treatment strategies. The 1996 CDC guidelines on the prevention of perinatal GBS infection also supported the use of intrapartum antibiotic prophylaxis to prevent neonatal GBS disease, and also did not declare one treatment strategy to be superior to another (i.e., screening vs risk-based strategies). The ACOG, AAP, and CDC recommendations were clearly having positive effects—from 1993 to 1998, invasive GBS infections decreased by more than 20%. The CDC tracked the results of the 1996 guidelines in order to refine their recommendations over time. The CDC found that although risk-based strategies were effective in determining which patients should receive intrapartum antibiotics, screening-based methods of determining the use of antibiotics were more effective in ultimately preventing neonatal GBS disease. This led the CDC to release the 2002 guidelines, primarily generated from evidence-based medicine, but from expert opinions when sufficient evidence was lacking.

RECOMMENDATIONS

Screening

"All pregnant women should be screened at 35–37 wk gestation for vaginal and rectal GBS colonization." The most significant change in the 2002 CDC GBS guidelines was the implementation of universal screening for all pregnant women for GBS colonization. At the time of the release of the 1996 guidelines, no data was available to evaluate the relative efficacy of screening-based vs risk-based strategy for the prevention of invasive GBS infection of the newborn. Although theoretical models suggested that the screening-based method would be more effective, some researchers suggested that the risk-based approach would be significantly easier to implement. Thus, the 1996 guidelines suggested that either strategy was acceptable for GBS prevention. Although no head-to-head clinical trials were carried out, data collected from hospital analyses and multistate population-surveillance studies since 1996 have found the screening-based strategy to be more effective at preventing perinatal GBS disease.

The 2002 CDC guidelines contain very specific details regarding screening methods. These include instructions for sites and methods of specimen collection, as well as for sample isolation and susceptibility testing. Recommendations state that cultures should be collected from both the vagina and the rectum— both potential sites of GBS colonization. The vaginal swab should be collected from the lower vagina, not from the endocervix, and a speculum should not be used. The rectal sample must be collected through the anal sphincter. Because the location of colonization is not significant with respect to the treatment strategy, one swab may be used for both sites, or two swabs may be used with both placed into the same culture medium to be sent for analysis.

The specification of testing at 35–37 wk gestation is owing to the transient nature of GBS infection. Colonization early in pregnancy is not predictive of neonatal invasive infection. Also, screening must be carried out in each pregnancy, as prior GBS colonization or lack thereof is not predictive for future pregnancies. It is important to note that GBS colonization in a previous pregnancy is not an indication for intrapartum prophylaxis. Women who are found to be colonized with GBS at 35–37 wk gestation should be treated in the intrapartum period (*see* Table 1). Early treatment is not indicated unless symptoms of infection are present, or GBS is detected in the urine (*see* below).

There are two groups of patients who will automatically receive prophylaxis, with no screening necessary—those with GBS bacturia and those with previous invasive GBS of a newborn. *"Women with GBS isolated from the urine in any concentration during their current pregnancy should receive intrapartum chemoprophylaxis (IAP)."* Detectable GBS in the urine of a pregnant woman represents a high level of genital tract colonization. GBS bacturia has been associated with early-onset GBS disease of the newborn. Women who are found

Table 1
Indications for Intrapartum Antibiotic Prophylaxis to Prevent Perinatal GBS Disease

Intrapartum prophylaxis indicated	Intrapartum prophylaxis not indicated
• Previous infant with invasive GBS	• Previous pregnancy with a positive GBS screening culture
• GBS bacteriuria during current pregnancy	• Planned cesarean delivery performed in the absence of labor or membrane rupture
• Positive GBS screening during current pregnancy	• Negative GBS screening in late gestation during the current pregnancy, regardless of intrapartum risk factor

• Unknown GBS status and any of the following:
  ○ Delivery at <37 wk gestation
  ○ Amniotic membrane rupture ≥18 h
  ○ Intrapartum temperature (°F)	

to have GBS bacturia at any time in pregnancy do not need screening at 35–37 wk, as they are known carriers of the bacteria. Both symptomatic and asymptomatic women should be treated at the time the GBS bacturia is detected, as well as in the intrapartum period.

"Women who have previously given birth to an infant with invasive GBS disease should receive IAP." Previous pregnancies with invasive GBS infection may increase the risk of GBS infection in subsequent pregnancies. GBS screening is thus not necessary in subsequent pregnancies, as these patients will be automatically treated with intrapartum prophylactic antibiotics.

COMMUNICATION OF RESULTS

"Health care providers should inform women of the GBS screening test result and recommend interventions." Fundamental to the process of universal screening is the reporting of the results of this screening. This is specifically stated in the guidelines as reporting to the patient, but it is contingent on accurate, timely collection and specimen labeling by the clinician, culturing, processing, and testing by the laboratory, reporting from the laboratory to the clinical facility, subsequent reporting within the facility to whomever is responsible for the patient, and ultimately reporting to the patient.

WHEN GBS SCREENING RESULTS ARE NOT KNOWN AT THE TIME OF LABOR

In some cases, GBS status is not known at the onset of labor. *"If the result of GBS culture is not known at the onset of labor, IAP should be administered* *to women with the following risk factors: gestation <37 wk, duration of membrane rupture ≥18 h, or a temperature of ≥100.4 (38°C)."* These criteria were used in the 1996 guidelines in the "risk-based" algorithm. Although the screening-based method was shown to be superior, using these criteria in the risk-based method is an effective way to reduce neonatal infection when no screening results are known.

SPECIAL CASES

"Women with threatened preterm delivery should be assessed for the need for intrapartum prophylaxis to prevent perinatal GBS disease." There is not sufficient data to define a particular strategy, but the CDC does provide a suggested approach in the event of preterm labor. If culture results are known to be negative from a specimen collected within the previous 4 wk, antibiotic prophylaxis should not be started. If cultures have been collected, but the results are not available, antibiotic prophylaxis should be initiated until culture results can be found. If cultures have not been collected within the previous 4 wk, cultures should be obtained, and intravenous penicillin should be started. If cultures remain negative at 48 h, penicillin can be stopped. If cultures are positive, penicillin should continue for at least 48 h. Prophylaxis can continue beyond 48 h if delivery has not occurred. Data are not available to dictate the duration of prophylaxis if the delivery is postponed. It is important to note that if a woman is GBS-positive and was treated with antibiotics for preterm labor, intrapartum prophylaxis should be reinitiated when labor likely to proceed to delivery occurs.

"GBS-colonized women who have a planned cesarean delivery performed before rupture of membranes and early onset of labor are at low risk for having an infant with early-onset GBS disease." GBS can cross intact amniotic membranes, so a cesarean section does not prevent transmission of GBS to the neonate; however, the risk of transmission is extremely low. In this case, risk to the neonate and mother from the use of intrapartum antibiotics is likely greater than that of the risk of transmission of GBS. It is therefore not recommended to initiate antibiotics in planned cesarean deliveries performed before rupture of membranes. Additionally, GBS colonization is not an indication to perform a cesarean delivery, and cesarean delivery is not an acceptable alternative to antibiotic prophylaxis for GBS prevention.

ANTIBIOTIC REGIMENS

"For IAP, penicillin is the preferred agent for use in women without penicillin allergy." Intravenous penicillin remains the treatment of choice for GBS prophylaxis as there has been no detection of penicillin- or ampicillin-resistant isolates to date. The intravenous route provides the highest intra-amniotic dose of antibiotic, and is the only recommended route of administration. The regimens recommended by the CDC divide women on the basis of presence or absence of penicillin

Table 2
Recommended Antibiotic Regimens for Perinatal GBS Prevention

No penicillin allergy	Penicillin G, 5 million U intravenously initial dose, then 2.5 million U⁻ every 4 h until delivery or Ampicillin, 2 g i.v. initial dose, then 1 g i.v. every 4 h until delivery
Penicillin allergy	
Patients not at high risk for anaphylaxis	Cefazolin, 2 g i.v. initial dose
Patient at high risk for anaphylaxis GBS susceptible to clindamycin and erythromycin	1 g i.v. every Clindamycin, 900 mg i.v. every 8 h until delivery or Erythromycin, 500 mg i.v. every 6 h until delivery
GBS resistant to clindamycin or erythromycin, or susceptibility unknown	Vancomycin, 1 g every 12 h until delivery

GBS, Group B streptococcal; i.v., intravenous

allergy, and the nature of their penicillin allergy. In GBS-colonized women who have no penicillin allergy, the recommended regimen is 5 million U of penicillin G initially, followed by 2.5 million U every 4 h until delivery. Ampicillin is listed as an appropriate alternative, with 2 g given intravenously initially followed by 1 g intravenously every 4 h until delivery (*see* Table 2).

GBS-colonized women with penicillin allergy are divided in the treatment algorithm based on the nature of their penicillin allergy. In women with penicillin allergy who are not at high risk for anaphylaxis, cefazolin should be given, 2 g intravenously initially, followed by 1 g intravenously every 8 h until delivery. In women who are at risk for an anaphylactic response, treatment with clindamycin or erythromycin is indicated (*see* below).

"IAP for penicillin-allergic women takes into account increasing resistance to clindamycin and erythromycin among GBS isolates." Increasing resistance of GBS isolates to these antibiotics requires that sensitivity testing be done for isolates collected from penicillin-allergic women. The CDC guidelines again stress that careful labeling of the samples as being drawn from penicillin-allergic pregnant patients helps to ensure that lab results are reported more rapidly. Regimens for the use of clindamycin and erythromycin are clindamycin, 900 mg i.v. every 8 h until delivery, or erythromycin, 500 mg i.v. every 6 h until delivery. Vancomycin is only recommended in penicillin-allergic

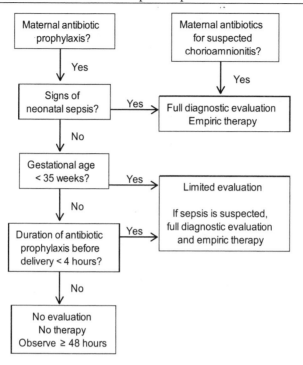

Fig. 1.

patients in two cases—resistance to both clindamycin and erythromycin, or unknown susceptibility to them. Vancomycin can be dosed at 1 g i.v. every 12 h until delivery.

MANAGEMENT OF NEWBORNS OF MOTHERS WHO HAVE RECEIVED IAP

"Routine use of antimicrobial prophylaxis for newborns whose mothers received IAP for GBS infection is not recommended." The 2002 guidelines for newborn care are aimed at decreasing unnecessary septic diagnostic evaluations, and unnecessary antibiotic use. A full diagnostic evaluation and empiric therapy should be initiated if a newborn born from a GBS-positive woman develops signs of sepsis, or if a newborn is born from a woman who was treated for chorioamnionitis, regardless of the newborn's clinical condition (*see* Fig. 1).

Current guidelines take into account whether a newborn's mother received "adequate" treatment. Penicillin, ampicillin, or cefazolin given at least 4 h prior to delivery will all reach appropriate levels in the amniotic fluid for prophylaxis. Other agents, such as those used in the event of penicillin allergy, have not been studied.

CONCLUSIONS

The 2002 CDC guidelines on the prevention of perinatal GBS disease are based on the fundamental principal that universal screening of pregnant women is more effective than risk factor-based strategies in preventing neonatal GBS infection. Universal screening for GBS is a safe, cost-effective technique of stratifying patients into treatment groups. Few side effects, such as antibiotic allergies, resistance to antibiotics, or increased incidence of other pathogens have been detected. Ultimately, universal screening may be replaced by other methods of prevention, such as GBS vaccination or rapid detection methods, which could be carried out on presentation during labor. Until these other methods are universally accepted as standard of care, universal screening at 35–37 wk gestation must be carried out for all patients, including those utilizing additional techniques of GBS prevention.

SOURCES

1. Prevention of Perinatal Group B Streptococcal Disease. MMWR, August 16, 2002/51(RR111); pp. 122.

13   Adult Immunizations

Brett Fissell, MD and Neil S. Skolnik, MD

INTRODUCTION

This chapter summarizes the Advisory Committee on Immunization Practices (ACIP) Adult Immunization Schedule for 2005 and 2006. Each vaccine is addressed in a similar manner—vaccine-preventable disease characteristics are briefly discussed, candidates for vaccination are discussed, followed by specifics of vaccination (dosage and administration, efficacy, side effects, and contraindications and cautions). Figures 1 and 2 are a copy of the Centers for Disease Control (CDC) Adult Immunization Schedules with footnotes.

From: *Current Clinical Practice: Essential Practice Guidelines in Primary Care*
Edited by: N. S. Skolnik © Humana Press, Totowa, NJ

Recommended Adult Immunization Schedule, by Vaccine and Age Group
UNITED STATES, OCTOBER 2005–SEPTEMBER 2006

Vaccine ▼ / Age group ▶	19–49 years	50–64 years	≥ 65 years
Tetanus, diphtheria (Td)[1]*	1-dose booster every 10 yrs		
Measles, mumps, rubella (MMR)[2]*	1 or 2 doses	1 dose	
Varicella[3]*	2 doses (0, 4–8 wks)	2 doses (0, 4–8 wks)	
Influenza[4]*	1 dose annually	1 dose annually	
Pneumococcal (polysaccharide)[5,6]	1–2 doses		1 dose
Hepatitis A[7]*	2 doses (0, 6–12 mos, or 0, 6–18 mos)		
Hepatitis B[8]*	3 doses (0, 1–2, 4–6 mos)		
Meningococcal[9]	1 or more doses		

- - - Vaccines below broken line are for selected populations - - -

NOTE: These recommendations must be read along with the footnotes.
*Covered by the Vaccine Injury Compensation Program.

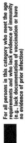

For all persons in this category who meet the age requirements and who lack evidence of immunity (e.g., lack documentation of vaccination or have no evidence of prior infection)

Recommended if some other risk factor is present (e.g., based on medical, occupational, lifestyle, or other indications)

This schedule indicates the recommended age groups and medical indications for routine administration of currently licensed vaccines for persons aged ≥19 years. Licensed combination vaccines may be used whenever any components of the combination are indicated and when the vaccine's other components are not contraindicated. For detailed recommendations, consult the manufacturers' package inserts and the complete statements from the ACIP (www.cdc.gov/nip/publications/acip-list.htm).

Report all clinically significant postvaccination reactions to the Vaccine Adverse Event Reporting System (VAERS). Reporting forms and instructions on filing a VAERS report are available by telephone, 800-822-7967, or from the VAERS website at www.vaers.hhs.gov.

Information on how to file a Vaccine Injury Compensation Program claim is available at www.hrsa.gov/osp/vicp or by telephone, 800-338-2382. To file a claim for vaccine injury, contact the U.S. Court of Federal Claims, 717 Madison Place, N.W., Washington D.C. 20005, telephone 202-357-6400.

Additional information about the vaccines listed above and contraindications for vaccination is also available at www.cdc.gov/nip or from the CDC-INFO Contact Center at 800-CDC-INFO (232-4636) in English and Spanish, 24 hours a day, 7 days a week.

DEPARTMENT OF HEALTH AND HUMAN SERVICES
CENTERS FOR DISEASE CONTROL AND PREVENTION

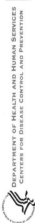

Fig. 1. Adult immunization schedule, 2005–2006. (http://www.cdc.gov/nip/recs/adult-schedule-bw-pss.pdf, accessed January 2, 2006)

Recommended Adult Immunization Schedule, by Vaccine and Medical and Other Indications

UNITED STATES, OCTOBER 2005–SEPTEMBER 2006

Vaccine ▼ / Indication ▶	Pregnancy	Congenital immunodeficiency;[10] leukemia; lymphoma; generalized malignancy; cerebrospinal fluid leaks; therapy with alkylating agents, antimetabolites, radiation, or high-dose, long-term corticosteroids	Diabetes; heart disease; chronic pulmonary disease; chronic liver disease, including chronic alcoholism	Asplenia[10] (including elective splenectomy and terminal complement component deficiencies)	Kidney failure, end-stage renal disease, recipients of hemodialysis or clotting factor concentrates	Human immunodeficiency virus (HIV) infection[10]	Healthcare workers
Tetanus, diphtheria (Td)[1]*	1-dose booster every 10 yrs						
Measles, mumps, rubella (MMR)[2]*			1 or 2 doses				
Varicella[3]*			2 doses (0, 4–8 wks)				2 doses
Influenza[4]*	1 dose annually		1 dose annually				
Pneumococcal (polysaccharide)[5,6]	1–2 doses		1–2 doses				1–2 doses
Hepatitis A[7]*			2 doses (0, 6–12 mos, or 0, 6–18 mos)				
Hepatitis B[8]*		3 doses (0, 1–2, 4–6 mos)					3 doses (0, 1–2, 4–6 mos)
Meningococcal[9]		1 dose	1 dose				1 dose

NOTE: These recommendations must be read along with the footnotes.
*Covered by the Vaccine Injury Compensation Program.

☐ For all persons in this category who meet the age requirements and who lack evidence of immunity (e.g., lack documentation of vaccination or have no evidence of prior infection)

☐ Recommended if some other risk factor is present (e.g., based on medical, occupational, lifestyle, or other indications)

 Contraindicated

Approved by the Advisory Committee on Immunization Practices (ACIP), the American College of Obstetricians and Gynecologists (ACOG), and the American Academy of Family Physicians (AAFP)

Fig. 2. Adult immunization schedule, 2005–2006. (http://www.cdc.gov/nip/recs/adult-schedule-bw-pss.pdf, accessed January 2, 2006)

TETANUS AND DIPTHERIA;
TETANUS–DIPHTHERIA–ACELLULAR PERTUSSIS

Once common in the United States, diptheria is now rare, thanks to high rates of vaccination—97% of children entering school had three or more doses of diptheria, tetanus, and pertussis (DTP). Prior to immunization, diptheria was a common and often deadly infection; for instance, in 1921 more than 200,000 cases were reported in the United States—the majority children, with a 5–10% fatality rate. Only 24 cases of respiratory diptheria were reported between 1980 and 1989, 75% of which occurred in adults who were inadequately vaccinated. Successful vaccination campaigns have apparently led to a dramatically decreased number of circulating oxygenic strains of *Corynebacterium diphtheriae*. However adults' protection based on serosurveys decreases (demographically speaking) with advancing age; a full 41–84% of those older than 60 may lack protective levels of circulating antitoxin to diptheria. This emphasizes the need to continue to periodically revaccinate adults against diptheria. A complete vaccination series not only drastically decreases one's chances of infection, but also decreases the severity of illness if one is infected; protection from vaccination lasts for at least 10 yr.

Because of widespread use of tetanus toxoid, tetanus prophylaxis in emergency rooms, and better wound care, the incidence of tetanus infection in the United States has decreased from 560 cases in 1947 to 48 cases in 1987. Serosurveys indicate that like diptheria protection, protection against *Clostridium tetani* decreases demographically with advancing age—up to 50% or more of those older than 60 lack adequate protection. Consequently, most recent cases of tetanus have occurred in those older than 50 who have unknown or inadequate vaccination to tetanus—case fatality is about 21%. Because tetanus is ubiquitous, and because no natural immunity has been demonstrated among Americans, it is essential to continue to immunize adults against tetanus. Similar to diptheria vaccination, a primary series of vaccines against tetanus is highly effective in preventing illness, and protection provided by boosters lasts for at least 10 yr.

Candidates for Tetanus and Diptheria Vaccination

The primary tetanus series is three doses, with the first two doses administered 4 wk apart, and the third dose 6–12 mo after the second. Adults, including pregnant women, with an uncertain history of vaccination should receive the primary series. If the primary series was given, but 10 yr have elapsed since the most recent dose, a single tetanus and diptheria (Td) dose should be administered. Once the primary Td series has been received, a booster is recommended for every 10 yr after 19 yr of age. A second option endorsed by the American College of Physicians Task Force on Adult Immunization involves a single Td dose given at age 50, if the primary pediatric series was completed (including an adolescent/early adult Td).

Table 1
Tetanus Wound Prophylaxis

Clean, minor wounds	All other wounds	Vaccination	History	Administer
Td	TIG			
Td	TIG			
Unknown or less than three doses				
Yes	No			
Yes	Yes ≥3 doses	No[a]	No No[b]	No

[a]Yes, if more than 10 yr since last dose.
[b]Yes, if more than 5 yr since last dose.

Tetanus Prophylaxis in Wound Management

In managing a wound, the patient's tetanus immunization status and the severity, or contamination of the wound, should be assessed (*see* Table 1). No assumptions about a person's immunity status should be made, with the possible exception that those having served in the military since 1941 have had at least one dose of Td.

All wounds should be adequately cleansed and debrided. If one has had the primary immunization series, Td or tetanus–diphtheria–acellular pertussis (Tdap; *see* section regarding Tdap) is recommended for a clean wound if 10 yr or more have elapsed since the most recent previous dose; for a contaminated wound the interval is shortened to 5 yr. For a contaminated wound, if one's tetanus immunity status cannot be determined, Td and (tetanus immune globulin TIG; 250 U i.m.) should be administered simultaneously at different sites. If primary vaccination has not occurred, it is recommended that adults receive three doses of Td—the second dose timed 4–8 wk after the first, and the third timed 6–12 mo after the second; Td should be administered subsequently thereafter every 10 yr.

Td Vaccine Characteristics

Td toxoids are made by treating their respective toxins with formaldehyde—the US standardizes the various vaccines' potency. Adverse reactions to diptheria toxoid are directly related to the amount of antigen present, and to the age and previous vaccine history of the recipient—because of this, and because adults form an adequate immune response to smaller antigen presentation, adult formulations contain less diptheria toxoid concentration than pediatric formulations. Td is intended for those 7 yr of age and older—a standard dose is 0.5 mL, injected intramuscularly.

The only contraindications to Td vaccine are severe allergic or neurological reactions to a previous dose. Local reactions do not warrant forgoing future doses. If anaphylaxis to tetanus toxoid is suspected, intradermal test dosing of appropriately diluted toxoid can be considered before making decisions regarding future Td boosters. Those who mount a febrile response more than 103°F, or those who have an Arthus-type hypersensitivity reaction as a result of Td vaccination should not be given booster doses, even for contaminated wounds, not more frequently than every 10 yr—these individuals generally have very high protective titers of tetanus antitoxin. TIG may be used as passive prophylaxis for contaminated wounds for individuals who have a contraindication to tetanus toxoid. There is no evidence that Td is teratogenic, but it is generally recommended to wait until the second trimester of pregnancy to administer the vaccine to women who are due for a booster. Routine Td boosters are not indicated more frequently than every 10 yr, and more frequent dosing may result in more (and more severe) reactions. Giving booster doses at 25, 35, 45, and so on, might help to prevent the too frequent dosing.

A newly licensed Tdap vaccine is now available for adults. Two tetanus toxoid, reduced diphtheria toxoid, and acellular pertussis vaccine, adsorbed Tdap products were licensed by the food and drug administration (FDA) in 2005 as single-dose booster vaccines to provide protection against tetanus, diphtheria, and pertussis. GlaxoSmithKline's BOOSTRIX® is indicated for persons 10–18 yr of age, and ADACEL™ (Sanofi Pasteur, Inc., Swiftwater, PA) is indicated for persons 19–64 yr of age.

On June 30, 2005 the ACIP voted to recommend the routine use of Tdap vaccines in adolescents 11–18 yr of age in place of Td toxoid vaccine. On October 26, 2005, the ACIP recommended routine use of a single dose of Tdap for adults 19–64 yr of age to replace the next booster dose of Td toxoid vaccine. These recommendations were subsequently approved. The recommendations, taken directly from the CDC website, are as follows.

The following recommendations for a single dose of Tdap (ADACEL) apply to adults 19–64 yr of age who have not yet received Tdap *(1–18)*.

- *Routine:* Adults should receive a single dose of Tdap to replace a single dose of Td for booster immunization against tetanus, diphtheria, and pertussis if they received their most recent tetanus toxoid-containing vaccine (e.g., Td) 10 or more years earlier.
- *Shorter intervals between Td and Tdap:* Tdap may be given at an interval shorter than 10 yr since receipt of the last tetanus toxoid-containing vaccine to protect against pertussis. The safety of intervals as short as approx 2 yr between administration of Td and Tdap is supported. The dose of Tdap replaces the next scheduled Td booster.
- *Prevention of pertussis among infants younger than 12 mo of age by vaccinating adult contacts:* Adults who have or who anticipate having close contact with an infant less than 12 mo of age (e.g., parents, child care providers, and health care providers) should receive a single dose of Tdap. An interval of 2 yr or more since the most recent tetanus toxoid-containing vaccine is suggested; shorter intervals may be used. Ideally, Tdap should be given at least 1 mo before beginning close contact with the infant. Women should receive a dose

of Tdap in the immediate postpartum period if they have not previously received Tdap. Any woman who might become pregnant is encouraged to receive a single dose of Tdap.

• *Simultaneous administration:* Tdap should be administered with other vaccines that are indicated during the same visit when feasible. Each vaccine should be administered using a separate syringe at different anatomic sites.

Special Situations

• *Tetanus prophylaxis in wound management:* Adults 19–64 yr of age who require a tetanus toxoid-containing vaccine as part of wound management should receive Tdap instead of Td if they have not previously received Tdap. If Tdap is not available or was administered previously, Td should be administered.

• *Incomplete or unknown vaccination history:* Adults who have never received Td toxoid-containing vaccine should receive a series of three vaccinations. The preferred schedule is a single dose of Tdap, followed by Td more than 4 wk later, and a second dose of Td 6–12 mo later. Tdap may substitute for Td for any one of the three doses in the series.

• *History of pertussis:* Adults with a history of pertussis generally should receive Tdap according to the routine recommendations.

• *Pregnancy:* Pregnancy is not a contraindication to Tdap or Td vaccination. Guidance on the use of Tdap during pregnancy is under consideration by ACIP. At this time, women who received the last tetanus toxoid-containing vaccine less than 10 yr earlier should receive Tdap in the postpartum period, according to the routine recommendations for vaccinating adult contacts of infants younger than 12 mo of age. Women who received the last tetanus toxoid-containing vaccine more than 10 yr earlier should receive Td during pregnancy in preference to Tdap, and pregnant women who have not received the primary three-dose vaccination series for tetanus should begin the series during pregnancy. If Td is indicated during pregnancy, vaccinating during the second or third trimester is preferred when feasible.

Future Considerations

Recommendations for use of Tdap among health care providers, pregnant women, and adults over the age of 65 will be considered at a future ACIP meeting.

PERTUSSIS

Until recently, pertussis vaccination for those older than 7 yr of age was not recommended. The recommendations are being changed because adults and adolescents with waning immunity are major reservoirs for pertussis transmission. In 2004, US adolescents 11–18 yr of age made up 34% (8897) of the total 25,827 reported cases; reported cases underestimate the true burden of pertussis in adolescents. The clinical presentation of pertussis in adolescents ranges from mild cough illness to classic pertussis (i.e., paroxysms of cough, posttussive emesis, and inspiratory whoop). The morbidity of pertussis in adolescents can be substantial with prolonged cough illness lasting weeks to months. Hospitalization and complications (e.g., pneumonia and rib fractures) occur in up to 2% of reported cases. (*See* also recommendations for Tdap listed above.)

Adolescents 11–18 yr of age should receive a single dose of Tdap instead of Td for booster immunization against tetanus, diphtheria, and pertussis. The preferred age for Tdap vaccination is 11–12 yr; routinely administering Tdap to young adolescents will reduce the morbidity associated with pertussis in adolescents.

Adolescents 11–18 yr of age who received Td, but not Tdap, are encouraged to receive a single dose of Tdap to provide protection against pertussis. An interval of at least 5 yr between Td and Tdap is encouraged to decrease the risk of local or systemic reactions after Tdap vaccination; however, intervals shorter than 5 yr between Td and Tdap may be used. The benefit of using Tdap at shorter intervals to protect against pertussis generally outweighs the risk of local or systemic reactions after vaccination in settings with increased risk of pertussis or its complications. Tdap (or Td) and tetravalent meningococcal conjugate vaccine ([MCV4] Menactra™) (which contains diphtheria toxoid) should be administered during the same visit if both vaccines are indicated and available. Tdap (or Td) should be administered with other vaccines that are indicated during the same visit when feasible. Each vaccine should be administered using a separate syringe at different anatomic sites. Women who received the last tetanus toxoid-containing vaccine less than 10 yr earlier should receive Tdap in the postpartum period, according to the routine recommendations for vaccinating adult contacts of infants younger than 12 mo of age.

INFLUENZA

Influenza epidemics in the United States typically occur each winter, and worldwide pandemics can also occur. Influenza-related deaths in the United Sates has recently averaged 36,000 per year, which is higher than the 19,000 or so per year between 1976 and 1990, possibly resulting from the aging of the US population—most flu-related deaths occur among those aged or older 65. Currently, the best way to prevent transmission and spread of influenza is through vaccination, usually timed in October and November of each year. Because of different flu strains and subtypes, and because of antigenic drift, vaccination yearly is needed to confer protection.

Candidates for Influenza Vaccination

Influenza vaccination is recommended annually for the following individuals:

- Individuals aged 50 or older.
- Individuals aged 19–49 with certain medical or occupational conditions.
- Those with chronic cardiovascular or pulmonary conditions including asthma, chronic metabolic disorders such as diabetes mellitus, renal dysfunction,

hemoglobinopathies, or immunosuppression—including that caused by medications or HIV infection.

- Pregnant women expected to be in their second or third trimester during flu season—for women with chronic diseases/conditions, vaccinate at any time during pregnancy.
- Health care workers as well as workers in long-term care facilities.
- Residents of long-term care facilities or nursing homes.
- Individuals likely to transmit influenza to persons at high risk (i.e., in-home household contacts and caregivers of children newborn through 23 mo of age, or persons of all ages with high-risk conditions).
- Anyone who wishes to be vaccinated.

Individuals between the ages of 5 and 49 without chronic conditions who are not contacts of severely immunocompromised persons, may receive either the inactivated injectible vaccine or the attenuated live intranasal vaccine.

INFLUENZA VACCINE CHARACTERISTICS

The inactivated injectible influenza vaccine is made up of inactivated or killed, highly purified hen's egg-grown virus hemagglutinins (usually two from type A and one from type B influenza strains) to reflect the strain of flu most likely to be in circulation in the United States during the upcoming winter season. The efficacy of the vaccine depends on the recipient's age and health status, as well as the degree of matching of the vaccine's antigens and the antigens expressed by the actual circulating virus. Most immunized healthy adults develop high antibody titers and when the vaccine is well-matched to the circulating strain of flu, 70–90% efficacy can be achieved among healthy persons less than 65 yr of age. Efficacy of vaccine-prevented influenza is estimated to be much lower among nursing home patients aged 65 or more, and may only be 30–40%. However, the vaccine is effective in preventing severe illness and complications—efficacy is estimated between 50 and 60% in preventing influenza-related pneumonia and hospitalization, and 80% effective in preventing death related to flu.

Injectible inactivated flu vaccine is administered to adults preferably in the lateral deltoid muscle (intramuscularly)—local soreness is common and lasts generally less than 2 d. Patients should be educated that the vaccine contains inactivated, killed virus, and cannot cause the flu; because cold virus illness is common, patients may make a "causal" connection between the vaccine and their cold—they should be informed that vaccination will not prevent their next cold. Myalgia, fever, and malaise can occur beginning 6–12 h after vaccination, and can persist for 1–2 d—most often in those being vaccinated for the first time. Immediate, allergic-type reactions rarely occur, and most are likely because of residual egg protein in egg-sensitive individuals. Those with history of anaphylaxis to egg protein should discuss the risk–benefit of proceeding with flu vaccine with a physician. Protocols exist for desensitization to egg before administration of influenza vaccine, but further discussion of this issue is beyond the scope of this chapter.

In 1976, the swine influenza vaccine was associated with higher-than-expected rates of Guillain-Barré syndrome (GBS)—according to epidemiological studies since that time, subsequent vaccines likely are not associated with such risk—and if they have been, it is on the order of one additional case per million; clearly, the benefits of vaccination outweigh this possible risk. For those who have experienced GBS within 6 wk after influenza vaccination, it may be prudent to forgo vaccination in those at low risk for complications of influenza—for those at high risk of flu-related complications, benefits outweigh the risks, and they should be vaccinated. Alternatively, chemoprophylaxis against influenza could be considered.

In an attempt to match the strain of flu likely to be circulating during the upcoming winter season, live attenuated influenza vaccines (LAIV) are formulated like the injected vaccine. They are administered intranasally, and animal studies show that the viruses replicate in nasopharyngeal mucosa, but inefficiently in the lower airways and lungs—the mechanism of host-developed immunity is not fully understood, but seems to involve both serum and nasal secretory antibodies. This vaccine is also developed using hen's eggs. It is indicated only for healthy persons between the ages of 5 and 49; it is more expensive than injectible influenza vaccine.

LAIV comes in a single-dose nasal inhaler that must be stored at 15°C or colder and should not be stored in a frost-free freezer, unless a special box provided by the manufacturer is used (frost-free freezers can cycle more than 15°C). It is intended for yearly intranasal administration. The vaccine is thawed, and half the dose is administered in each nostril. Because the vaccine is made up of live virus, person-to-person transmission can occur—the estimated risk of close contact of contracting vaccine virus is 0.58–2.4%. Transmitted vaccine virus has been shown to remain phenotypically stable. Because active viral replication is needed for vaccine efficacy, it should not be coadministered with antiviral medicines (it can be given 2 d after cessation of antiviral therapy, and antiviral therapy can be given 2 wk after the vaccine has been administered).

Side effects of LAIV reported more often than placebo among adults may include nasal congestion or runny nose, sore throat, cough, headache, chills, and tiredness/weakness. A serious adverse event among healthy adult recipients of LAIV is less than 1%.

Contraindications to LAIV include health status other than healthy, age younger than 5 or older than 49, anaphylaxis to egg protein, children receiving aspirin or other salycilate therapy, pregnancy, or a history of GBS. Killed injected vaccine is preferred for those in close contact with persons who are at high risk for developing influenza-related complications because of the theoretical risk of transmitting live vaccine-related virus. It may be prudent to postpone LAIV if a recipient has significant nasal congestion, so that adequate mucosal contact of vaccine can be assured.

PNEUMOCOCCAL PNEUMONIA AND DISEASE

Streptococcus pneumoniae (also referred to as "pneumococcus") is a bacteria that causes significant illness and death among children and adults alike. After colonizing the upper respiratory tract, pneumococcus can cause otitis media and sinusitis. It can also cause pneumonia and other lower respiratory tract infections and can cause invasive illnesses including bacteremia and meningitis. Demographics of this pathogen are impressive—pneumococcus causes each year in the United States an estimated 3000 cases of meningitis, 50,000 cases of bacteremia, 500,000 cases of pneumonia, and 7 million cases of otitis media. The burden of annual cases of invasive disease is highest among children younger than 2, followed by adults older than 65. About 60–87% of pneumococcal bacteremia in those aged 65 or older is associated with pneumonia; the primary site of infection is often not identified among children 2 yr or younger.

In addition to being elderly or very young, other risk factors for invasive pneumococcal disease include diabetes, cardiovascular disease, chronic obstructive pulmonary disease, asplenism, malignancy, chronic renal disease, chemotherapy, HIV, or other causes of immunocompromise (congenital immunodeficiency), and chronic liver disease. Complicating the issue of invasive disease is the emergence of drug-resistant strains of pneumococcus.

Candidates for Pneumococcal (Polysaccharide) Vaccination

Pneumococcal vaccine is recommended:

- Once at age 65.
- For individuals between 2 and 65 yr with certain medical conditions.
- For individuals with chronic pulmonary disorders (excluding asthma—note asthma is an indication for influenza vaccination, but not for pneumococcal vaccination); cardiovascular diseases; diabetes mellitus; chronic liver diseases; nephrotic syndrome or chronic renal failure; functional or anatomical asplenia (sickle cell disease and splenectomy); immunosuppressive disorders (such as congenital immunosuppression, HIV infection, malignancy, bone marrow, or organ transplants).
- For individuals undergoing chemotherapy with antimetabolites and alkylating agents.
- For individuals using long-term systemic corticosteroids.
- Alaska natives, certain Native American populations (and non-natives living within such a population).
- Residents of nursing home and long-term care facilities.
- For individuals undergoing elective splenectomy, administer pneumococcal vaccine at least 2 wk prior to the procedure.

- Vaccinate HIV-positive persons as soon after diagnosis as possible (when CD4 counts are highest).

One-time revaccination is recommended for those less than 65 yr of age if more than 5 yr have elapsed since initial vaccination. Revaccination with a single dose is recommended for those 65 or older if more than 5 yr have elapsed since first vaccination and they were aged less than 65 at the time of original vaccination. Administration of more than two total doses of pneumococcal vaccine is not currently recommended—the need for subsequent booster doses will be assessed as more data becomes available, but as yet, the safety and efficacy of three or more doses is not known.

Pneumococcal (Polysaccharide) Vaccine Characteristics

The currently licensed 23-valent vaccine replaced a previously available 14-valent vaccine, and helps prevent invasive pneumococcal illnesses, but may be less efficacious in preventing other pneumococcal disease. It incorporates 85–90% of the serotypes that cause invasive pneumococcal illness in US children and adults. Type-specific antibody response to vaccination is generally strong among healthy adults (vaccine effectiveness is about 75% for healthy persons 65 or older), and vaccine protection lasts at least 5 yr. Less predictable efficacy is demonstrated for those with chronic illness, but has been estimated between 65 and 84% for those with diabetes, cardiovascular disease, congestive heart failure, chronic obstructive pulmonary disease, and anatomical asplenia. Effectiveness for those with other aforementioned risk factors is less well known (power of existing studies is lacking owing to lack of adequate numbers of patients with illnesses such as chronic renal failure, sickle cell disease, lymphomas, multiple myeloma, leukemia, or immunoglobulin deficiencies).

The pneumococcal polysaccharide vaccine is administered either intramuscularly or subcutaneously in a 0.5 mL dosage. About half of vaccine recipients experience (typically for 2 d or less) pain, erythema, and/or swelling at the injection site. More serious reactions such as fever, myalgias, and local induration are rare—as is anaphylaxis. Safety of the vaccine in the first trimester of pregnancy has not been established, but of those women who were inadvertently given pneumococcal vaccine during pregnancy, no adverse fetal outcomes have been attributed to the vaccine.

HEPATITIS B

As of 1991, approx 1–1.25 million Americans were chronically infected with hepatitis B, with the potential to infect others, and with the potential to develop chronic liver disease and/or hepatocellular carcinoma as a result of their infection. Each year, about 4000–5000 of these chronically infected persons die as a result of chronic liver disease. Treatment for those chronically infected with hepatitis B continues to evolve, but currently the best way to prevent infection and transmission of hepatitis B is through vaccination. Newborns in the United States are routinely vaccinated against hepatitis B, but there are many susceptible adolescents and adults, and the following section reviews those groups of people who should be immunized.

Candidates for Hepatitis B Vaccine

Generally speaking, risks of acquiring hepatitis B are similar to the risks of acquiring HIV. Candidates for hepatitis B vaccine include:

* All adolescents (because as a group they are at risk, and often are unlikely to divulge at-risk behaviors to health care workers).
* Persons at risk because of occupational exposure (health care workers, first responders, laboratory employees who have contact with blood). Medical students, dental students, and nursing students are vaccinated while in school, prior to exposure to patients, blood, or blood-contaminated body fluids.
* Clients and staff of institutions for the developmentally disabled.
* Hemodialysis patients and patients who have clotting disorders that require transfusion of clotting-factor concentrates.
* Sex partners and household contacts of hepatitis B carriers.
* Adoptees from countries where hepatitis B is endemic.
* Prostitutes.
* Inmates of long-term correctional facilities.
* Injection drug users.
* Men who have sex with men.
* Men and women who have had more than one sexual partner in the last 6 mo.
* Anyone treated for another sexually transmitted disease (STD).
* International travelers, especially those who plan to reside in an endemic region for longer than 6 mo, and who will have close contact with locals, should consider hepatitis B vaccination.

In addition, in October 2005, the ACIP included the following recommendations for hepatitis B vaccination:

* All unvaccinated adults at risk for hepatitis B virus (HBV) infection.
* All adults seeking protection from HBV infection. Acknowledgment of a specific risk factor is not a requirement for vaccination.

In settings in which a high proportion of adults are likely to have risk factors for HBV infection, all unvaccinated adults should be assumed to be at risk and should receive hepatitis B vaccination. These settings include STD treatment facilities, HIV testing facilities, HIV treatment facilities, facilities providing drug abuse treatment and prevention, correctional facilities, health care settings serving men who have sex with men, chronic hemodialysis facilities and end-stage renal disease programs, and institutions and nonresidential day care facilities for developmentally disabled persons.

Standing orders should be implemented to identify and vaccinate eligible adults in primary care and specialty medical settings. If ascertainment of risk for HBV infection is a barrier to vaccination in these settings, providers may use alternative vaccination strategies such as offering hepatitis B vaccine to all unvaccinated adults in age groups with highest risk for infection (e.g., <45 yr).

Hepatitis B Vaccine Characteristics

Three intramuscular doses of hepatitis vaccine are recommended, the second dose timed 1–2 mo after the first, and the third timed 4–6 mo after the first. If vaccine dosing is interrupted, the second dose should be given as soon as possible, and at least 2 mo should elapse between the second and third doses—if only the third dose is delayed, it should be subsequently administered when convenient. Hepatitis B vaccines produced by different manufacturers are regarded as interchangeable. In general, vaccine immunogenicity is strong, and hepatitis B susceptible vaccine recipients are 80–95% protected against acquiring infection—those who respond with protective antibody levels are virtually 100% protected. There are "nonresponders," but in general, titer testing and boosters are not recommended unless hepatitis immune status is critical to subsequent health care management. These would include HIV patients, hemodialysis patients, or occupationally exposed persons likely to be exposed to sharp objects because their immune status to hepatitis B would help guide postexposure prophylaxis. Antibody titer testing in these cases is recommended 1–6 mo after vaccine series completion, and nonresponders should receive one or more additional doses. About 15–25% develop antibody response after one additional dose, and 30–50% converts after three additional doses.

The currently available hepatitis B vaccine in the United States utilizes common baker's yeast into which the recombinant gene for hepatitis B surface antigen has been inserted. The initial vaccine produced from the serum of chronically infected persons is no longer available. Neither pregnancy nor lactation are considered contraindications for hepatitis B vaccination. Pain at the injection site and low-grade fever are the most common side effects of hepatitis B vaccination, and occur up to 29 and 6% of the time, respectively (although these "reactions" occurred at the same rate among recipients of placebo). No serious adverse reactions have been definitively attributed to hepatitis B vaccine.

HEPATITIS A

Hepatitis A virus infection is transmitted by the fecal–oral route by contaminated food or water sources, or by person-to-person contact, and causes about 100 deaths per year in the United States, as a result of acute liver failure. About 11–22% of those infected with hepatitis A are hospitalized and those who are ill miss an average of 27 d of work.

Candidates for Hepatitis A Vaccine
Hepatitis A vaccine is indicated for the following individuals:

* Travelers to, or workers in, endemic regions.
* Men who have sex with men.
* Illegal drug users.
* Individuals who receive clotting factor concentrates for clotting disorders.
* Persons with chronic liver disease.
* Those who work with hepatitis A in a laboratory setting.
* Those who work with nonhuman primates.
* *Note:* those exposed to raw sewage in the United States have not been found to be at higher risk for infection, and do not need to be immunized.

Hepatitis A Vaccine Characteristics
Two US manufacturers currently produce hepatitis A vaccine. Both are inactivated vaccines and are administered via the intramuscular route (in the deltoid muscle). Hepatitis A vaccine is highly immunogenic, and after one dose of vaccine 94–100% of recipients develop protective antibody levels. It is given in two doses, the second dose timed 6–12 mo after the first. It can also be given at 0, 1, and 6 mo (three doses) if given with the combination hepatitis A/hepatitis B vaccine. Currently available data indicate that two doses of vaccine effectively protect one from contracting hepatitis A for at least 7, and perhaps up to 20 yr or more (recommendations regarding booster doses will be updated as more information becomes available). Tenderness or warmth at the injection site, headache, and malaise are the most commonly reported adverse reactions among adult recipients of hepatitis A vaccine. No serious adverse reactions have definitively been linked to hepatitis A vaccination. The only contraindication to vaccination is a serious adverse reaction possibly attributable to a previous dose of hepatitis A vaccine. Safety of hepatitis A vaccination has not been evaluated in pregnancy, but theoretically, it should pose no risk to mother or fetus; additionally, the vaccine can safely be given to immunocompromised individuals.

MEASLES, MUMPS, AND RUBELLA
Since the introduction of monovalent measles, mumps, and rubella (MMR) vaccines, the incidence of these illnesses has decreased to 99%. The elimination of US indigenous transmission of these illnesses now seems possible.

Clinical measles occurs after an incubation period of 7–14 d, and apart from its characteristic rash, it is often associated with diarrhea, pneumonia, and middle ear infection. Fatality of US measles (rubeola) cases runs between 1 and 2 per 1000 cases, and in developing countries can be up to 25%. Death most often results from pneumonia or encephalitis. Encephalitis complicates 1 in 1000 cases of measles—survivors of such usually suffer brain damage and mental retardation. Subacute sclerosing panencephalitis is a rare degenerative brain disorder that can manifest years after clinical measles—because of the relative success of measles vaccination; this disorder has virtually been eliminated in the United States. Premature labor, increased rates of spontaneous abortion, and low birthweight are associated with measles infection during pregnancy—causality of birth defects has not been definitively proved. Measles infection is most severe among the very young, among adults, and the immunocompromised—older children and adolescents in general have less severe infection.

Rubella occurs after a 12- to 23-d incubation period, and involves an exanthem that is often transient, erythematous, occasionally pruritic, and often similar to other viral exanthems. Low-grade fever, arthralgia, and postauricular or suboccipital lymphadenopathy can also occur. About 25–50% of infections are subclinical; its manifestations are similar to other illnesses caused by enteroviruses, parvoviruses, and adenoviruses. Rubella-infected adults often develop arthralgia and transient arthritis. Thrombocytopenia and encephalitis can also occur. Rubella's burden comes mostly from its teratogenicity and its ability to induce congenital rubella syndrome (CRS).

Rubella infection during pregnancy (especially in the first trimester) can lead to fetal anomalies, spontaneous abortion, and stillbirth. The fetal anomalies associated with CRS can be neurological (microencephaly, mental retardation, and menigoencephalitis), ophthalmic (chorioretinitis, cataracts, glaucoma, and microthalmia), auditory (sensorineural deafness), and cardiac (patent ductus arteriosis, atriol septal defect, ventricular septal defect, and peripheral pulmonary artery stenosis). Severe cases of CRS are usually recognized at birth, but milder cases may not be picked up for months or years. Rubella infection after gestational week 20 rarely causes congenital malformations—prior to the 12 wk, the rate of anomalies may be higher than 25%; maternal infection during the first 8 wk of pregnancy carries an 85% chance of CRS. Thankfully, because of vaccination strategies over the years, rubella and CRS cases have dramatically decreased. In 1969, there were more than 57,000 cases of measles, with 69 CRS cases reported in 1970. In the late 1990s, rubella cases per year were in the range of 200 and CRS cases per year were less than a handful.

The classic "chipmunk-cheek" look of bilateral parotitis from mumps infection happens in only 30–40% of cases, 15–20% of cases are asymptomatic, and 50% involve only nonspecific upper respiratory symptoms. The incubation period is 16–18 d. Prior to the onset of parotitis, patients may experience malaise, anorexia, fever, headache, and myalgias. Children between the ages of 2 and 9 are most likely to develop parotitis—adults are most likely to have subclinical infection, but are most likely to suffer complications. Orchitis affects as many as 38% of postpubertal men, but sterility is thought to be rare. About 4–6% of mumps patients develop (typically mild) aseptic meningitis; serious sequelae include cranial nerve palsies, paralysis, seizures, aqueduct narrowing, and hydrocephalus. Sensorineural deafness can be unilateral or bilateral, and can occur suddenly—prior to mumps vaccination, mumps was a major cause of childhood deafness. Increased rates of fetal demise occur in women infected during their first trimester of pregnancy, but mumps has not been otherwise associated with fetal anomalies. More than 185,000 mumps cases were reported in 1968 and 906 cases were recorded in 1995. Incidence should continue to decline with the continued administration of two doses of MMR to children.

Candidates for MMR Vaccination

Adult candidates for vaccination with MMR vaccine are discussed regarding each individual illness:

- Those born before 1957 are generally regarded as immune to measles.
- Those born in or after 1957 should receive at least one dose of MMR, unless there exists a contraindication.
- A second dose is recommended for international travelers, health care workers, students in postsecondary institutions, those previously vaccinated with a killed vaccine or unknown type of vaccine between 1963 and 1967, and those in an outbreak or exposure setting.
- One dose of mumps vaccine is considered as a adequate protection against mumps.
- All women of childbearing age who do not have evidence of immunity by prior disease, vaccination, or antibody status should receive one dose of MMR to protect against rubella and CRS—they should be counseled not to become pregnant for at least 3 mo after vaccination.
- A pregnant woman's rubella-immune status should be determined, and if not immune, she should receive one dose of MMR as soon after delivery as possible—do not vaccinate while pregnant, or if a woman intends to become pregnant in the next 3 mo.

Breast-feeding is not a contraindication for MMR vaccination. Those with anaphylaxis to egg protein may receive MMR. Topical allergic sensitivity to neomycin is not a contraindication to MMR vaccination, but anaphylaxis to neomycin is a contraindication. Extreme caution should be exercised when considering administration of MMR vaccine to those with an anaphylactic reaction to gelatin, as the vaccine contains traces of gelatin. Moderate or severe illness usually precludes MMR vaccination; the vaccine dose should be postponed until 1–2 wk after resolution of the illness—minor illness does not preclude MMR administration. Those who are severely immunocompromised have the potential for severe reaction to, or death from MMR vaccination, and should not receive MMR vaccine.

MMR Vaccine Characteristics

Each component of MMR vaccine is a live attenuated virus that induces among recipients, a mild noncommunicable, usually asymptomatic infection

that confers long-term, possibly lifelong immunity. Two total doses administered at least 28 d apart are recommended to ensure that the few vaccines (5%
or less) who do not respond to rubella or measles with protective antibody
after one dose, will convert with the second dose. The vaccine is administered
subcutaneously, and must be shipped, stored, and reconstituted appropriately.
The vaccine is shipped at 10°C, and stored at 2–8°C or colder; reconstituted
vaccine should not be frozen, and should be discarded if not used within 8 h.
Adverse events after MMR vaccination include local induration, edema, and
pain at the injection site, and rare cases of anaphylaxis have been reported (one
case per million vaccinations). About 7–12 d after MMR vaccination, about 5%
of recipients develop fever of 103°F or higher that lasts 1–2 d, likely most often
associated with the measles component. Measles and rubella components of the
vaccine can each induce a rash—usually 7–10 d after the vaccine in about 5% of
recipients; parotitis has rarely been reported. Transient lymphadenopathy may
also occur. Thrombocytopenia, usually mild, but rarely associated with hemorrhage, can occur about 2 mo after vaccination; however, the risk of thrombocytopenia from measles or rubella infection is much than MMR vaccine-induced
thrombocytopenia. Arthralgia and arthritis occurs in up to 25% of postpubertal
female vaccine recipients 1–3 wk after dosing, and can last 1–3 wk—chronic
arthropathy as a result of MMR vaccine seems unlikely, according to available
data. In general, those with reliable adequate vaccination history (i.e., two doses
of MMR) are considered immune to MMR and need not undergo titer testing to
ensure immunity.

VARICELLA (CHICKEN POX)

Varicella, caused by the varicella zoster virus (VZV) is a self-limited illness,
characterized by malaise, fever, and a vesicular rash—usually between 250 and
500 vesicles erupt. Prior to licensing of a varicella vaccine (in 1995), approx
4 million cases occurred per year in the United States, with 11,000 hospitalizations, and about 100 deaths per year. About 99% of infections were among children, but complications happen most often among infants, adolescents, adults,
and the immunocompromised. Complications include pneumonia, hepatitis,
bacterial infection of skin lesions, dehydration, and encephalitis. Attack rates
approach 90% among susceptible exposed persons, after an incubation period
usually 14–16 d. Infection is transmitted person-to-person by direct contact,
droplet or aerosol from lesions, or by respiratory secretions—and one is considered contagious 1–2 d prior to the onset of rash, and until all vesicles have
crusted over.

Natural infection usually induces life-long immunity, but VZV persists dor-
mant in sensory nerve ganglia, and can re-emerge as varicella zoster (also
known as shingles or herpes zoster)—a painful vesicular eruption affecting usually one or two contiguous dermatomes. About 15% of adults will eventually

develop herpes zoster—susceptible persons can contract primary varicella infection from contact with zoster lesions, but attack rates are much less for susceptible persons than for those exposed to a primary VZV infection.

Varicella can be a serious infection during pregnancy. Serological and epidemiological studies indicate that about 90–95% of US adults are immune to VZV, so it is relatively uncommon for a pregnant woman to be primarily infected with VZV. When infection occurs during the first half of gestation, congenital varicella syndrome occurs at a rate between 0.4 and 2%. Congenital varicella syndrome can manifest as low birthweight, cataracts, chorioretinitis, cutaneous scarring, limb hypoplasia, microencephaly, cortical atrophy, and other anomalies. The clinical onset of varicella in a susceptible woman from 5 d prior to delivery to 2 d after delivery can result in severe neonatal infection of chicken pox, which can be life-threatening.

Candidates for Varicella Vaccine

In June 2005, the ACIP expanded recommendations for varicella vaccine to promote wider use of the vaccine for adolescents and adults, HIV-infected children, and a second dose for outbreak control. The recommendations are currently under review. The updated recommendations include the following:

1. *Middle school, high school, and college requirements:* Official health agencies should take necessary steps, including developing school immunization requirements, to ensure that students at all grade levels including college and children in child-care facilities are protected against vaccine-preventable diseases, which include varicella. For varicella, this recommendation adds middle school, high school, and college requirements to the child-care and elementary school entry requirements already covered by the 1999 recommendation.

2. *Varicella vaccination of HIV-infected children:* Asymptomatic or mildly symptomatic HIV-infected children aged 12 mo or older with age-specific CD4+ T-lymphocyte counts of 15% or higher and without evidence of varicella immunity should receive two doses of varicella vaccine 3 mo apart. Varicella vaccine was previously recommended for asymptomatic or mildly symptomatic HIV-infected children with age-specific CD4+ T-lymphocyte counts of 25% or more.

3. *Prenatal assessment and postpartum vaccination:* Women should be assessed prenatally for evidence of varicella immunity. On completion or termination of their pregnancies, women who do not have evidence of varicella immunity should receive the first dose of varicella vaccine before discharge from the health care facility. The second dose should be administered 4–8 wk later (at the postpartum or other health care visit). Standing orders are recommended for health care settings in which completion or termination of pregnancy occurs to ensure administration of varicella vaccine.

4. *Vaccination of persons aged 13 yr or older:* Varicella vaccine was previously recommended for persons without evidence of immunity in this age group who have close contact with persons at high risk for severe disease (health care

workers and family contacts of immunocompromised persons) or are at high
risk for exposure or transmission. The ACIP now recommends that all other
persons aged 13 yr or older without evidence of immunity being vaccinated
with two doses of varicella vaccine 4–8 wk apart.
5. *Second-dose varicella vaccine for outbreak control:* During a varicella outbreak, persons who have received one dose of varicella vaccine should receive
   a second dose as long as the minimum interval has elapsed since the first dose
   (3 mo for persons aged 12 mo–12 yr and at least 4 wk for persons aged ≥13 yr).

The revised definition for evidence of immunity to varicella includes any of
the following:
1. Written documentation of age-appropriate vaccination:
   a. Children vaccinated from 12 mo to 12 yr: one dose.
   b. Persons vaccinated at age 13 yr or older: two doses 4–8 wk apart.
2. Born in the United States before 1966.
3. History of varicella disease based on health care provider diagnosis or self- or
   parental report of typical varicella disease for non-US born persons born before
   1966, and all persons born during 1966–1997. For persons reporting a history
   of atypical mild case, health care providers should seek either:
   a. An epidemiological link to a typical varicella case (e.g., case occurred in the
      context of an outbreak or patient had household exposure in the previous 3 wk).
   b. Evidence of laboratory confirmation if it was performed at the time of acute
      disease. When such documentation is lacking, persons should not be consid-
      ered as having a valid history of disease because other diseases may mimic
      mild atypical varicella. For persons born during or after 1998, history of dis-
      ease is no longer considered as evidence of immunity, unless the illness was
      laboratory confirmed.
4. History of herpes zoster based on health care provider diagnosis.
5. Laboratory evidence of immunity or laboratory confirmation of disease.

Varicella Vaccine Characteristics

The US-licensed varicella vaccine is a live, attenuated strain of natural chicken
pox, of the Oka strain—it was first isolated from vesicle fluid of an otherwise
healthy varicella-infected child in Japan in the early 1970s. It was attenuated via
serial propagation in human embryonic lung cells, embryonic guinea pig cells,
and human diploid cells—for a total of 31 passages. The lyophilized vaccine must
be stored frozen at or less than 5°F, and must be used within 30 min of reconsti-
tution. A single 0.5 mL subcutaneously administered dose is about 97% effective
in inducing seroconversion in those aged 2–12 yr. Of those 13 yr and older, a
single dose induces an antibody response in 78% of recipients, so a second dose,
timed 4–8 wk after the first is recommended—99% seroconvert after the second
dose. Efficacy of the vaccine in preventing chicken pox is 70–90% for at least
7–10 yr, and the vaccine is 95% effective in preventing severe disease.

Breakthrough infection can occur, usually leading to less severe infection, without fever, and with 50 or fewer vesicles.

Up to one-third of adult varicella vaccine recipients develop local irritation with the first or second injection—this includes soreness, warmth, swelling, erythema, pruritis, rash, induration, hematoma, or numbness. Up to about 5% of vaccinees develop a varicella-like nonlocalized rash of about five vesicles within 3 wk of vaccination—most frequently after the first dose. No other serious adverse reactions have been definitively linked to varicella vaccination. Those who have received varicella vaccine can develop herpes zoster, but the incidence seems significantly less than that of those who have acquired chicken pox naturally—interestingly, some vaccinees' zoster-related virus is of the wild-type, and some is vaccine-associated virus. This may reflect antecedent natural varicella infection in vaccinated individuals.

Contraindications to varicella vaccination include sensitivity to gelatin, or anaphylaxis to neomycin (topical sensitivity to neomycin is not a contraindication). Transmission of vaccine-related virus is rare, and this risk in regard to immunocompromised household contacts is likely outweighed by benefits. The risk of transmission seems higher among those vaccine recipients who develop a rash; it seems prudent to advise vaccinees who develop a rash to avoid contact with immunosuppressed persons. Minor illness does not preclude varicella vaccination, but those with severe illness should postpone vaccination until after recovery. Varicella vaccine should not be administered to those with significant immunosuppression, including those receiving immunosuppressive doses of steroids, those with blood dyscrasias, leukemia, lymphoma, or other malignancies affecting the lymphatics or bone marrow. The vaccine should be avoided during pregnancy, and pregnancy should be avoided until at least 1 mo after vaccination. If a pregnant woman is inadvertently vaccinated with varicella vaccine, she should be counseled about theoretical risks to the developing fetus; however, natural wild varicella poses limited risk, and it is thought that vaccine-associated varicella poses even less risk, so varicella vaccination during pregnancy is not considered an indication for termination. Varicella-susceptible breast-feeding mothers may be considered for varicella vaccination.

MENINGOCOCCAL DISEASE

Neisseria meningitidis has become a leading cause of bacterial meningitis in the United States, since decreases in the incidence of *S. pneumoniae* and *Haemophilus influenzae* type B has occurred after the widespread use of conjugate vaccines. An estimated 1400–2800 cases of meningococcal disease occurs in the United States annually, a rate of 0.5–1.1/100,000 population. *N. meningitidis* colonizes mucosal surfaces of nasopharynx and is transmitted through direct contact with large droplet respiratory secretions from patients or asymptomatic carriers. Humans are the only host. Meningococcal disease also causes substantial mortality and morbidity, with a mortality rate of 11–14% and 11–19% of survivors have sequelae (e.g., neurological disability, limb loss, and hearing loss). During 1991–2002, the highest rate of meningococcal disease (9.2/100,000) occurred among infants aged 0–1 yr; the rate for persons aged 11–19 yr (1.2/100,000) was higher than that for the general population. Although rates of disease are highest among children aged below 2 yr, 62% of meningococcal disease in the United States occurs among persons aged 11 yr or older.

In the United States, more than 98% of cases of meningococcal disease are sporadic; however, since 1991, the frequency of localized outbreaks has increased. Of all cases of meningococcal disease among persons aged no younger than 11 yr, 75% are caused by serogroups (C, Y, or W-135), which are included in vaccines available in the United States.

There are two types of meningococcal vaccine available, tetravalent polysaccharide vaccine (MPSV4) and tetravalent conjugate vaccine (MCV4). MPSV4 is a tetravalent meningococcal polysaccharide vaccine (Menomune-A, C, Y, W-135, Sanofi Pasteur). Each dose consists of the four (A, C, Y, W-135) purified bacterial capsular polysaccharides (50 µg each). MPSV4 (Menomune) is available in single-dose (0.5 mL) and 10-dose (5-mL) vials.

Meningococcal Tetravalent Conjugate Vaccine

MCV4 is a tetravalent meningococcal conjugate vaccine (Menactra, Sanofi Pasteur) that was licensed for use in the United States in January 2005. A 0.5-mL single dose of vaccine contains 4 µg each of capsular polysaccharide from serogroups A, C, Y, and W-135 conjugated to 48 µg of diphtheria toxoid. MCV4 is available only in single-dose vials.

Adverse Reactions

Approximately 50% of patients have adverse systemic reactions, with 3–4% having severe reactions. Reactions include pain at the site of injection as well as fever. In the 6 mo after the administration of vaccine, the events reported were consistent with events expected among healthy adolescent and adult populations. The FDA and the CDC in an October 14, 2005 issue of *MMWR* alerted health care providers to preliminary information of a possible relation between the administration of MCV4 and GBS. The *MMWR* reported on five cases that developed within 6 wk of receiving the vaccine.

Recommendations for Use of Meningococcal Vaccines

Recommendations for the use of meningococcal vaccine are summarized in (Table 2). In 2000, ACIP and the Committee on Infectious Diseases of the American Academy of Pediatrics concluded that college students, especially those living in dormitories, are at moderately increased risk for meningococcal disease compared with other persons their age. ACIP and American Academy

Table 2
Meningococcal Vaccine Use Among Persons Not Vaccinated Previously

Population group <2 yr 2–10 yr, 11–19, 20–55, >55 General population	Not recommended	Not recommended
A single dose of MCV4 at age 11–12 yr, or at high school entry (~15 yr)	Not recommended	Not recommended
Groups at increased risk[a] A single dose of MPSV4 A single dose of MCV4 is preferred (MPSV4 is an acceptable alternative A single dose of MCV4 is preferred (MPSV4 is an acceptable alternative A single dose of MPSV4	Not usually recommended[b]	

[a]Group's at increased risk include college freshman living in dormitories; those who travel to or reside in the "meningitis belt" may benefit from vaccination (the meningitis belt in sub-Saharan Africa extends from Senegal to Ethiopia—epidemics recur typically in the dry season between December and June. Travelers to or US residents of Mecca or Saudi Arabia should also consider vaccination because these regions are considered hyperendemic for meningococcal disease); microbiologists with exposure to *N. menigitidis*; certain populations experiencing an outbreak of meningococcal disease; military recruits; persons with increased susceptibility such as those with terminal complement deficiencies and those with anatomic or functional asplenia.

[b]MPSV4 (two doses, 3 mo apart) can be considered for children aged 3–18 mo to elicit short-term protection against serotype A disease (a single dose should be considered for children aged 19–23 mo). MCV4, meningococcal conjugate vaccine; MPSV4, meningococcal polysaccharide vaccine.

of Pediatrics recommended that (1) college students and their parents be informed by health care providers of the risks of meningococcal disease and of the potential benefits of vaccination with MPSV4; (2) college and university health services facilitate implementation of educational programs about meningococcal disease and the availability of vaccination services; and (3) MPSV4 be made available to those persons requesting vaccination.

Routine Vaccination of Adolescents

The ACIP recommends routine vaccination of young adolescents (defined as persons aged 11–12 yr) with MCV4 at the preadolescent health care visit (i.e., a visit to a health care provider at age 11–12 yr). For those adolescents who have not previously received MCV4, the ACIP recommends vaccination before high school entry (~15 yr) as an effective strategy to reduce meningococcal disease incidence among adolescents and young adults. By 2008, the goal will be routine vaccination with MCV4 of all adolescents beginning at age 11 yr.

Other adolescents who wish to decrease their risk for meningococcal disease may elect to receive vaccine.

Revaccination

Revaccination might be indicated for persons previously vaccinated with MPSV4 who remain at increased risk for infection (e.g., persons residing in areas in which disease is epidemic), particularly children who were first vaccinated below age 4 yr. Such children should be considered for revaccination after 2–3 yr if they remain at increased risk. Although the need for revaccination among adults and older children after receiving MPSV4 has not been determined, antibody levels decline rapidly after 2–3 yr, and if indications still exist for vaccination, revaccination might be considered after 5 yr.

The ACIP expects that MCV4 will provide longer protection than MPSV4; however, studies are needed to confirm this assumption. More data will likely become available within the next 5 yr to guide recommendations on revaccination for persons who were previously vaccinated with MCV4.

Precautions and Contraindications

Recommended vaccinations can be administered to persons with minor acute illness. Because both MCV4 and MPSV4 are inactivated vaccines, they may be administered to persons who are immunosuppressed as a result of disease or medications; however, response to the vaccine might be less than optimal. Studies of vaccination with MPSV4 during pregnancy have not documented adverse effects among either pregnant women or newborns. On the basis of these data, pregnancy should not preclude vaccination with MPSV4, if indicated. MCV4 is safe and immunogenic among nonpregnant persons aged 11–55 yr, but no data are available on the safety of MCV4 during pregnancy. Women of childbearing age who become aware that they were pregnant at the time of MCV4 vaccination should contact their health care provider or the vaccine manufacturer.

ANTIMICROBIAL CHEMOPROPHYLAXIS

In the United States, the primary means for prevention of sporadic meningococcal disease is antimicrobial chemoprophylaxis of close contacts of a patient with invasive meningococcal disease (see Table 3). Close contacts include household members, child-care center contacts, and anyone directly exposed to the patient's oral secretions (e.g., through kissing, mouth-to-mouth resuscitation, endotracheal intubation, or endotracheal tube management). For travelers, antimicrobial chemoprophylaxis should be considered for any passenger who had direct contact with respiratory secretions from an index patient or for anyone seated directly next to an index patient on a prolonged flight (i.e., one lasting ≥8 h). The attack rate for household contacts exposed to patients who have sporadic meningococcal disease was estimated to be 4 cases per 1000 persons exposed,

Table 3
Schedule for Chemoprophylaxis Against Meningococcal Disease

Drug age Group Dosage Duration Rifampin[a] Children aged <1 mo
Children aged ≥1 mo
Adults 5 mg/kg q 12 h
10 mg/kg q 12 h
600 mg q 12 h2 d
2 d
2 d Ciprofloxacin[b] Adults 500 mg Single dose Ceftriaxone Children aged <15 yr 125 mg Single i.m. dose Ceftriaxone Adults 250 mg Single i.m. dose

[a]Rifampin is not recommended in pregnancy; because oral contraceptive reliability may be effected by rifampin, additional contraceptive measure should be considered.

[b]Usually not recommended for persons less than 18 yr, or pregnant or lactating women. Can be used in children when not acceptable alternative is available.

which is 500–800 times more than the rate for the total population. In the United Kingdom, the attack rate among health care workers exposed to patients with meningococcal disease was determined to be 25 times higher than among the general population.

Because the rate of secondary disease for close contacts is highest immediately after onset of disease in the index patient, antimicrobial chemoprophylaxis should be administered as soon as possible (ideally <24 h after identification of the index patient). Conversely, chemoprophylaxis administered more than 14 d after onset of illness in the index patient is probably of limited or no value.

Rifampin, ciprofloxacin, and ceftriaxone are 90–95% effective in reducing nasopharyngeal carriage of *N. meningitidis* and are all acceptable antimicrobial agents for chemoprophylaxis. Systemic antimicrobial therapy of meningococcal disease with agents other than ceftriaxone or other third-generation cephalosporins might not reliably eradicate nasopharyngeal carriage of *N. meningitidis*. If other agents have been used for treatment, the index patient should receive chemoprophylactic antibiotics for eradication of nasopharyngeal carriage before being discharged from the hospital.

One recent study has reported that a single 500-mg oral dose of azithromycin was effective in eradicating nasopharyngeal carriage of *N. meningitidis*. Azithromycin, in addition to being safe and easy to administer, is also available in a suspension form and is approved for use among children. Further evaluation is warranted.

SOURCES

1. CDC (2003) Notice to Readers: Recommended Adult Immunization Schedule—United States, 2003–2004. MMWR 52(40):965–969.

2. CDC (1991) Diptheria, tetanus, and pertussis: Recommendations for vaccine use and other preventative measures. Recommendations of the Immunization Practices Advisory Committee (ACIP) MMWR 40(No. RR-10).

3. CDC (2003) Prevention and control of influenza: Recommendations of the Advisory Committee for Immunization Practices. MMWR 52(No. RR-8).

4. CDC (2003) Using live, attenuated influenza vaccine for the prevention and control of influenza: Supplemental recommendations of the Advisory Committee on Immunization Practices (ACIP). MMWR 52(No. RR-13).

5. CDC (1997) Prevention of pneumococcal disease: Recommendations of the Advisory Committee on Immunization Practices (ACIP). MMWR 47(No. RR-8).

6. CDC (1991) Hepatitis B virus: a comprehensive strategy for eliminating transmission in the United States through universal childhood vaccination. Recommendations of the Immunization Practices Advisory Committee (ACIP). MMWR 40(No. RR-13).

7. CDC (1999) Prevention of hepatitis A through active or passive immunization: Recommendations of the Advisory Committee on Immunization Practices (ACIP). MMWR 48(No. RR-12).

8. CDC (1998) Measles, mumps, and rubella—vaccine use and strategies for elimination of measles, rubella, and congenital rubella syndrome and control of mumps: Recommendations of the Advisory Committee on Immunization Practices (ACIP). MMWR 47(No. RR-8).

9. CDC (1996) Prevention of varicella: Recommendations of the Advisory Committee on Immunization Practices (ACIP). MMWR 45(No. RR-11).

10. CDC (1999) Prevention of varicella: Updated recommendations of the Advisory Committee on Immunization Practices (ACIP). MMWR 48(No. RR-6).

11. CDC (2000) Prevention and control of meningococcal disease and meningococcal disease and college students: Recommendations of the Advisory Committee on Immunization Practices (ACIP). MMWR 49(No. RR-7).

12. CDC (1999) Vaccine-preventable diseases: improving vaccination coverage in children, adolescents, and adults. MMWR 48(No. RR-8).

13. CDC (2003) Facilitating influenza and pneumococcal vaccination through standing orders programs. MMWR 52:68–69.

14. Prevention and Control of Meningococcal Disease (May 27, 2005) MMWR 54(RR07):1–21.

15. Guillain-Barré Syndrome among Recipients of Menactra® Meningococcal Conjugate Vaccine—United States, June–July 2005. MMWR. October 14, 2005/54(40):1023–1025.

16. ACIP Votes to Recommend Routine Use of Tetanus Toxoid, Reduced Diphtheria Toxoid and Acellular Pertussis Vaccines (Tdap) for Adolescents http://www.cdc.gov/nip/vaccine/tdap/tdap_child_recs.pdf (accessed December 22, 2005).

17. ACIP Votes to Recommend Use of Combined Tetanus, Diphtheria and Pertussis (Tdap) Vaccine for Adults. http://www.cdc.gov/nip/vaccine/tdap/tdap_adult_recs.pdf (accessed December 26, 2005).

18. Prevention of Varicella—Provisional Updated ACIP Recommendations for Varicella Vaccine Use. http://www.cdc.gov/nip/vaccine/varicella/varicella_acip_recs.pdf (accessed December 26, 2005).

APPENDIX

FOOTNOTES—RECOMMENDED ADULT IMMUNIZATION SCHEDULE, UNITED STATES, OCTOBER 2005–SEPTEMBER 2006

1. **Td vaccination.** Adults with uncertain histories of a complete primary vaccination series with diphtheria and tetanus toxoid-containing vaccines should receive a primary series using combined Td toxoid. A primary series for adults is three doses; administer the first two doses at least 4 wk apart and the third dose 6–12 mo after the second. Administer one dose if the person received the primary series and if the last vaccination was received more than 10 yr previously. Consult ACIP statement for recommendations for administering Td as prophylaxis in wound management (www.cdc.gov/mmwr/preview/mmwrhtml/00041645.htm). The American College of Physicians Task Force on Adult Immunization supports a second option for Td use in adults: a single Td booster at age 50 yr for persons who have completed the full pediatric series, including the teenage/young adult booster. A newly licensed Tdap vaccine is available for adults. ACIP recommendations for its use will be published.

2. **MMR vaccination.** *Measles component:* adults born before 1957 can be considered immune to measles. Adults born during or after 1957 should receive more than one dose of MMR unless they have a medical contraindication, documentation of more than one dose, history of measles based on health care provider diagnosis, or laboratory evidence of immunity. A second dose of MMR is recommended for adults who (1) were recently exposed to measles or in an outbreak setting, (2) were previously vaccinated with killed measles vaccine, (3) were vaccinated with an unknown type of measles vaccine during 1963–1967, (4) are students in postsecondary educational institutions, (5) work in a health care facility, or (6) plan to travel internationally. Withhold MMR or other measles-containing vaccines from HIV-infected persons with severe immunosuppression. *Mumps component:* one dose of MMR vaccine should be adequate for protection for those born during or after 1957 who lack a history of mumps based on health care provider diagnosis or who lack laboratory evidence of immunity. *Rubella component:* administer one dose of MMR vaccine to women whose rubella vaccination history is unreliable or who lack laboratory evidence of immunity. For women of childbearing age, regardless of birth year, routinely determine rubella immunity and counsel women regarding CRS. Do not vaccinate women who are pregnant or might become pregnant within 4 wk of receiving the vaccine. Women who do not have evidence of immunity should receive MMR vaccine on completion or termination of pregnancy and before discharge from the health care facility.

3. **Varicella vaccination.** Varicella vaccination is recommended for all adults without evidence of immunity to varicella. Special consideration should be

given to those who (1) have close contact with persons at high risk for severe disease (health care workers and family contacts of immunocompromised persons) or (2) are at high risk for exposure or transmission (e.g., teachers of young children; child-care employees; residents and staff members of institutional settings, including correctional institutions; college students; military personnel; adolescents and adults living in households with children; nonpregnant women of childbearing age; and international travelers). Evidence of immunity to varicella in adults includes any of the following: (1) documented age-appropriate varicella vaccination (i.e., receipt of one dose before age 13 yr or receipt of two doses [administered at least 4 wk apart] after age 13 yr); (2) born in the United States before 1966; (3) history of varicella disease based on health care provider diagnosis or self- or parental report of typical varicella disease for non-US born persons born before 1966 and all persons born during 1966–1997 (for a patient reporting a history of an atypical, mild case, health care providers should seek either an epidemiological link with a typical varicella case or evidence of laboratory confirmation, if it was performed at the time of acute disease); (4) history of herpes zoster based on health care provider diagnosis; or (5) laboratory evidence of immunity. Do not vaccinate women who are pregnant or might become pregnant within 4 wk of receiving the vaccine. Assess pregnant women for evidence of varicella immunity. Women who do not have evidence of immunity should receive dose 1 of varicella vaccine on completion or termination of pregnancy and before discharge from the health care facility. Dose 2 should be given 4–8 wk after dose 1.

4. **Influenza vaccination.** *Medical indications:* chronic disorders of the cardiovascular or pulmonary systems, including asthma; chronic metabolic diseases, including diabetes mellitus, renal dysfunction, hemoglobinopathies, or immunosuppression (including immunosuppression caused by medications or by HIV); any condition (e.g., cognitive dysfunction, spinal cord injury, seizure disorder or other neuromuscular disorder) that compromises respiratory function or the handling of respiratory secretions or that can increase the risk of aspiration; and pregnancy during the influenza season. No data exist on the risk for severe or complicated influenza disease among persons with asplenia; however, influenza is a risk factor for secondary bacterial infections that can cause severe disease among persons with asplenia. *Occupational indications:* health care workers and employees of long-term care and assisted living facilities. *Other indications:* residents of nursing homes and other long-term care and assisted living facilities; persons likely to transmit influenza to persons at high risk (i.e., in-home household contacts and caregivers of children birth through 23 mo of age, or persons of all ages with high-risk conditions); and anyone who wishes to be vaccinated. For healthy nonpregnant persons aged 5–49 yr without high-risk conditions who are not contacts of severely immunocompromised persons in special care units, intranasally administered influenza vaccine (FluMist®) may be administered in lieu of inactivated vaccine.

5. **Pneumococcal polysaccharide vaccination.** *Medical indications:* chronic disorders of the pulmonary system (excluding asthma); cardiovascular diseases; diabetes mellitus; chronic liver diseases, including liver disease as a result of alcohol abuse (e.g., cirrhosis); chronic renal failure or nephrotic syndrome; functional or anatomic asplenia (e.g., sickle cell disease or splenectomy [if elective splenectomy is planned, vaccinate at least 2 wk before surgery]); immunosuppressive conditions (e.g., congenital immunodeficiency, HIV infection [vaccinate as close to diagnosis as possible when CD4 cell counts are highest], leukemia, lymphoma, multiple myeloma, Hodgkin's disease, generalized malignancy, organ or bone marrow transplantation); chemotherapy with alkylating agents, antimetabolites, or high-dose, long-term corticosteroids; and cochlear implants. *Other indications:* Alaska Natives and certain Native American populations; residents of nursing homes and other long-term care facilities.

6. **Revaccination with pneumococcal polysaccharide vaccine.** One-time revaccination after 5 yr for persons with chronic renal failure or nephrotic syndrome; functional or anatomic asplenia (e.g., sickle cell disease or splenectomy); immunosuppressive conditions (e.g., congenital immunodeficiency, HIV infection, leukemia, lymphoma, multiple myeloma, Hodgkin's disease, generalized malignancy, organ or bone marrow transplantation); or chemotherapy with alkylating agents, antimetabolites, or high-dose, long-term corticosteroids. For persons over 65 yr, one-time revaccination if they were vaccinated more than 5 yr previously and were younger than 65 yr at the time of primary vaccination.

7. **Hepatitis A vaccination.** *Medical indications:* persons with clotting factor disorders or chronic liver disease. *Behavioral indications:* men who have sex with men or users of illegal drugs. *Occupational indications:* persons working with hepatitis A virus (HAV)-infected primates or with HAV in a research laboratory setting. *Other indications:* persons traveling to or working in countries that have high or intermediate endemicity of hepatitis A (for list of countries, visit www.cdc.gov/travel/diseases.htm#hepa) as well as any person wishing to obtain immunity. Current vaccines should be given in a two-dose series at either 0 and 6–12 mo, or 0 and 6–18 mo. If the combined hepatitis A and hepatitis B vaccine is used, administer three doses at 0, 1, and 6 mo.

8. **Hepatitis B vaccination.** *Medical indications:* hemodialysis patients (use special formulation [40 µg/mL] or two 20 µg/mL doses) or patients who receive clotting factor concentrates. *Occupational indications:* health care workers and public-safety workers who have exposure to blood in the workplace; and persons in training in schools of medicine, dentistry, nursing, laboratory technology, and other allied health professions. *Behavioral indications:* injection-drug users; persons with more than one sex partner in the previous 6 mo; persons with a recently acquired STD; and men who have sex with men. *Other indications:* household contacts and sex partners of persons with chronic HBV infection; clients and staff of institutions for the developmentally disabled; all clients of STD clinics; inmates of correctional facilities; or international travelers who will be in countries with

high or intermediate prevalence of chronic HBV infection for more than 6 mo (for list of countries, visit www.cdc.gov/travel/diseases.htm#hepa).

9. **Meningococcal vaccination.** *Medical indications:* adults with anatomic or functional asplenia, or terminal complement component deficiencies. *Other indications:* first-year college students living in dormitories; microbiologists who are routinely exposed to isolates of *Neisseria meningitidis;* military recruits; and persons who travel to or reside in countries in which meningococcal disease is hyperendemic or epidemic (e.g., the "meningitis belt" of sub-Saharan Africa during the dry season [December–June]), particularly if contact with the local populations will be prolonged. Vaccination is required by the government of Saudi Arabia for all travelers to Mecca during the annual Haj. Meningococcal conjugate vaccine is preferred for adults meeting any of the above indications who are younger than 55 yr, although meningococcal polysaccharide vaccine (MPSV4) is an acceptable alternative. Revaccination after 5 yr may be indicated for adults previously vaccinated with MPSV4 who remain at high risk for infection (e.g., persons residing in areas in which disease is epidemic).

10. **Selected conditions for which *H. influenzae* type B vaccine may be used.** *H. influenzae* type B conjugate vaccines are licensed for children aged 6 wk–71 mo. No efficacy data are available on which to base a recommendation concerning use of Hib vaccine for older children and adults with the chronic conditions associated with an increased risk for Hib disease. However, studies suggest good immunogenicity in patients who have sickle cell disease, leukemia, or HIV infection, or have had splenectomies; administering vaccine to these patients is not contraindicated.

14   Rabies Prevention

Doron Schneider, MD

CONTENTS

INTRODUCTION

Rabies is a viral infection transmitted through the saliva of infected mammals. The virus enters the central nervous system and causes encephalomyelitis, which is almost always fatal. Human cases of rabies are rare in the United States (average of two cases per year); however, international travelers to areas where canine rabies is still endemic have a greatly increased risk of exposure. Rabies among wildlife (raccoons, skunks, and bats) has been increasing in prevalence since the 1950s, accounting for 85% of all reported cases of animal rabies. Rabies among the wildlife occurs throughout the continental United States; Hawaii remains rabies free. Since 1980, 58% of the 36 human cases of rabies in the United States have been associated with bats. In most other countries, dogs remain the most common source of rabies transmission to humans.

Although no controlled human trials have been performed, extensive field experience indicates that postexposure prophylaxis combining wound treatment, passive immunization, and vaccination is uniformly effective when appropriately

From: *Current Clinical Practice: Essential Practice Guidelines in Primary Care*
Edited by: N. S. Skolnik © Humana Press, Totowa, NJ

administered. Rabies has occasionally developed in humans when key elements of the rabies postexposure prophylaxis regimen were omitted or incorrectly administered (1).

Rabies Biologics

Two types of rabies interventions are available in the United States. Rabies vaccine leads to an immune response with antibody production. The antibody response requires 7–10 d to develop and lasts for more than 2 yr. Rabies immune globulin (RIG) provides rapid, passive immunity that persists for only a short period with a half-life of approx 21 d. For postexposure prophylaxis in persons who were previously not immunized, both active and passive prophylaxis should be used.

Immunizations

Rabies vaccine induces an active immune response that produces neutralizing antibodies. Antibody response requires 7–10 d to develop and usually persist for no less than 2 yr. Four forms of three inactivated rabies vaccines are currently licensed for pre- and postexposure prophylaxis in the United States. They are all equally safe and efficacious (see Table 1). Only the Imovax rabies intradermal vaccine (human-diploid cell vaccine [HDCV]) has been approved for intradermal use. All other rabies vaccines are for intramuscular administration.

PRIMARY PRE-EXPOSURE VACCINATION

Primary pre-exposure vaccination should be offered to people at high risk for contacting rabies sources either through bite, nonbite, or aerosolization. This includes individuals such as veterinarians, animal handlers, and certain laboratory workers, as well as those who potentially are in contact with rabid bats, raccoons, skunks, cats, dogs, or other species at risk for having rabies. In addition, international travelers might be candidates for pre-exposure vaccination if they might be in contact with animals in areas where dog rabies is enzootic and access to medical care might be limited. Persons with continuous or frequent exposure risks should have periodic serological testing and booster doses given if needed.

Pre-exposure vaccination eliminates the need for RIG after rabies exposure and decreases the number of vaccine doses needed. In addition, pre-exposure prophylaxis might protect people whose postexposure vaccines are delayed, and may also protect persons after inapparent exposure to rabies (Table 2).

Pre-Exposure Booster Doses and Serological Testing

Routine serological testing is recommended for individuals at continuous or frequent exposure risk. Routine serological testing to confirm seroconversion after primary vaccination is not necessary unless the individual may be

Table 1
Rabies Biologics

Human diploid cell vaccine (Imovax rabies):

• Supplied in two forms, intramuscular (i.m.) and intradermally (id)
• A single-dose vial in the form of i.m., which is reconstituted to a final volume of 1 mL
• A single-dose syringe in the form of id that is reconstituted to a final volume of 0.1 mL
• Manufacturer: Pasteur-Merieux Serum et Vaccins, Connaught Laboratories, Inc., phone: (800) vaccine (822-2463)

Rabies vaccine absorbed (RVA):

• Approved for i.m. administration in a 1 mL dose
• Manufacturer: BioPort Corporation, phone: (517) 335-8120

Purified chick embryo cell (PCEC) vaccine (Rabavert):

• Approved for i.m. administration in a 1 mL dose
• Manufacturer: Chiron Corporation, phone: CHIRON8 (800) 244-7668

Rabies immune globulin (RIG):

• Provide rapid passive immunity that persists for a short time (half-life of about 21 d)
• In all postexposure prophylaxis regiments, except for persons previously immunized, both products (vaccine and RIG) should be used
• Two products licsensed for use in the United States, BayRab™ and Imogram Rabies-HT
• Both contain rabies neutralizing antibody at a concentration of 150 U/mL and are equally efficacious
• Recommended dose is 20 U/kg body weight
• Manufacturers: (1) Imogam Rabies-HT—Pasteur-Merieux Serum et Vaccins, Connaught Laboratories, Inc. phone: (800) vaccine (822-2463) (2) BayRab—Bayer Corporation Pharmaceutical Div. phone: (800) 288-8370

immunosuppressed. If a patient is suspected of being immunosuppressed by disease or medication, primary rabies vaccination should be postponed and activities that may place the patient at risk for rabies should be avoided. If this is not possible, primary vaccination should be initiated and checked for the antibody titers. Those individuals who fail to seroconvert after the third dose should be managed with consultation to the appropriate public health officials.

Persons at continuous risk for rabies exposure (e.g., rabies research lab workers and rabies biological production workers) should have a serum sample tested for rabies antibody every 6 mo. Single intramuscular or intradermal booster doses should be administered, if reduced serum antibody level is seen with complete virus neutralization at one-fifth dilution by the rapid flourescent focus inhibition test.

Persons at frequent risk for rabies exposure (e.g., rabies diagnostic lab workers, spelunkers, veterinarians and staff, animal-control and wildlife workers in

Table 2
Primary Vaccination

Intramuscular primary vaccination:

- Three 1 mL injections of HDCV, RVA, or PCEC administered intramuscularly in the deltoid area.
- One dose is administered on days 0, 7, and 21 or 28.

Intradermal primary vaccination:

- Three 0.1 mL injections of HDCV administered intradermally over the deltoid area
- One dose is administered per day on days 0, 7, and 21 or 28
- The 1 mL HDCV vial is not approved for multidose id use, only the 0.1 mL HDCV syringe can be used for single id use
- Do not administer id HDCV to individuals traveling to malaria endemic areas who will be receiving chloroquione related antimalarials (e.g., mefloquine). There is a decreased immune response
- If both malaria prophylaxis and primary rabies vaccination must be administered, start id HDCV at least 1 mo prior to travel to complete three doses prior to antimalarial prophylaxis. If this is not possible, then the i.m. regimen should be followed

---

HDCV, human-diploid cell vaccine; RVA, rabies vaccine absorbed; PCEC, purified chick embryo cell.

enzootic areas) should have a serum sample tested for rabies antibody every 2 yr. Single intramuscular or intradermal booster doses should be administered if reduced serum antibody level is seen with complete virus neutralization at one-fifth dilution by the rapid flourescent focus inhibition test.

Persons at infrequent risk for rabies exposure (e.g., veterinarians, veterinary students, and animal-control and wildlife officers working in areas with low rabies rates, and at-risk international travelers) do not require routine serological testing or booster doses of vaccine.

Postexposure Therapy for Previously Vaccinated Persons

Previously vaccinated individuals exposed to rabies should receive two intramuscular doses of vaccine. One dose should be administered on day 0 (immediately) and one dose on day 3. RIG is unnecessary and should not be administered to previously vaccinated individuals.

POSTEXPOSURE VACCINATION

General Issues With Postexposure Management

There are two types of exposure to rabies virus, bite and nonbite exposures. Administration of RIG and vaccine after exposure is a medical urgency and not a medical emergency. Physicians should evaluate each possible rabies exposure on an individual basis and if necessary, should consult local public health officials. In assessing the risk of rabies exposure, general animal rabies guidelines, as well as local incidence of rabies in the animal population should be considered. This can be done with the consultation of the local health department.

Essential components of rabies postexposure prophylaxis are wound treatment and immunization with both RIG and vaccine for previously unvaccinated patients. Individuals who have been bitten by an animal suspected or proven to have rabies should begin postexposure prophylaxis immediately. In assessing the risk of rabies exposure, general animal rabies, as well as local incidence of rabies in the animal population (may consult local health department) should be considered.

When a likely or documented exposure has occurred, postexposure prophylaxis is indicated regardless of the length of delay in starting, provided that clinical signs of rabies are not present. Rabies virus is transmitted by introduction of the virus into bite wounds, open skin cuts, or onto mucous membranes. The virus is transmitted via saliva or any neural tissue. Bite exposures are any penetration of the skin by teeth. All bites from high-risk animals pose potential risk of transmitting rabies, regardless of location or severity of the wound. Some animal bites may inflict minimal injury and go undetected (e.g., bat bites).

Nonbite exposures are potential sources of exposure through means other than a bite. Nonbite exposures from terrestrial animals rarely cause rabies; however, the existence of such cases is the reason to consider postexposure prophylaxis. The highest risk of transmission from nonbite exposures is among individuals exposed to large amounts of aerosolized rabies virus (e.g., spelunkers in caves with millions of bats and rabies lab workers) and surgical recipients of corneas from donors who died from rabies. Saliva or neural tissue from a rabid animal contaminating an open wound, abrasion, mucous membrane, or scratch constitutes a nonbite exposure. Simply petting a rabid animal or contact with blood, urine, or feces does not constitute an exposure and prophylaxis is not recommended.

ANIMAL RABIES EPIDEMIOLOGY

The circumstances of biting incident and vaccination status of animal influence the risk of the bite being rabies. An unprovoked bite is much more likely than a provoked bite to indicate a rabid animal. Feeding or handling the animal is considered provocation.

Currently vaccinated dogs, cats, and ferrets are unlikely to become infected with rabies.

Domestic Dogs, Cats, and Ferrets

The likelihood of rabies in domestic animals varies by region. In the United States, it is most commonly reported along the US–Mexico border and sporadically in the United States in enzootic areas. During most of the 1990s, more cats than dogs in the United States were reported as rabid, probably because of fewer cat vaccination laws. In developing countries, dogs are the major vector for rabies. After a dog, cat, or ferret bite, the animal should be confined and observed for a period of 10 d. Any illness in the animal prior to release should be evaluated by a veterinarian and reported to the local public health department. If rabies is suspected, the animal should be euthanized and tested. The patient should begin rabies prophylaxis after the animal shows the first signs of rabies.

Bats

All 49 continental states have documented rabid bats. Bats are an important wildlife reservoir for rabies. In all human exposures with bats, the bat should be safely collected and submitted for rabies diagnosis. Postexposure prophylaxis is recommended for all individuals with bat exposure unless the bat is available for testing and tested negative or unless the individual can be certain that no bite, scratch, or mucous membrane exposure occurred. Postexposure prophylaxis should be considered for individuals who were in the same room with a bat and who might be unaware that a bite or direct contact had occurred (e.g., sleeping child, mentally disabled, or intoxicated).

Wild Terrestrial Carnivores

Raccoons, skunks, foxes, and coyotes are the terrestrial animals most commonly infected with rabies. All bites from these animals should be considered an exposure and postexposure prophylaxis should be initiated as soon as possible unless the animal has already been tested and proved negative. If captured, the animal should be immediately euthanized and submitted for testing. If negative for rabies, postexposure prophylactic regime can be stopped. Symptoms of rabies among wildlife cannot be interpreted reliably. If caught, the animals head should be submitted for testing, and prophylaxis should be initiated.

Other Wild Animals

Small rodents (e.g., squirrels, hamsters, guinea pigs, gerbils, chipmunks, rats, and mice) and lagomorphs (rabits and hares) are almost never infected with rabies and are not known to transmit rabies to humans. Woodchucks accounted for 93% of rodent rabies from 1990 to 1996 in areas of the country where racoon rabies was enzootic. All potential rabies exposure cases involving rodents should be handled in consult with the local health department. Offspring of wild animals crossbred with domestic dogs and cats are considered wild animals. Since the time period of rabies virus shedding in these animals is unknown, they should be euthanized and tested rather than confined and observed in any exposure case.

WOUND TREATMENT

All bite wounds and scratches should be washed immediately with soap and water and a virucidal agent like providone–iodine solution irrigation. Tetanus prophylaxis and measures to control bacterial infection also should be administered.

IMMUNIZATION

Unvaccinated Individuals

• RIG and vaccine is recommended for both bite and nonbite exposures in previously unvaccinated patients.
• RIG is administered only once in previously unvaccinated persons to provide immediate antibody protection, until the patient responds to the vaccine.
• If RIG was not given when vaccination was begun, it can be administered up to 7 d after the first dose of vaccine.
• Recommended dose of RIG is 20 U/kg body weight. This is applicable to all age groups including children.
• If possible, the full dose of RIG should be infiltrated into and around the wound. Any remaining RIG should be administered intramuscularly at a distant site from where the vaccine will be administered.
• RIG should never be administered in the same syringe or in the same anatomical site as the vaccine.
• Five 1 mL doses of HDCV, rabies vaccine absorbed (RVA), or purified chick embryo cell vaccine (PCEC) should be administered intramuscularly one dose per day on days 0, 3, 7, 14, and 28 for all previously unvaccinated exposures.
• The first dose of vaccine should be given as soon as possible after exposure.
• For adults, the vaccines should be administered in the deltoid area. For children, the anterolateral thigh is also acceptable. The gluteal area should never be used for HDCV, RVA, or PCEC injections because of low-resulting antibody titers.

Vaccinated Individuals

• Do not administer RIG.
• Two 1 mL doses of HDCV, RVA, or PCEC should be administered intramuscularly in the deltoid area, one dose per day on days 0 and 3.

ADVERSE REACTIONS TO VACCINES

Adverse reactions to HDCV, RVA, and PCEC immunizations are less common and less serious compared with previously available vaccines. Local reactions (e.g., pain, errythema, smelling, or itching at the injection site) to HDCV injections have been reported in 30–74% of recipients. Systemic reactions (e.g., headache, nausea, abdominal pain, muscle aches, and dizziness) have been reported among 5–40% of recipients. Three cases of neurological illness resembling Guillain-Barre syndrome that resolved without sequelae in 12 wk were reported.

RIG administration may be followed by local pain and low-grade fever. There is no evidence that any viruses have ever been transmitted by commercially available RIG in the United States. Once initiated, rabies prophylaxis should not be interrupted or discontinued because of local or mild systemic reactions. These reactions should be managed with anti-inflammatory and antipyretic agents.

If a patient with a history of serious hypersensitivity to rabies vaccine must be revaccinated, antihistamines can be administered. Epinephrine should be available and the patient must be observed carefully after vaccination. If a patient receiving rabies vaccine develops serious systemic, anaphylactic, or neuroparalytic reactions, then the individual's risk of aquiring rabies from the exposure must be carefully considered before discontinuation of the vaccination. Advice regarding management of serious adverse reactions can be obtained from the state health department or Center for Disease Control and Prevention. All serious systemic, neuroparalytic, or anaphylactic reactions should be reported to the Vaccine Adverse Event Reporting System *(2)*.

PRECAUTIONS AND CONTRAINDICATIONS

Corticosteroids, immunosuppressive agents, antimalarials, and immunosuppresive illnesses can all interfere with the development of immunity after vaccination. Immunosuppressive agents should not be administered during postexposure therapy unless essential for the treatment of other conditions. If postexposure prophylaxis is administered to an immunosuppressed patient, serum samples must be tested for rabies antibody to ensure seroconversion. Pregnancy is not a contraindication to either pre-exposure or postexposure prophylaxis.

SOURCES

1. Human Rabies Prevention—United States (1999) Recommendations of the Advisory Committee on Immunization Practices (ACIP). MMWR January 08, 48(RR-1):1–21.
2. Vaccine Adverse Event Reporting System (800) 822–7967.

15 Practice Guidelines for the Management of Infectious Diarrhea

Pam Fenstemacher, MD

CONTENTS

INTRODUCTION

One to two times a year every person in the United States has an episodic increase in the water content of their normal bowel movement, which then leads to an increase in the volume, frequency, or liquidity of their stools. It has been estimated that in the United States people have these diarrheal episodes up to 375 million times each year, resulting in 73 million physician consultations, 1.8 million hospitalizations, and 3100 deaths. When the Centers for Disease Control and Prevention (CDC) surveyed a population about their diarrheal illness, an estimated 31% used an antidiarrheal medication, 12% telephoned the physician or provider's office, 8% visited a physician's or other provider's office, 5% used an antimicrobial agent, and 0.6% were hospitalized. In addition to the acute morbidity and mortality of diarrhea, some causes of infectious diarrhea result in serious long-term sequelae such as hemolytic uremic syndrome (HUS) with renal failure, Guillain-Barré syndrome, and malnutrition.

From: *Current Clinical Practice: Essential Practice Guidelines in Primary Care*
Edited by: N. S. Skolnik © Humana Press, Totowa, NJ

183

The number of different enteric pathogens associated with illnesses of the gastro-intestinal (GI) tract is quickly multiplying as our food supply is rapidly being expanded to the world's markets. Diarrheal illness is spread as organisms are easily transmitted through food or water or from one person to another. In 1988 alone, an estimated $23 billion was spent on 99 million cases of diarrhea. In order to develop a cost-effective approach to the evaluation and management of infectious diarrhea, available diagnostic methods, therapies, and preventive measures must be carefully targeted to the clinical scenarios in which they will yield the greatest benefits for the individual, as well as the public's health. When clinicians aid public health practitioners by obtaining appropriate pathogen-specific diagnoses, the subtyping of bacterial isolates through public health surveillance lowers transmission rates by the timely detecting and controlling of outbreaks. Although clinicians and public health practitioners have different agendas, in order to reduce the morbidity and mortality associated with infectious diarrhea, it will be important for the clinical and public health practitioner communities to work closely together so that optimal diagnostic, treatment, and prevention methods can be identified. These guidelines contain recommendations aimed at both groups.

Although not all populations are equally at risk for contracting diarrhea or from its morbidity and mortality, in the United States an estimated $6 billion is spent each year on medical care and lost productivity from food-borne diseases alone. Young children are more at risk than other age groups for having episodes of diarrhea, as seen in a study of families in Charlottesville, Virginia with an average of 2.46 illnesses per year per child younger than 3 yr old and with a peak in the winter when rotavirus and other enteric viruses predominate. If that young child is attending a day-care center, the risk of contracting diarrhea is even higher with an average of five illnesses per year as seen in a study from Arizona. When different types of child-care settings have been compared, a 2.2- to 3.5-fold greater relative risk of contracting diarrhea is seen among children younger than 3 yr of age who are attending child-care centers vs those same children cared for at a child-care home. Even with this increased diarrhea seen in children cared for outside of a home, young children in the United States still do not suffer as much as those in developing tropical areas of the world, where young children usually have 6–10 illnesses each year. There is a growing awareness of the potentially huge impact of these repeated early childhood enteric infections during the critical years of children's development. In the developing world, diarrhea has been shown to cause long-term disability and may also have a lasting impact on the physical and cognitive development of effected children.

Worldwide, 3.1 million deaths result from diarrhea each year or more than 8400/d. Most of dead are young children in developing areas, which is a 1000-fold higher rate than in the United States where the elderly are more likely to succumb to diarrheal illness. Lew et al. reviewed the National Center for Health Statistics data from a 9-yr period (1979–1987) and found 28,538 deaths (with an average of 3171 deaths per year) in which diarrhea was listed as the immediate or underlying cause. Elderly people over the age of 74 accounted for 51% of the deaths, whereas, only 27% who died were 55–74 yr old and 11% were less than 55 yr old. When the McDonnell-Douglas Health Information System database was reviewed by Gangarosa et al., they found that 25% of all hospitalizations and 85% of all mortality associated with diarrhea involved the elderly as well. Individuals not in high-risk age groups who develop a compromised immune systems or structural abnormalities of the GI tract can also be devastated by diarrhea illness.

THE ROLES OF CLINICIANS
AND PUBLIC HEALTH PRACTITIONERS

Clinicians who promptly diagnose an episode of acute diarrhea desire to alleviate the patient's symptoms and prevent transmission to others. Public health practitioners on the other hand want to diagnose acute episodes of diarrhea to promptly identify the sources of any epidemics, which can spread. Diarrhea resulting from an infectious etiology is often accompanied by symptoms of nausea, vomiting, or abdominal cramps. When diarrhea lasts 14 d or less it is considered *acute*, more than 14 d it is considered *persistent*, and more than 30 d it is considered *chronic* diarrhea. In a 1997 CDC population survey, an estimated 6 million fecal specimens were submitted for stool culture and 3 million were submitted for examination for ova and parasites from 374 million people. Physicians surveyed from different geographic areas and specialties, when seeing the same patient with a diarrheal illness, obtain a stool culture with significant variability. When stool cultures are requested, their usefulness has been questioned because the yield of such cultures is often thought to be quite low. Obtaining a history that includes the patient's exposure, immune status, severity, and duration of the illness, and determining whether the process is inflammatory or hemorrhagic is helpful in improving the yield of stool testing. Even positive stool cultures seem an unnecessary expense for many clinicians because most diarrheal illnesses are self-limited and test results are often available only after the illness has been resolved, thereby providing little information directly relevant to the clinical care of the patient. Stool cultures, therefore, are often viewed by clinicians as a test with little value. But even when a stool culture result does not help the original patient who was tested, the result may have great public health importance.

In 1994 there was an outbreak of illnesses because of *Salmonella enteritidis* serotype. During this outbreak, an elevated number of *Salmonella* isolates were sent to the state public health laboratory from one region of Minnesota. Although individual patients continued to receive supportive care without antibiotics (as is recommended for infections with this organism), the submitted cultures led to the detection of an ongoing nationwide outbreak of this organism from contaminated commercially distributed ice cream, which was then removed from the market. Almost 250,000 people were affected by this outbreak, widely dispersed to more than 41 states. Only because clinicians ordered stool cultures while evaluating 15 ill persons, instead of empirically treating them, was the reason for the outbreak to get recognized. When public health investigators are attempting to detect and control outbreaks, each positive stool culture can be potentially important. Only 0.3% of the outbreak cases were confirmed by culture and reported to health authorities during this outbreak, as it is common and demonstrates the insensitivity of our surveillance system for enteric diseases.

THE UTILITY OF STOOL TESTING

In the United States each year, agents such as enterohemorrhagic *Escherichia coli, Salmonella, Shigella, Cyclospora, Cryptosporidium, Giardia, Campylobacter jejuni, Clostridium difficile,* caliciviruses, and other enteric viruses cause more than 200 million cases of diarrheal illnesses. Enterohemorrhagic *E. coli* is referred to as Shiga toxin-producing *E. coli* (STEC). All stool culture yields for all enteric pathogens have been reported to be between 1.5 and 5.8%. *C. jejuni* is typically the most common organism detected, followed by *Salmonella, Shigella,* and STEC. In one study in which laboratories reported processing 233,212 stools, crude yield estimates of 1.4% for *Campylobacter,* 0.9% for *Salmonella,* 0.6% for *Shigella, and* 0.3% for *E. coli* O157 were obtained. When Slutsker et al. looked at 10 US hospital laboratories that were culturing all stools for STEC O157 (30,463), they found that specimens yielding STEC O157 were overtly bloody 63% of the time and came from patients with a history of bloody diarrhea in 91% of cases. Patients with stool cultures positive for STEC O157 had less severe fever but more abdominal pain than patients whose stool yielded *Campylobacter, Salmonella,* or *Shigella* spp. Since it was first calculated in 1980 by Koplan et al., the price of a positive stool culture result has been shown to be between $952 and $1200 USD. But the cost per positive stool culture is an incomplete and misleading measure of the value of diagnostic testing because the information obtained from diagnostic stool testing is used for both individual patient care and public health purposes. The cost per positive stool culture will decrease as improvements are made in stool culture sensitivity for likely pathogens and the selection of specimens to be tested.

STRATEGIES FOR IMPROVING THE YIELD OF STOOL CULTURE

Three methods of improving the yield of stool testing have been proposed, *selective testing,* the *3-d rule* for hospitalized patients, and *screening for inflammatory diarrhea.* The first method for improving the yield of stool culture and examination uses selective criterion to determine which patient's stool needs to be tested. Some current examples of using selective criterion include the CDC recommendation that all persons with acute bloody diarrhea or HUS, are tested for STEC O157 because of the higher the yield of stool testing in these individuals. If a patient has severe bloody diarrhea or HUS with a negative stool culture, testing of stool or culture supernatants can be used to increase detection of non-O157 species of STEC toxin. Even better yield of STEC is seen when these stool samples are tested with an enzyme immuno assay (EIA) kit for shiga toxin after broth enrichment. Stool cultures were performed for *Vibrio* on thiosulfate-citrate-bile salts medium in persons who have ingested shellfish in the 3 d before a diarrheal illness. The cultures were also performed for *Yersinia enterocolitica* in fall or winter for at-risk Asian-Americans in California and African-American infant populations.

The second method, the 3-d rule, improves the yield of fecal specimens from hospitalized patients with diarrhea. Patients who develop diarrhea after 3 d of hospitalization have fecal specimens with a very low yield when cultured for standard bacterial pathogens (*Campylobacter, Salmonella, Shigella*, etc.) or examined for ova and parasites. The 3-d rule does not recommend these stool studies in patients who have developed diarrhea after being hospitalized for 3 d. Implementing this rule in 1996 would have saved $20–$73 million because these specimens accounted for an estimated 15–50% of all specimens submitted in the United States that year. This rule does not apply to patients admitted to the hospital for a diarrheal illness. In these patients, appropriate cultures should be performed for all indicated pathogens, irrespective of the date of hospital admission (whereas multiple stool examinations for ova and parasites are of low yield even in these patients). This rule also does not apply to any patient who seems involved in a nosocomial outbreak of a diarrheal illness (e.g., because of *Salmonella*) either. A European study involving multiple centers suggests that the elderly, those with comorbid disease, neutropenia, or HIV infection are at high risk for infectious diarrhea and should be exempt from the 3-d rule because they might have a positive stool culture even if onset of diarrhea occurs for more than 3 d after hospitalization. Therefore, unless there are extenuating circumstances, patients who begin to have diarrhea after 3 d in the hospital should not have stool submitted for routine stool culture. But submitting specimens for *Clostrium difficile* toxin(s) in any patient who develops diarrhea in the hospital (or who has taken antimicrobial agents recently) will yield *C. difficile* in 15–20%. The yield of *C. difficile* is even higher if the patient is severely ill or has inflammatory diarrhea.

The last suggested method for limiting specimens processed in the laboratory advises culturing specimens screened first for diarrheal illnesses that are inflammatory or invasive. Inflammatory or invasive diarrheal illnesses are more likely to be caused by pathogens for which culture or toxin testing is usually available.

Several studies have already shown that fecal specimens screened for evidence of an inflammatory process have a substantially increased yield of culture for invasive pathogens. If fever, tenesmus, or bloody stools are seen, this method recommends that a stool sample should first be evaluated for inflammatory markers such as fecal polymorphonuclear leukocytes or the neutrophil marker lactoferrin (Leukotest, TechLab). Lactoferrin testing is somewhat costly (at about $3.75 per test kit) and has false-positive results for breast-fed infants, but some studies suggest that it may be more sensitive than screening for inflammatory diarrhea with microscopy that requires fresh-cup specimens and an experienced microscopist. One draw back to the testing of all stools for an inflammatory response before culturing is that noninvasive toxin-mediated infections such as those because of STEC or enterotoxic *E. coli* will often not have an inflammatory response. More refined diagnostic algorithms and screening tests need to be developed through research because a potential source of cost-savings without sacrifice of diagnostic specificity is the use of improved algorithms.

STOOL CULTURE VS EMPIRIC ANTIBIOTICS

If stool examination is not pursued and empiric antibiotic therapy is used to treat acute infectious diarrhea, the lack of a specific diagnosis may result in the use of unnecessary antibiotics that can hinder appropriate management and treatment of an infection or a disease. On one hand, patients with severe abdominal cramps or bloody stools can avoid unnecessary colonoscopy, surgery, or corticosteroid treatment for presumed ulcerative colitis when a diagnosis of *E. coli* O157:H7, *C. jejuni*, or *Entamoeba histolytica* infection is discovered. On the other hand, inflammatory diarrhea is not always infectious as is the case with inflammatory bowel diseases (IBD). The diagnosis of IBD is greatly aided when a thorough microbiological assessment is negative. When metronidazole or vancomycin is used for possible *C. difficile* diarrhea during hospitalization, colonization with and spread of vancomycin-resistant *Enterococci* is enhanced. The use of certain antibiotics to treat the initial diarrhea in patients with *E. coli* O157:H7 infections increases the likelihood of HUS and clinical relapse. Prolonged carrier states are seen when salmonellosis is treated with any antibiotics. Empiric antibiotic use during an acute diarrheal illness can cause increased susceptibility to overt infection and symptomatic illness of *Salmonellosis*, when selective pressure converts the silent carriage of *Salmonella*. If infectious diarrhea is not tested, the lack of knowledge of the local patterns of susceptibility will hinder the initial choosing of antibiotic treatment because there will be no isolation of pathogens from recent clinical specimens. Organisms such as *Shigella* can develop drug resistance during treatment failures with broad-spectrum antimicrobials and can spread easily from person to person. The frequent use of antimicrobial agents causes resistant strains to emerge and more common treatment failures will result in an increasing need for determinations of antimicrobial susceptibility.

Obtaining stool cultures for the organism-specific diagnosis of infectious diarrheal diseases allows clinicians to administer antimicrobial therapy more appropriately and helps to avoid secondary transmission to others. During a nursing home outbreak of *E. coli* O157:H7, several staff members became secondarily infected. This was discovered because of the use of stool testing for an organism-specific diagnosis. An organism-specific diagnosis allows clinicians and public health authorities to provide the appropriate follow-up recommendations for patients who are ill with infectious diarrhea. If specific pathogens are detected, disease surveillance, outbreak detection, and other public health measures can operate to protect the public health. Ill food-handlers and health care workers may need to stay home from work and submit follow-up stool samples after infection with a particular pathogen has been diagnosed. On identification of a case of *E. coli* O157 in a child attending a day-care center or shigellosis in a person working in a restaurant, physicians who notify public health authorities promptly and give advice about initial clinical management and any subsequent public health actions protect others to whom the infection might spread. When *E. coli* O157:H7 infections are discovered public health authorities and clinicians can detect HUS. Serotyping and molecular subtyping of isolates and the appropriate use of stool culturing and reporting helps to detect the outbreaks. When new diarrheal pathogens emerge, they are likely to be detected first among outbreak-associated cases, as was the case with *Salmonella* isolates submitted to health departments that led to detection and characterization of an emerging multidrug-resistant *Salmonella typhimurium* DT 104. The public health cannot be as easily protected when there is a lack of a specific diagnosis that then impedes disease surveillance, outbreak detection, and other critical measures.

THE GUIDELINE

The observed geographic and interspecialty variability in the treatment and diagnosis of infectious diarrhea has illustrated the need for diagnostic guidelines that are evidence-based and cost-effective. Enteric infections that require specific therapy or are responsive to control measures need to be identified with clear guidelines that apply diagnostic methods. The guideline contains testing and treatment recommendations intended to aid clinicians and public health practitioners in the management of acute infectious diarrhea. It also addresses which patients to test and what steps will ensure appropriate public health actions. Information about the diagnosis and management of acute diarrheal diseases is scattered among disease-specific articles and textbooks. This is the first single reference that comprehensively addresses both clinical and public health issues dealing with management of diarrheal diseases. Key research questions that remain unanswered relating to the diagnosis, treatment, and prevention of diarrheal diseases are identified. The guideline "is intended to provide a working framework for clinicians and public health providers and should not ride or be construed as a substitute for sound clinical decision making."

The six recommendations in the guideline address oral rehydration, clinical and epidemiological evaluation, when to obtain fecal studies, when to give antimicrobial and antidiarrheal therapy, and when to immunize. Because diarrheal illness has substantial regional variation throughout the world, in its prevalence of specific pathogens, the availability of means of diagnosis and treatment, and the degree of prevention achieved, these recommendations focus on the industrialized world. These recommendations focus in particular on the United States where diagnostic capacities are widespread. The diagnosis and management of diarrheal illness in the developing world where major epidemic enteric infections such as cholera and typhoid fever have not been controlled is discussed in the 1993 guidelines published by the World Health Organization (WHO).

Clinical Recommendations

These recommendations are aimed at optimizing the care of the individual patient and the needs of the community. Published practice guidelines in the pediatric, gastroenterology, and clinical laboratory literature agree with these recommendations. They are divided into two sections that give separate recommendations for clinical practice and for public health management. The complete public-health management of all diarrheal illnesses is beyond the scope of this guideline, but management has been summarized for each infection. The need for specific fecal testing, pathogen isolation, and patient intervention for optimal clinical care and to protect the public health is discussed in the recommendations. "Wherever possible the recommendations are evidence-based and provide indications regarding the quality of available evidence (on a scale of I–III) and the degree of certainty for a given recommendation (on a scale of A–E; Table 1 http://www.journals.uchicago.edu/CID/journal/issues/v32n3/ 001387/001387.text.html—tb2#tb2http://www.journals.uchicago.edu/CID/ journal/issues/v32n3/001387/001387.text.html—fg1#fg1)."

REHYDRATION

Because dehydration usually occurs with diarrheal illness, initial treatment must include rehydration. If a patient has mild diarrhea, dehydration can be prevented by ingesting extra fluids in clear juices and soups. When diarrhea becomes more significant with postural light-headedness and reduced urination, rehydration fluids with an oral glucose or starch-containing electrolyte solution can be used in the vast majority of cases (A–I). Local pharmacies carry oral

Table 1
Strength of Recommendations and the Quality of Evidence

Category	Definition	Category	Definition
Strength of evidence to support a recommendation	–	Quality of evidence	–
A	Good for use	I	Evidence from at least one properly randomized, controlled trial
B	Moderate for use	II	Evidence from at least one well-designed clinical trial without randomization, from cohort or case-controlled analytic studies (preferably from more than one center), from multiple time-series studies, or from dramatic results in uncontrolled experiments
C	Poor for or against use	III	Evidence from opinions of respected authorities, based on clinical experience, descriptive studies, or reports of expert committees
D	Moderate against use		
E	Good against use		

rehydration solutions that approach the WHO-recommended electrolyte concentrations (e.g., ceralyte, pedialyte, or generic solutions) or it can be prepared by mixing the ingredients listed in Table 2. Oral rehydration therapy was hailed in 1978 as "potentially the most important medical advance of this century" because it has been used throughout the world. It is more readily available and safer, as well as less painful and costly than intravenous fluids. Lifesaving administration of this solution in those able to take oral fluids with severe diarrhea is superior to administration of intravenous fluids because decreasing thirst with rehydration protects against hydration. Nutritional deficiencies of vitamin

Table 2
WHO Recommended Oral Rehydration Solution

1. 3.5 g of NaCl and 2.5 g of NaHCO$_3$ (or 2.9 g of Na citrate): Na 90 mM and HCO$_3$ 30 mM
2. 1.5 g of KCl: K 20 mM and Cl 80 mM
3. 20 g of glucose or glucose polymer (e.g., 40 g of sucrose or 4 Tbl of sugar or 5060 g of cooked cereal flour such as rice, maize, sorghum, millet, wheat, or potato): glucose 111 mM
4. One liter (1.05 qt) of clean water

A and zinc should be considered and repleted if necessary. The ingestion of food-based oral rehydration helps reduce stool output, whereas the incorporation of glutamine and its derivatives speeds up repair of the mucosa. Incorporation of glutamine and its derivatives is one of the new approaches to oral rehydration and nutrition therapy being investigated.

EVALUATION

During a patient's evaluation for a diarrheal illness, obtaining a thorough history (Table 3) should be the first priority. When evaluating a diarrheal illness that has fever, dehydration, bloody or profuse stools, both clinical and epidemiological features of the illness should be sought. This is especially important at the extremes of age and in immunocompromised patients (A–II). Because AIDS patients continue to frequently struggle with significant diarrhea despite aggressive antiretroviral therapy, algorithms modified for AIDS patients are available with recommendations tailored to their diagnosis and therapy.

After a thorough history, a directed physical examination will help elucidate the appropriate management of any acute diarrheal illness. Any abnormal vital signs, evidence of volume depletion, abdominal tenderness, or altered sensorium are important to investigate. Common infectious diarrheal illnesses' predominant clinical features are reviewed in Table 4. Usually it is difficult to predict an enteric pathogen based on the clinical features of a diarrheal illness. Inflammatory diarrheas that can be diagnosed by stool culture (shigellosis, salmonellosis, and campylobacteriosis) have in common the inflammatory features of fever, abdominal pain, bloody stools, and the presence in stools of leukocytes, fecal lactoferrin, and/or occult blood (II).

STOOL TESTING

The guidelines recommended a selective algorithmic approach that combines both clinical and epidemiological features of diarrheal illness (Fig. 1). Developing better algorithms is an area for future research. Enteric illnesses are first placed into one or more categories for which specific testing is suggested. Community-acquired or traveler's diarrhea; nosocomial diarrhea that occurs 3 d after the

Table 3
History (A–II)

Clinical	Epidemiological
When and how the illness began	Travel to a developing area
1. Abrupt	Day-care center attendance or employment
2. Gradual onset	
Stool characteristics	*Consumption of unsafe foods or water*
1. Watery	1. Raw meats, eggs, or shellfish
2. Bloody	2. Unpasteurized milk or juices
3. Mucous	3. Swimming in or drinking untreated fresh
	surface water
4. Purulence	
5. Greasy	
Stool volume and frequency	*Animal contact*
Presence of dysenteric symptoms	
1. Fever	1. Visiting a farm or petting zoo
2. Tenesmus	2. Contact with reptiles
3. Blood and/or pus in the stool	3. Pets with diarrhea
	Knowledge of other ill persons (such as in a
	dormitory or office or a social function)
Symptoms of volume depletion	*Recent or regular medications*
or dehydration	
1. Thirst	1. Antibiotics
2. Tachycardia	2. Antacids
3. Orthostasis	3. Antimotility agents
4. Decreased urination	4. Other
5. Lethargy or obtundation	*Predisposing medical conditions*
6. Decreased skin turgor	1. AIDS
7. Dry mucous membranes	2. Immunosuppressive medications
	3. Prior gastrectomy
	4. Extremes of age
Associated symptoms and their	*Receptive anal intercourse or oral–anal*
frequency and intensity	*sexual contact*
1. Nausea	*Occupation as a food-handler or caregiver*
2. Vomiting	
3. Abdominal pain	
4. Cramps	
5. Headache	
6. Myalgias	
7. Altered sensorium	

start of hospitalization; and persistent diarrhea are the three categories (B–II). Table 4 is a summary of the common organisms associated with diarrheal illness, their clinical and stool characteristics as well as treatment suggestions. For community-acquired diarrhea that lasts more than 1 d, especially if the diar-

Table 4
Organisms, Clinical Evaluation, and Treatment

Organism	Clinical characteristics	Stool sample characteristics	Stool evaluation	Treatment of immunocompetent (see Table 5 for dosing recommendations)
Traveler's diarrhea	Recent travel history	If bloody test for shiga toxin, if recent antibiotic exposure test for *C.difficile*	Not recommended	Treatment with fluoroquinolones —adults, TMP-SMZ—children
Bacteria				
Aeromonas/ plesiomonas	*Aeromonas* mild diarrhea, though sometimes chronic; *Plesiomonas* should be suspected with any diarrhea illness following travel or shellfish consumption	Occult blood in about 40%, sometimes bloody	*Plesiomonas*—Stool culture for other enteric organisms should be negative	TMP-SMZ (B-III)
Campylobacter species	Fever > abdominal tenderness > blood in stool; can cause Guillain-Barré syndrome	Occult >> visible blood	White blood counts (WBCs), fecal lactoferrin positive	Treatment with fluoroquinolones— adults, TMP-SMZ— children—shortens course B–II; Can see symptomatic relapse with resistance to quinolones, erythromycin can also be used

194

	Clinical features	Stool blood	Diagnosis	Treatment
Clostridium difficile toxigenic	Recent antibiotics, 1/4 with fever and abdominal pain	—	WBCs, fecal lactoferrin positive, Screen for toxins A & B	Stop antibiotics and begin metronidazole (B–II)
E. coli species Enterotoxigenic	—	—	—	Empiric antibiotics, fluoroquinolones—adults, TMP-SMZ—children (B–III)
Enteropathogenic	—	—	—	As above (B–III)
Enteroinvasive	—	—	—	As above (B–III)
Enteroaggregative	Can cause malnutrition	Visible blood 1/3	—	Consider above treatment (B–I)
Enterohemorrhagic (STEC)	Most common with visible blood in stool and right sided Abdominal tenderness >> fever (1/3), rare Tenesmus; can cause HUS	Occult or visible blood	No fecal lactoferrin, check for with Shiga toxin with any bloody stool, and check for toxin and culture in HUS, testing *E. coli* O157 on sorbitol-MacConkey agar or by sending *E. coli* isolates to the state public health laboratory	No antimotility agents E–II; Antibiotics are not syndrome routinely used, increases HUS risk and Shiga toxin production (esp. fluoroquinolones)
Salmonella	Fever > than blood in stool or abdominal tenderness, nausea and vomiting	Occult >> visible blood	WBC's, fecal lactoferrin positive	If severe or patient is <6 mo or >50-yr-old or has prostheses, valvular heart disease, severe

(Continued)

Table 4 (Continued)

Organism	Clinical characterisics	Stool sample characteristics	Stool evaluation	Treatment of immunocompetent (see Table 5 for dosing recommendations)
				atherosclerosis, malignancy, or uremia use TMP-SMZ (if susceptible) or in adults may use fluoroquinolone therapy, in *Nontyphi* species antibiotics, may prolong shedding of *Salmonella*. A vaccine for typhoid is recommended if traveling to endemic areas. (B–III)
Shigella species	Fever > blood in stool > abdominal tenderness, Tenesmus	Occult >> visible blood	Most with WBC's, fecal lactoferrin positive	Treatment with fluoroquinolones – adults, TMP-SMZ– vchildren, shortens course AI, use a macrolide if resistance is suspected
Yersinia species	Fever and abdominal pain > vomiting and nausea	Visible blood 1/4	WBC's, use cold enrichment for *Yersinia* in anyone with fever and abdominal pain	Antibiotics are not usually required (B–III). In severe infections or associated bacteremia treat as for immunocompromised hosts, using combination

therapy with doxycycline, aminoglycoside, TMP-SMZ, or fluoroquinolone (B–III) with-hold deferoxamine therapy (B–II)

Organism	Clinical features		Diagnosis	Treatment
Vibrio cholerae O1 or O139	Seafood or seacoast exposure	—	—	Doxycycline, tetracycline, TMP-SMZ, or fluoroquinolones (A–I)
Traveler's diarrhea	—	—	—	Empiric antibiotics shortens course, fluoroquinolones—adults, TMP-SMZ—children (A–I)
Mycobacterium	—	—	Acid-fast stain & culture for *Mycobacterium avium*	Test for in HIV
Other				
Cyclospora species	Fever and abdominal pain, vomiting and nausea, weight loss, Marked fatigue	—	Acid-fast stain	TMP/SMZ (A–I)
Cryptosporidium parvum	Fever and abdominal pain, vomiting and nausea, weight loss and malnutrition	Occasional bloody stool	Fluorescence and EIA or acid-fast stain	If severe, consider paromomycin (C–III), In immunocompromised paromomycin (B–I), add highly active antiretroviral therapy including a protease inhibitor for AIDS

(Continued)

Table 4 (*Continued*)

Organism	Clinical characterisics	Stool sample characteristics	Stool evaluation	Treatment of immunocompetent (see Table 5 for dosing recommendations)
E. histolytica	Fever occasionally	Occult blood	patients (A–II) WBC's	Metronidazole, plus either diiodohydroxyquin or paromomycin (A–II)
Giardia	Travel or water exposure, diarrhea > 14 d	—	Negative stool cultures, found by fluorescence and EIA	If negative stool culture may treat empirically with metronidazole (A–I)
Isospora species	—	—	Acid-fast stain	TMP-SMZ (B–III), in immunocompromised followed by TMP-SMZ thrice weekly, or weekly sulfadoxine and pyrimethamine indefinitely for patients with AIDS (A–I)
Microsporidium species	—	—	Test for in HIV Special chromotrope or other microsporidia stains	Not determined, unless immunocompromised Albendazole; highly active antiretroviral therapy including a protease inhibitor is warranted for patients with AIDS (A–II)

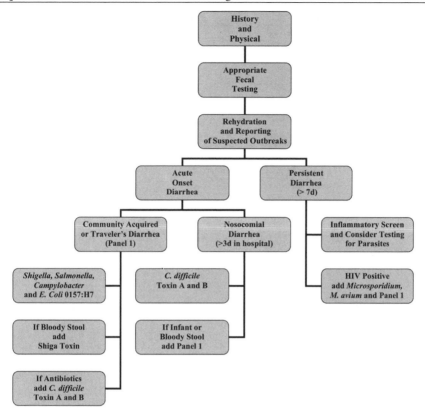

Fig. 1. Clinical algorithm for testing in acute diarrheal illness.

rhea is bloody or is accompanied by fever; stool culture for enteric pathogens (*Shigella, Salmonella, Campylobacter, and E. coli O157:H7*) is recommended. In 87% of patients with 3 or more days of diarrhea and fever, vomiting, myalgias or headache, stool cultures had positive results for *Salmonella, Shigella*, or *Campylobacter*. Day-care center attendance and dehydration should prompt evaluation of a fecal specimen as well. Although experts recommend that traveler's diarrhea should not be tested for enteric pathogens unless it has not responded to empirical therapy with a quinolone or trimethoprim-sulfamethoxazole (TMP-SMZ), some experts recommend avoiding administration of antimicrobial agents to persons in the United States with bloody diarrhea. If either community-acquired or traveler's diarrhea is bloody, it should be tested for shiga toxin. If the abdominal pain is predominantly right-sided, without high fever, regardless of blood in the stool, culture for STEC O157. (If the shiga toxin is positive and if STEC is negative, stools isolates need sent to a reference laboratory.) HUS occurring after a diarrhea illness should also cause stools to be tested for STEC O157 and shiga toxin. When the patient's history reveals seafood or seacoast exposure, stool culture should be performed for *Vibrio* spp. as well. Anyone with diarrhea, fever, and persistent abdominal pain should be cultured for *Yersinia enterocolitica* with cold enrichment. If antibiotics or chemotherapy were recently used as a screen for *C. difficile*, toxins A and B should be performed on the stool.

If an outbreak of gastroenteritis is suspected, special studies of stool specimens and *E. coli* isolates may be indicated. During outbreaks of diarrheal illness the performance of stool testing is crucial for tracking antibiotic resistance and determining serotypes and subtypes of bacteria. Not only should outbreaks of acute diarrhea illness be promptly reported to health department, but if there is an outbreak it is suggested that culture plates and isolates are saved and that whole stools or swabs are frozen at −70°C. Commercial assays are able to detect rotavirus infection, which is a leading cause of diarrhea in young children (especially in temperate climates in the winter months), but Norwalk-like virus infections can only be diagnosed with research assays.

In those patients who have been hospitalized for more than 3 d, especially if abdominal pain is present, fecal testing should be done for *C. difficile* toxins A and B. Hospitalized patients whose initial workup was incomplete or those patients in whom diarrhea is suspected to be nosocomial in origin should be tested for other pathogens as suggested by their clinical circumstances. When the stool is noted to be bloody or the patient is an infant, the testing for community-acquired diarrhea should also be done on their stool samples.

At times, clinical and epidemiological features or disease severity suggests the need for additional diagnostic evaluations in selected cases. Serum chemistry analysis, complete blood cell count, blood cultures, urinalysis, abdominal radiography, anoscopy, and flexible endoscopy need to be considered when appropriate. Sigmoidoscopy can diagnose proctitis in symptomatic homosexual men in whom involvement in only the distal 15 cm suggests herpesvirus, gonococcal, chlamydial, or syphilitic infection. Tenesmus can be a prominent feature of sexually transmitted proctitis. When colitis in these men extends more proximally, *Campylobacter*, *Shigella*, *Clostridium difficile*, or chlamydial (LGV serotype) infection are suggested, whereas noninflammatory diarrhea in homosexual men suggests giardiasis. Although the presence of fecal leukocytes or lactoferrin further suggests an inflammatory diarrhea illness, experts differ in their opinions on whether the initial testing of patients with community, travelers, or nosocomial diarrhea should include screens for inflammatory disease as well. Invasive colitis with *Salmonella*, *Shigella*, or *Campylobacter* usually has inflammation that can be documented with fecal lactoferrin testing or microscopy. On one hand, screens for inflammatory disease are also frequently positive with more severe *C. difficile* colitis, and with inflammatory bowel disease. On the other hand, even though patients infected with STEC often have bloody diarrhea, they may have negative or low levels of lactoferrin.

When the diarrhea illness persists for more than 7 d, especially in the immunocompromised host, testing of fecal specimens for inflammation and parasitic infection is useful. The parasites that need to be tested for are *Cyclospora, Isospora belli, Giardia,* and *Cryptosporidium. Cyclospora* and *Isospora* are seen on acid-fast stain, whereas *Giardia* is seen by fluorescence and EIA and *Cryptosporidium* is seen by fluorescence and EIA or acid-fast stain. New techniques are rapidly being developed that are aimed at improving the sensitivity of EIA and DNA probe nonculture techniques. In patients with HIV, investigation for *Microsporidia* and *Mycobacterium* spp. are needed as well as stool culture for enteric pathogens (*Shigella, Salmonella, Campylobacter, and E. coli O157:H7*). *Mycobacterium* spp. are evaluated with acid-fast stains as well as culture for *Mycobacterium avium* complex and microsporidia is discovered with special chromotrope or other microsporidia stains. When appropriate in HIV patients, based on history and physical status, the testing for *C. difficile* and Shiga toxin should be added as well.

If a patient has unexplained persistent or recurrent diarrhea with negative fecal studies but a positive inflammatory screen, ulcerative colitis, or Crohn's disease could be the cause. A gastroenterologist could be very helpful in determining the diagnosis of possible IBD. Other noninfectious or extraintestinal causes of diarrhea should be considered as well when all of the recommended diagnostic tests are completed and a diagnosis has not been made. Some of the more common diagnoses that should be considered are irritable bowel syndrome, Whipple's disease, celiac sprue, pernicious anemia, malabsorption, ischemic bowel disease (especially if the patient is 50 and/or has peripheral vascular disease), obstruction, diabetes, scleroderma, rectosigmoid abscess, and small-bowel diverticulosis.

TREATMENT

Although the empiric treatment of a diarrheal illness with antimicrobial agents can be problematic because of antimicrobial-resistant infections, side effects of treatment, suprainfections when normal flora are eradicated, and the induction of disease-producing phage, at times it is the best avenue of treatment. Antibiotics for the treatment of acute diarrhea illnesses are reviewed in Table 5. Traveler's diarrhea is one indication for empiric antibiotic treatment without cultures because it is usually caused by enterotoxigenic *E. coli* or other bacterial pathogens that respond well to treatment. Fluoroquinolones or in children, TMP-SMZ can reduce the duration of traveler's diarrhea from 3–5 d to less than 1–2 d (A–I). Resistance to TMP-SMZ is seen in up to 20% of *Shigella* isolates from foreign travelers but fluoroquinolones are not approved for treatment of children in the United States. In persons with a history of travel or water exposure, and diarrhea that lasts more than 10–14 d with negative stool examinations, suspect giardiasis and consider empirical treatment with metronidazole. Prior to stool results empiric treatment is recommended for anyone with a febrile diarrhea illness and moderate or more invasive disease. Using empiric treatment can reduce the duration and shedding of susceptible *Shigella* and *Campylobacter* spp. when

Table 5
Antibiotics Recommended in the Treatment of Acute Diarrheal Illness

Treatment	Organisms	Immunocompetent adults	Immunocompetent children	Immunocompromised patients
Antibiotics				
All antibiotics	Enterohemorrhagic (STEC)	Avoid (C–II)	Avoid (C–II)	Avoid (C–III)
Aminoglycoside	*Yersinia* spp.	Severe infections or associated bacteremia treat as in immuno-compromised	–	Doxycycline in combination with aminoglycoside (B–III)
Albendazole	*Microsporidium* spp.	Not determined	Not determined	400 mg bid × 3 wk (B–I); highly active antiretroviral therapy including a protease inhibitor is warranted for patients with AIDS (A–II)
Azithromycin	*Shigella* spp. Nontyphi species of *Salmonella*	1 g/d × 5 d	Same	1 g/d × 7–10 d × 14 d (or longer if relapsing)
Ceftriaxone	*Shigella* spp. Nontyphi species of *Salmonella*	1 g/d × 5 d	Same	If <6 mo 100 mg/kg/d in one or two divided doses × 5–7 d 1 g/d × 7–10 d × 14 d (or longer if relapsing)

202

Drug	Organism/Condition	Dosing		Comments
Doxycycline	*Yersinia* spp. *Vibrio cholerae* O1 or O139	Severe infections or associated bacteremia treat as in immunocompromised 300 mg single dose (A–I)	—	Doxycycline in combination with aminoglycoside or TMP-SMZ or fluoroquinolone (B-III
Erythromycin	*Campylobacter* spp.	500 mg bid × 5 d, more effective if used early (B-II)	—	Same (but may require prolonged treatment)
Fluoroquinolone	Traveler's diarrhea *Shigella* spp. *Aeromonas/Plesiomonas E. coli* spp.: Enterotoxigenic Enteropathogenic Enteroinvasive Enteroaggregative *Yersinia* spp. Nontyphi species of *Salmonella Vibrio cholerae* O1 or O139	(Dosing listed below with each drug) (A–I) preferred TMP-SMZ (B-III) (A–I) (B, II) (B, II) unknown (C–III) usually not (C–II), Severe infections or associated bacteremia treat as in immunocompromised not recommended routinely (E–I), but if severe or >50 yr old or has prostheses, valvular heart disease, severe atherosclerosis, malignancy, or uremia × 5–7 d (B–III) (A–I)		Not recommended in children (drug dosing the same for all organisms unless listed below) × 7–10 d (B–III) (B–III) (B–III) (B–III) (B–III) (B–III) (B–I) in combination with doxycycline (B–III) × 14 d (or longer if relapsing) (B–III)
Ciprofloxacin	As above	500 mg bid. × 3 d	Single-dose for *Vibrio cholerae*	Not recommended 500 mg bid × 3 d
Norfloxacin	As above	400 mg bid. × 3 d	Single-dose for *Vibrio cholerae*	Not recommended 400 mg bid × 3 d

(Continued)

Table 5 (Continued)

Treatment	Organisms	Immunocompetent adults	Immunocompetent Children	Immunocompromised Patients
Ofloxacin	As above	300 mg bid × 3 d,	Single-dose for *Vibrio cholerae*	Not recommended 300 mg bid × 3 d 5 and 25 mg/kg,
TMP-SMZ	Same as fluoroquinolones, but second choice for traveler's diarrhea (2nd to 20% resistance) *Isospora* spp. *Cyclospora* species Nontyphi species of *Salmonella*	160 and 800 mg, respectively, bid × 3 d 160 and 800 mg, respectively, bid × 7–10 d (B–III)	TMP/SMZ, 160 and 800 mg, respectively, bid × 7 d (A–I) 160 and 800 mg, respectively, bid × 5–7 d (B–III)	respectively, bid × 3 d 160 and 800 mg, respectively, bid × 3 d 160 and 800 mg, respectively, q.i.d. × 10 d, followed by 3 wk, indefinitely for patients with AIDS (A–I) TMP-/SMZ, 160 and 800 mg, respectively, q.i.d. × 10 d, followed by TMP-SMZ thrice weekly indefinitely (A–II) 160 and 800 mg, respectively, bid × 14 d (or longer if relapsing)
Metronidazole	Toxigenic *Clostridium difficile Giardia*	250 mg q.i.d. to 500 mg t.i.d × 10 d (A–I) 250–750 mg t.i.d. × 7–10 d (A–I) 1 g/d × 5 d	—	250 mg q.i.d. to 500 mg t.i.d. × 10 d (B–III)
Nalidixic acid	*Shigella* spp.		55 mg/kg/d × 5 d	—

Agent	Organism			
Paromomycin	Cryptosporidium spp.	If severe, consider paromomycin, 500 mg t.i.d. × 7 d (C–III)	500 mg t.i.d. × 14–28 d, then bid if needed (B–I)	—
Pyrimethamine	Isospora spp.	—	—	Weekly sulfadoxine and pyrimethamine (25 mg) indefinitely for patients with AIDS (A–I)
Sulfadoxine	Isospora spp.	—	—	After treatment, weekly sulfadoxine (500 mg) and pyrimethamine indefinitely for patients with AIDS (A–I)
Tetracycline	Vibrio cholerae O1 or O139	500 mg q.i.d. × 3 d; (A–I)	—	500 mg q.i.d. × 3 d (A–I)
Treatment Antibiotics	Enterohemorrhagic (STEC)	administration should be avoided (C–II)	—	Same (C–III)
Antimotility agents	Enterohemorrhagic (STEC)	Avoid (E–II)	Avoid (E–II)	Avoid (C–III)
Antiretroviral therapy	Cryptosporidium spp.	—	—	Highly active antiretroviral therapy including a protease inhibitor is warranted for patients with AIDS (A–II)
Deferoxamine therapy	Yersinia spp.	Withhold (B–II)	Withhold (B–II)	Withhold (B–II)
Remove Antibiotics	Toxigenic Clostridium difficile	(B–II)	(B–II)	(B–III)

Letters indicate the strength of the recommendation and Roman numerals indicate the quality of evidence supporting it, respectively (see Table 1).

a quinolone antibiotic or for children TMP-SMZ, is used. Although quinolones are recommended for empiric treatment of diarrhea illness in adults, resistance to them is becoming increasingly problematic. Quinolone-resistant *Campylobacter* infections can be worsened when quinolones destroy normal flora and its prevalence is increasing worldwide (10.2% in Minnesota). Quinolone resistance can also develop during treatment of *Campylobacter* and be accompanied by symptomatic relapse. These changing patterns of antimicrobial resistance make knowledge of local patterns of antibiotic resistant key when making decisions about antimicrobial therapy.

Quinolones may be the preferred antibiotic to use with traveler's diarrhea, but *Aeromonas* responds best to TMP-SMZ. *Aeromonas* is an enteric pathogen found in the healthy host that is usually associated with mild, although sometimes chronic and/or bloody diarrhea. TMP-SMZ might also decrease the duration of symptoms of *Plesiomonas*. *Plesiomonas* has less evidence to support its pathogenicity, but it should be considered a pathogen in the setting of a diarrheal illness following travel or shellfish consumption when no other pathogens are found.

In severe infection or extremes of age, organisms like *salmonella* may warrant quinolone or other antimicrobial therapy; however, antibiotics can prolong shedding of nontyphi species of *Salmonella*. Quinolones can also create problems by inducing a shiga-toxin phage in STEC infection. Illness that could be because of STEC O157 should only be treated with an antimicrobial agent as a last resort because treatment may worsen the risk of HUS developing and has not been shown to improve illness outcomes. Not only can antimicrobial agents increase the production of Shiga toxin in STEC infections, but animal studies have demonstrated harmful effects of antibiotic treatment of STEC infections. Fosfomycin has been shown in nonrandomized studies of patients and in vitro research done in Japan, that it may improve the clinical course of STEC infections (C–III). Antimotility agents in suspected or documented STEC infections are also contraindicated (E–II).

New treatments to which resistance cannot develop and that ameliorate symptoms by blocking secretory or inflammatory toxins or enhancing electrolyte absorption and intestinal repair are being investigated. New vaccines can help reduce the spread of illness as well as reducing symptoms. Currently vaccines such as the parenteral (Vi) or oral (Ty21a) typhoid vaccines are recommended for travelers in endemic typhoid areas and those not staying at the usual tourist hotels, making them high risk for infection. The old (often toxic) heat-phenol-inactivated parenteral vaccine is still available for typhoid fever. Because typhoid fever in the United States is usually acquired during international travel and is potentially severe and largely preventable, the guidelines recommend the Vi or Ty21a (or, only for children <2 yr old, the heat-phenol-inactivated) vaccine for those with significant likely exposure (B–II). Although not available in the United States, new live and killed oral cholera vaccines are being made. Only the old parenteral cholera vaccine is licensed for use in the United States and it is not recommended because of the extremely low risk of cholera to the traveler and the limited efficacy of the vaccine. New oral live (CVD 103HgR) and killed (whole-cell B-subunit) vaccines are licensed outside the United States and are occasionally used by some travelers. A vaccine has been developed for rotavirus as well, but although the rotavirus vaccine is effective, it is not recommended or marketed because of rare cases of intussusception.

PUBLIC HEALTH RECOMMENDATIONS

Health departments provide information to educate the general public or persons at increased risk on disease prevention for diarrheal diseases, and handle inquiries from the media. Many websites from a number of sources give educational information on food safety. Preventing diarrheal illnesses and outbreaks through education is crucial to the public's health. When personal hygiene is encouraged, many diarrheal diseases can be prevented. People who are involved in food handling need to follow simple rules of personal hygiene and safe food preparation. Using hand sanitizer or hand-washing with soap are both effective in preventing spread of illness and should be emphasized for caregivers and people preparing food. Human waste is always potentially hazardous and diarrhea or microbial studies are not needed to justify the need for meticulous attention to hand cleansing.

Educating certain groups about the best way to prevent the spread of a diarrheal disease to others once they are infected is also important. If a food-handler in a food service establishment or a health care worker involved in direct patient care develops diarrhea, they should be tested for bacterial pathogens because they can transmit their infection to large numbers of people.

GI illnesses in a day-care attendee or employee, or resident of any institutional facility should be evaluated for bacterial or parasitic infection because disease outbreaks occur in day-care frequently, prisons, psychiatric institutions, and nursing homes centers. Appropriate diagnostic testing should be requested for the suspected clinical illness in order to facilitate identification of the etiological agent and to define the extent of the outbreak to be reported to public health authorities. The earlier an outbreak is discovered through prompt reporting and investigation of possible sources, the more additional illnesses will be prevented.

Health care providers can play an important role in educating high-risk groups about food safety and how to protect themselves by learning about foods to avoid and how to follow safe food-handling and preparation practices. *Salmonella* and *E. coli* are both particularly dangerous organisms for young children and the elderly to contract and their transmission can be avoided with following safe food-handling practices. Enteric pathogens are also more likely to cause illness of greater severity and with more frequent complications in individuals susceptible to infection because of immunocompromise (e.g., persons receiving long-term oral steroids, immunosuppressive agents, or cancer chemotherapy, and HIV-infected patients). *Listeria monocytogenes* is seen in soft cheeses, unheated deli meats, and raw dairy products and can cause infection in the immunocompromised as well in pregnant women, who should avoid these foods. Pregnancy is a time for women to avoid undercooked meats as well, because of the risk of infection with *Toxoplasma gondii*, which along with *Listeria* is associated with miscarriage. *Vibrio vulnificus* is seen in raw shellfish and causes infections in alcoholics and persons with chronic liver disease (hemachromatosis or cirrhosis) when they ingest raw shellfish.

The regulations on food-handlers and health care workers vary between jurisdictions and by pathogen, so providers should contact their local public health office before advising individual workers. Once people in these job categories become infected with a bacterial or parasitic diarrheal disease it is important to determine when they are cured and are no longer fecal carriers. Because food-handlers and health care workers can transmit disease even when they are asymptomatic, when they are symptomatic they should be excluded from working with food or high-risk patients. Before these workers resume their jobs, it is recommended that 48 h or more after resolution of symptoms they have two or more consecutive negative stool samples taken 24 h apart. When the worker is given antibiotics, the first stool specimen should be obtained at least 48 h after the last dose of antibiotics is taken. *E. coli* O157:H7 and *Shigella sonnei* frequently cause diarrheal illnesses in day-care centers and easily spread from person to person. Public health officials may be able to assist by obtaining follow-up samples and providing patient education. Some of the approaches to preventing and controlling the spread of diarrheal disease in day-care settings include the education of the community, keeping any ill children at home, and placing all of the recovering children together within the center. Controlling the spread of diarrheal illnesses in day-care centers needs the cooperation of physicians who are able to first detect the organism and the local public health personnel who can help identify potential outbreaks and control the spread of disease.

The cornerstone of public health surveillance is the reporting of specific infectious diseases to the appropriate public health authorities for outbreak detection, and control efforts. Clinicians and clinical laboratories need to report to the local or state health department when a notifiable infection is diagnosed. The requirements and procedures for reporting differ by jurisdictions. The reporting of disease requirements can be obtained from the website of the Council of State and Territorial Epidemiologists: http://www.cste.org or the state or local health department. Once local health departments are notified, they can notify and counsel individual patients, conduct outbreak investigations, and follow up with patients involved in disease outbreaks.

In 1997, a national network was developed for molecular subtyping of isolates of enteric bacterial organisms in the state public health laboratories for public health surveillance, as well as detection and investigation of outbreaks. This network of state public health laboratories called Pulse Net began performing standardized pulsed-field gel electrophoresis on isolates of STEC O157 and comparing the patterns they identified with a national database maintained at the CDC in order to define the success of control measures. Pulse Net has since been expanded to include serotyping of isolates of *Salmonella*, *Shigella*, and *Listeria*, which is critical during outbreaks of food-borne illness in which early detection and termination are so important. Public health surveillance has led to outbreak prevention by this network. Not only are molecular subtyping strategies developed for bacteria but for viral pathogens as well, hepatitis A and caliciviruses isolates may soon be available for public health surveillance.

"Initial rehydration, clinical and epidemiological evaluation, and selecting appropriate fecal studies and therapy are key to optimal diagnosis and management, and reporting suspected outbreaks and cases of notifiable illnesses to local health authorities is vital in order to allow measures to be taken to investigate threats of enteric infection arising from our increasingly global and industrialized food supplies."

SOURCES

1. Practice Guidelines for the Management of Infectious Diarrhea (2001) Clin Inf Dis 32:331–351.

Tuberculosis Testing and Treatment
of Latent Infection

Pam Fenstemacher, MD

CONTENTS

BACKGROUND

Overview

Worldwide, there are more than 8 million new cases of *Mycobacterium tuberculosis* (TB) and 3 million deaths each year. In the United States, approx 15 million people are infected with TB. In 1965, shortly after isoniazid was found to be effective for the treatment of TB, the first recommendation for treating latent *M. tuberculosis* infection (LTBI) in the general population was given. The American Thoracic Society recommended that all persons with evidence of previously untreated TB, with recent tuberculin test conversions, and all children younger than 3 yr of age with a positive tuberculin skin test (TST) should be treated with isoniazid. Despite broadened recommendations in 1967 and a more widespread number of people being treated with an inexpensive drug that was thought to have few side effects, the morbidity from TB never dramatically fell as had been projected. When the hepatotoxicity of isoniazid began to be recognized in the early

From: *Current Clinical Practice: Essential Practice Guidelines in Primary Care*
Edited by: N. S. Skolnik © Humana Press, Totowa, NJ

1970s a controversy erupted over what would be the appropriate age cutoff in low-risk people that would ensure the benefits of therapy for LTBI and outweigh the risks of treatment. Rifampin (RIF) was introduced for the treatment of LTBI in the early 1980s because the real and perceived problems with isoniazid's hepatotoxicity and the long period of treatment required with isoniazid had impaired isoniazid's widespread usefulness.

In 1989, the strategic plan developed by the Centers for Disease Control and Prevention (CDC) gave the responsibility for detection and treatment of LTBI in high-risk groups to public health agencies. Because of the advent of managed-care organizations and other changes in delivery of clinical services to populations at high risk for TB in 1995, health departments were encouraged by the CDC to begin assisting local providers with TB screening programs appropriate for their communities. Neighborhood health centers, jails, homeless shelters, methadone and syringe/needle-exchange programs are all examples of community-based social-service organizations with high-risk populations that have been evaluated for targeted testing.

Transmission and the Tuberculin Reaction

TB is spread through the air by suspended droplets produced when an infected person sneezes or coughs. After infection, the organisms grow and reproduce for 2–12 wk until cell-mediated immunity occurs to stop the progression of illness. Because there is often little immune response at first, the purified protein derivative (PPD) tuberculin does not immediately turn positive. The PPD response is a delayed-type hypersensitivity reaction that may also be seen in various nontuberculous *Mycobacterium* or with vaccination from *Mycobacterium bovis* (Bacille Calmette Guerin [BCG] vaccine). In addition, the majority of TB infections are clinically and radiologically silent. Individuals with latent TB but no active disease are not infectious.

Natural History and Efficacy of Treatment

Of all individuals who are infected with TB and who do not receive preventive treatment, 10% will eventually develop active disease. The greatest risk for developing disease is concentrated in the first 1–2 yr after infection, when the rate of developing active disease among people whose skin test has converted from negative to positive is approx 1–2% per year, compared with 0.1–0.2% per year in subsequent years. Groups of persons at increased risk for recently being infected with TB include those in close contact with persons with infectious pulmonary TB, persons with a conversion of their skin test in the past 2 yr, persons who have recently emigrated (>5 yr ago) from a country with a high-endemic rate, and children under 5 yr of age. Other people at high risk for acquiring a recent TB infection are homeless persons, injection drug users, and persons with HIV infection because of high rates of transmission. Anyone who works or resides in an institutional setting (e.g., homeless shelters, correctional facilities, nursing homes, and residential homes for patients with AIDS) is also at ongoing risk for developing TB infection, but the risk of transmission varies greatly among institutions and their sites.

Children under 5 yr of age with skin-test conversion are not only at high risk for recent conversion but especially are also at high risk of progressing to active TB and potentially disseminating. The risk of developing active TB is also high in adolescents and young adults. Persons with illnesses that cause relative immunosuppression have a greater likelihood of developing active disease as well. Rates of progression to active TB among HIV-infected persons are the highest, especially if the person is an injection drug user. Injection drug users without HIV infection are also at increased risk for progression to active TB. Other clinical conditions associated with a high risk of progression to active TB include fibrotic lesions on chest X-rays (presumed from previous untreated TB), silicosis, diabetes especially if poorly controlled, and chronic renal failure on hemodialysis. When a person is underweight by 15% or more, or has had gastrectomy with weight loss and malabsorption or a jejunoileal bypass, they are at greater risk of developing active TB. Immunosuppression induced by immunosuppressive agents or prolonged therapy with steroids needed for solid organ transplant or other disease states, and neoplasms (e.g., lung cancer, lymphoma, and leukemia), especially carcinoma of head or neck, also place a person at increased risk of activating TB.

Most people with active TB have pulmonary TB characterized by cough and systemic signs of fever, anorexia, weight loss, weakness, night sweats, and general malaise. Of note, patients with coexisting HIV have a higher incidence of nonpulmonary TB.

DIAGNOSIS

Who Should Be Tested?

A decision to test is a decision to treat, if the test is positive. Tuberculin testing should be concentrated on those people who are at high risk of developing active TB, and who would benefit from treatment of a LTBI. Persons who have had recent exposure to TB and those who have risk factors for being exposed to TB are at risk. Screening of low-risk persons for administrative purposes such as at school entrance and school employees should be discouraged. Groups with a high risk of exposure to TB include homeless persons, people with HIV infection, injection drug users, persons who work or reside in institutional settings (hospitals, homeless shelters, correctional facilities, nursing homes, etc.), where TB transmission occurs. Testing is discouraged unless it is possible to arrange for the evaluation and treatment of LTBI in the individuals being tested, with the appropriate medical supervision.

Testing

Two tests can be used for the detection of LTBI and TB infection, the new in vitro test, QuantiFERON®-TB Gold (QFT-G, manufactured by Cellestis Limited, Carnegie, Victoria, Australia), that has recently received final approval from the US Food and Drug Administration (FDA) and the traditionally used test, the PPD, or Mantoux test. The PPD places 0.1 mL of five tuberculin units of PPD of tuberculosis intradermally on the volar or dorsal surface of the forearm, producing a wheal. If administration does not produce a wheal, another test dose can be administered a few centimeters away from the first dose. TB infection produces a delayed-type hypersensitivity reaction to tuberculins in the PPD. The hypersensitivity reaction begins 5 h after injection with PPD and reaches a maximum at 48–72 h. The TST should be read 48–72 h after the test is placed, and the transverse diameter of induration should be recorded in millimeters. Tests read after 72 h tend to underestimate the size of induration (1–4).

The QFT-G enzyme-linked immunosorbent assay test is an aid in diagnosing *M. tuberculosis* infections; it detects the release of interferon-γ in fresh heparinized whole blood from sensitized persons. Recommendations were given on use of the test in late 2005. These antigens impart greater specificity than is possible with tests using PPD as the TB antigen. In direct comparisons, the sensitivity of QFT-G was statistically similar to that of the TST for detecting infection in persons with untreated culture-confirmed tuberculosis. The performance of QFT-G in certain populations targeted by TB control programs in the United States for finding latent TB infection is under study.

Criteria for a Positive Test

In patients with active TB, because of associated poor nutrition and severe medical illness, the TST can have a false-negative rate up to 25%, and cannot be used to rule out the possibility of active TB. When testing asymptomatic individuals for latent TB, to maximize both the sensitivity and specificity of the test, three cutoff levels have been recommended for defining a positive test based on the risk of an individual having been exposed to TB. They are defined in Table 1. For individuals who receive annual testing, an increase in reaction size of more than 10 mm within a 2-yr period is considered a skin-test conversion consistent with recent infection with TB. No available method can distinguish tuberculin reactions caused by vaccination with BCG from those caused by TB; therefore "it is usually prudent to consider a positive reaction as indicating infection." The BCG vaccine is not likely to cause a reaction of 20 mm or less of induration. Anergy testing is not recommended for several reasons including that selective nonreactivity to TST can occur, and mumps reactivity may remain after loss of PPD reactivity. Over time, in individuals who have been exposed to TB, the size of the skin test might diminish, and even disappear. In these individuals, if a TST is given, the initial test may be negative, but a repeat may

Table 1
Criteria for a Positive PPD Test

Reaction >10 mm is a positive test

- HIV+ persons
- Recent contacts of TB patients
- Patients with fibrotic changes on chest X-ray consistent with prior TB
- Patients with organ transplants or otherwise immunosuppressed

Reaction >10 mm is a positive test

- Recent immigrants from high-prevalence countries (within the last 5 yr)
- Injection drug users
- Residents and employees of high-risk settings (prisons, nursing homes, hospitals, and homeless shelters)
- *Mycobacterium* lab personnel
- Persons with clinical conditions that place them at high risk: silicosis, diabetes mellitus, chronic renal failure, some hematological disorders (leukemias and lymphomas); other specific malignancies (cancer of head, neck, or lung); weight loss of >10% of ideal body weight, gastrectomy, jejunoileal bypass
- Children younger than 4 or infants, children, and adolescents exposed to adults at high risk

Reaction >15 mm is a positive test

- Persons with no risk factors for TB

then be positive. This is called the "booster effect" and is not a skin-test conversion. Persons with a booster effect were exposed to TB many years ago placing them in a group that is at much lower risk for conversion to active TB and that is not recommended for LTBI treatment. Therefore, in people who will likely get annual testing such as health care workers or individuals living in institutions, a two-step test is recommended, in which individuals who have a negative initial TST get a second PPD 1–3 wk later. The results of the second test are considered to reflect the person's true tuberculin status.

QFT-G testing is also indicated for diagnosing infection with *M. tuberculosis*, including both TB disease and LTBI. The test can be positive, negative, or indeterminant. QFT-G sensitivity for LTBI might be less than that of the TST. QFT-G, as with the TST, cannot differentiate infection associated with TB disease from LTBI. A diagnosis of LTBI requires that TB disease be excluded by medical evaluation, which should include checking for suggestive symptoms and signs, a chest radiograph, and, when indicated, examination of sputum or other clinical samples for the presence of *M. tuberculosis*. Similar to any other diagnostic test, the predictive value of QFT-G results depends on the prevalence of *M. tuberculosis* infection in the population being tested. The performance of QFT-G, in particular its sensitivity and its rate of indeterminate results, has not been determined in persons who, because of impaired immune function, are at increased risk for *M. tuberculosis* infection progressing to TB disease.

QFT-G can be used in all circumstances in which the TST is used, including contact investigations, evaluation of recent immigrants who have had BCG vaccination, and TB screening of health care workers and others undergoing serial evaluation for *M. tuberculosis* infection. QFT-G usually can be used in place of (and not in addition to) the TST. An indeterminate QFT-G result does not provide useful information regarding the likelihood of *M. tuberculosis* infection. The optimal follow-up of persons with indeterminate QFT-G results has not been determined. The options are to repeat QFT-G with a newly obtained blood specimen, administer a TST, or do neither. For persons with an increased likelihood of *M. tuberculosis* infection who have an indeterminate QFT-G result, administration of a second test, either QFT-G or TST, might be prudent. The potential for TST to cause boosting and the need for two-step testing in settings conducting serial testing should be considered. For persons who are unlikely to have *M. tuberculosis* infection, no further tests are necessary after an indeterminate QFT-G result.

TESTS USED TO DIAGNOSE ACTIVE TB

Chest Radiograph

Usually, the chest radiograph is normal in persons with LTBI, although it may show abnormalities suggestive of a previous TB infection. If TB is healed, dense pulmonary nodules that may be calcified are often seen in the upper lobes or hilum. The nodules seen in the upper lobes are usually smaller and if accompanied by fibrotic scars often have associated upper-lobe volume loss. All the lesions seen in healed TB are well demarcated with sharp margins. Noncalcified nodules and fibrotic scars are more likely to have tubercle bacilli that are still slowly multiplying and putting their host at substantial risk for progression to active TB. Basal pleural thickening and bronchiectasis of the upper lobes can also be seen from prior TB, but both are less specific to TB.

Sputum Examination

If acid-fast bacilli (AFB) are found in the sputum, a confirmatory culture needs to identify *M. tuberculosis* in patients suspected of having active pulmonary TB. Three to six sputum specimens should be collected on different days in order to make the diagnosis of TB. Culture is more sensitive than AFB stains; it is able to detect as few as 10 bacteria per mililiter, compared with AFB stain, which needs 5000–10,000 bacteria per mililiter to detect TB. Culture also helps to determine species identifications and drug susceptibility of the organism. AFB testing is positive in 50–80% of patients with positive TB cultures. If chest radiograms are normal, tubercle bacilli are not usually found in sputum smear or culture, except in some HIV-infected persons. Currently, nucleic acid amplification testing has the same sensitivity and specificity as AFB testing, but this technique that is expected to evolve rapidly over the next few years.

DIAGNOSIS OF LATENT TB INFECTION

Chest Radiograph

A decision to test for latent TB is a decision to treat if the test is positive. All persons with a positive PPD need a posterior–anterior chest radiograph to exclude active TB. Children younger than 5 yr old also need to have a lateral chest radiograph. Pregnant women with either a positive PPD or recent exposure to someone with active TB need a chest radiograph, even if they are in their first trimester, because of the risk of progression to active TB and/or congenital TB. If a chest radiograph is negative for active TB and the person does not have symptoms of active TB, then he or she is a candidate for treatment for LTBI. When the chest radiograph is abnormal and pulmonary or extrapulmonary TB is suspected, further evaluation, which may include sputum examination, medical evaluation, and comparison of any old chest radiographs, should be done to determine if the person needs treatment for active TB.

Sputum Examination

Sputum culture is not indicated for most patients with a positive PPD being considered for treatment for LTBI. However, persons with a chest radiograph consistent with prior healed TB infection (except only calcified pulmonary nodules) should have three consecutive sputum samples obtained on different days for AFB smear and culture. HIV-infected persons with respiratory symptoms should also have sputum cultures completed before being treated for LTBI, even if their chest radiograph is negative. Treatment for LTBI should not be undertaken until active TB is excluded, which may require bronchoscopy or needle biopsy, in some cases in which bacteriology is negative but the chest radiograph in questionable. In situations in which there is a positive PPD and a significant chance of active disease, multidrug treatment for active disease can be started until active TB has been ruled out with negative sputum cultures. A repeat chest radiograph that shows improvement with treatment would suggest active TB even if cultures are negative.

TREATMENT

Treatment of Latent Tuberculosis Infection

STANDARD TREATMENT: ISONIAZID

Isoniazid (Table 2) is a bactericidal, relatively nontoxic, easily administered, and inexpensive agent that when given daily for 9 mo is the current standard

Table 2
Drug Regimens for Treatment of Latent TB:
Doses, Adverse Reactions, Monitoring

Isoniazid

Preferred: Isoniazid dose: adults—5 mg/kg/d to maximum 300 mg daily; pediatrics—*see* literature, daily for 9 mo

Alternatives

- Isoniazid with twice weekly dosing 15 mg/kg per dose to maximum 900 mg per dose for 9 mo (directly observed therapy [DOT] must be used with twice-weekly dosing), pediatrics—*see* literature
- Isoniazid dose: adults—up to 300 mg daily for 6 mo
- Isoniazid up to 900 mg twice weekly for 6 mo with DOT

  ○ 6-mo course is not indicated for

    – Persons with fibrotic lesions on chest X-ray
    – Children
    – HIV-infected persons

Monitoring

- Clinical monitoring monthly
- Liver tests (AST, ALT, and serum bilirubin) at baseline

  ○ In HIV, pregnancy, alcoholism, and with any history of liver disease
  ○ Repeat if abnormal, in the immediate postpartum period, or the patient is at risk for abnormal liver tests or has symptoms of an adverse reaction

Adverse reactions

- Rash
- Increased liver enzymes and hepatitis
- Peripheral neuropathy and CNS side effects
- Increases levels of phenytoin and disulfram

Monitoring

- Clinical monitoring monthly
- Liver tests (AST, ALT, and serum bilirubin) at baseline

  ○ In HIV, pregnancy, alcoholism, and with any history of liver disease
  ○ Repeat if abnormal, in the immediate postpartum period, or the patient is at risk for abnormal liver tests or has symptoms of an adverse reaction

Comments

- Hepatitis risk increases with age and alcohol use
- Pyridoxine (vitamin B_6, 10–25 mg/d) might decrease peripheral neuropathy and CNS side effect
- Only drug with efficacy studies in children, need to use for 9 mo in HIV-positive or -negative children

(Continued)

Rifampin with pyrazinamide

- Rifampin up to 600 mg plus pyrazinamide up to 2 g daily for 2 mo:
    - Recommendations were revised on August 31, 2001 to no longer include this as one of the preferred treatments except in HIV-infected persons *(5)*
    - May also be offered to persons who are contacts of isoniazid-resistant, rifampin-susceptible TB
    - Rifampin is contraindicated or should be used with caution in HIV-infected patients taking protease and NNRT inhibitors
- Rifampin plus pyrazinamide twice weekly with DOT
    - Recommendations were revised on August 31, 2001 to no longer include this as one of the preferred treatments except in HIV-infected persons *(5)*
    - Less efficacious alternative, use only if daily therapy cannot be used

Rifampin

- Rifampin 10 mg/kg/d to maximum of 600 mg daily; or with twice weekly dosing 10 mg/kg/dose to maximum of 600 mg per dose; pediatrics (*see* literature) daily for 4 mo (for persons who cannot tolerate pyrazinamide)
- Rifampin is contraindicated or should be used with caution in HIV-infected patients taking protease and NNRT inhibitors

Monitoring

- Clinical monitoring at 2, 4, and 8 wk when given with pyrazinamide
- Complete blood count, platelets, and liver tests (AST, ALT, and serum bilirubin) at baseline
    - In HIV, pregnancy, alcoholism, and with any history of liver disease
    - Repeat if abnormal or the patient has symptoms of an adverse reaction

Adverse reactions

- Rash
- Hepatitis
- Fever
- Thrombocytopenia
- Flu-like symptoms
- Orange-colored body fluids (secretions, tears, and urine)

Comments

- Rifampin is contraindicated or should be used with caution in HIV-infected patients taking protease and NNRT inhibitors
- Decreases levels of many drugs (Table 3)
- Might permanently discolor soft contact lenses

Pyrazinamide

- Given with rifampin, adults—15–20 mg/kg/d to maximum of 2 g daily; or with twice weekly dosing 50 mg/kg per dose to maximum 4 g per dose; pediatrics—*see* literature

(Continued)

Table 2 *(Continued)*

Monitoring

- Clinical monitoring at 2, 4, and 8 wk when given with pyrazinamide
- Liver tests (AST, ALT, and serum bilirubin) at baseline
  - In HIV, pregnancy, alcoholism, and with any history of liver disease
  - Repeat if abnormal or the patient has symptoms of an adverse reaction

Adverse reactions

- Astrointestinal upset
- Hepatitis
- Rash
- Arthralgias
- Gout (rare)

Comments

- Treat hyperuricemia only if patient has symptoms
- Might make glucose control more difficult in diabetes
- Should be avoided in pregnancy but can be given after the first trimester

AST, aspartate aminotransferase; ALT, amino alanine transferase; CNS, central nervous system; INH, isoniazid; NNRT, non-nucleoside reverse transcriptase.

recommendation for the treatment of latent TB. The absorption from the GI tract of isoniazid is nearly complete (peak concentrations occurring 0.5–2 h after a single 300-mg dose) with excellent penetration of the drug into all body fluids and cavities, where it is highly active against *M. tuberculosis*. Hepatitis is the most severe toxic effect of isoniazid, with alcohol consumption increasing its toxicity. Mild central nervous system effects are common with isoniazid, necessitating adjustments in the timing of administration. In those patients at risk for a peripheral neuropathy (e.g., diabetes, uremia, alcoholism, malnutrition, and HIV infection), isoniazid's interference with pyridoxine metabolism should be treated with pyridoxine supplementation. Pyridoxine supplementation is also recommended during pregnancy and with seizure disorders and if nutritional deficiency is suspected. Because giving isoniazid and phenytoin together increases both of their levels, levels of phenytoin need to be monitored when giving this combination of drugs. A daily treatment with 300 mg of isoniazid for 9 mo provides substantially more effect than a 6 mo course of treatment. Daily treatment with isoniazid for 12 mo provides minimal additional benefit.

Rifampin and Pyrazinamide

Because more recent studies demonstrate an increased hepatotoxicity of the RIF–pyrazinamide (PZA) combination, the original guidelines were revised to include the following: "The 2-mo (RIF–PZA) treatment regimen (Table 2) for LTBI should be used with caution, especially in patients concurrently taking other medications associated with liver injury, and those with alcoholism, even if alcohol use is discontinued during treatment. RIF–PZA is not recommended for persons with underlying liver disease or for those who have had isoniazide-associated liver injury. No more than a 2-wk supply of RIF–PZA should be dispensed at a time. Patients should be reassessed in person at 2, 4, 6, and 8 wk of treatment. A serum ALT and bilirubin should be measured at baseline and at 2, 4, and 6 wk of treatment in patients taking RIF–PZA. The RIF–PZA combination was left on the preferred treatment list only for persons with HIV. RIF 600 mg with 2 mg of PZA daily is the recommended dosing for the 2 mo of treatment.

RIF is a rifamycin derivative that is also bactericidal for *M. tuberculosis*, quickly absorbed from the GI tract in 1.5–3 h, and although 75% protein bound, is able to penetrate well into tissues and cells. RIF can also cause hepatitis, but GI upset is the common adverse drug reaction seen. Infrequently, rashes and low platelet counts can also be seen with RIF. Because RIF induces microsomal enzymes in the liver it may increase the rate of metabolism of many drugs (Table 3). RIF thereby reduces the effectiveness of oral contraceptives, HIV protease inhibitors, and non-nucleoside reverse transcriptase (NNRT) inhibitors by reducing their levels. HIV protease and NNRT inhibitors will increase the level of RIF and subsequently its risk of toxicity; therefore, RIF should be avoided or used with caution in individuals on any of these drugs. Intermittent dosing of RIF with more than 10 mg/kg has been associated with thrombocytopenia, an influenza-like syndrome, hemolytic anemia, and acute renal failure, whereas lower doses uncommonly cause problems. When RIF is excreted in body fluids it colors them orange, which can permanently discolor soft contact lenses. RIF can be given alone at doses of up to 600 mg daily for 4 mo.

PZA is bactericidal in the acidic environment of macrophages. Absorption from the GI tract is nearly complete and occurs approx 2 h after ingestion. As with RIF, GI upset is the most common side effect, but hepatotoxicity is the most severe adverse side effect. Hyperuricemia with rare cases of gout can also occur with PZA treatment, as well as rash and arthalgias. GI upset is minimized if both medications are taken with food, and salicylic acid can be used for the arthalgias of PZA.

PRETREATMENT EVALUATION AND MONITORING

If a person is targeted for treatment of LTBI, there is an opportunity for health care providers to establish rapport with patient, discuss the details of the patient's risk for TB, emphasize the benefits of treatment and the importance of adherence to the treatment, review any side effects or drug interactions of the

Table 3
Drugs That Have Metabolism Increased by Rifampin

• Methadone
• Coumadin derivatives
• Glucocorticoids
• Hormonal contraceptives
• Oral hypoglycemic agents
• Digitalis
• Anticonvulsants
• Dapsone
• Ketoconazole
• Cyclosporin

regime, and establish an optimal follow-up regime. It is important to interview the patient in his or her primary language and to document risk factors before treatment for TB as well as to determine pre-existing medical conditions that make treatment contraindicated or increase the risk of adverse drug reactions. A detailed history of current and previous drug therapy should be taken to determine if there is a chance for adverse drug reactions or interactions with the drug regime being proposed. A physical examination looking for evidence of liver disease should be performed and the patient should be instructed to contact his or her provider immediately on the onset of suspicious symptoms or any unexplained illness. Treatment should be quickly stopped and a clinical evaluation of the patient should occur, if there is unexplained anorexia, nausea, vomiting, dark urine, icterus, rash, persistent paresthesias of the hands or feet, persistent fatigue, weakness, or fever lasting for more than 3 d, abdominal tenderness (especially the right upper quadrant), easy bleeding, and arthralgias. Baseline testing and monitoring should be performed according to Table 2. Subsequent evaluations are an opportunity for reinforcing the reasons for treatment and adherence to treatment and to discover any problems with adherence or adverse drug effects or interactions.

If the patient's transaminase levels are more than three times the upper limit of normal with symptoms, or five times the upper limit of normal without symptoms some experts recommend that isoniazide be withheld. "Practitioners and other health professionals should report serious adverse events associated with the treatment of LTBI to the US Food and Drug Administration's MedWatch program. Serious adverse events include those associated with hospitalization, permanent disability, or death. Reporting may be by mail, telephone (1-800-FDA-1088), fax (1-800-FDA-0178), or the internet site (www.fda.gov/medwatch)."

COMPLETION OF TREATMENT

Therapy is completed if enough doses are given in the correct amount of time. The 9-mo isoniazid treatment regime should consist of 270 doses given within 12 mo, allowing for interruptions in therapy. The 6-mo regime of isoniazid should consist of 180 doses given within 9 mo. The combination of RIF–PZA should include 60 doses within 3 mo, whereas daily RIF alone should consist of at least 120 doses administered within 6 mo. Depending on how long treatment was interrupted for, it may either be continued or must be restarted. If treatment is interrupted for more than 2 mo, a medical exam to exclude active TB disease is indicated.

SPECIAL CONSIDERATIONS

Treatment of HIV-infected patients is similar to that of non-HIV-infected patients except that a 6 mo regimen of isoniazid is not acceptable. RIF is often contraindicated or needs to be used with caution in patients on protease inhibitors or NNRT inhibitors. Experts recommend that persons using protease inhibitors or NNRT inhibitors can substitute rifabutin for RIF in some circumstances. Rifabutin can be safely used with indinavir, nelfinavir, amprenavir, ritonavir, and efavirenz, but not with hard-gel saquinavir or delavirdine. Caution must be used with soft-gel saquinavir or nevirapine because data is limited. There is no data on the efficacy of regimes using rifabutin-containing regimes in treating LTBI. Recommendations are based on use of rifabutin for treatment of active TB and studies in mice. Rifabutin can be administered at one-half the daily dose (150 mg/d) with indinavir, nilfinavir, or amprenavir or at one-fourth the usual dose with ritinovir. When efavirenz is being used with rifabutin, the dose of rifabutin should be increased to 450 or 600 mg/d, but can be used at 300 mg with nevirapine. The use of rifabutin is not recommended if more than one protease inhibitor or NNRT inhibitor or a combination of the two is being used. Rifapentine is not recommended in persons with HIV. Treatment of HIV patients who are tuberculin-negative is not recommended unless they have had recent contact with a patient with active TB.

With fibrotic lesions on chest radiograph and a TST of 5 mm or more, three regimens are acceptable: isoniazid daily for 9 mo, 2 mo of daily RIF plus PZA, or 4 mo of daily RIF, if infection with drug-resistant organism is unlikely. Anyone who has begun therapy for suspected pulmonary TB, but is later cleared of active disease, should complete at least a 2-mo regime containing RIF–PZA if the skin test is at least 5 mm and any radiographic abnormalities have been excluded. Persons with chest X-rays consistent with healed primary

TB (such as calcified solitary pulmonary nodules, calcified hilar lymph nodes, or apical pleural capping) are not at increased risk of TB compared with those with normal chest X-rays and their need for treatment should be determined by their other risk factors and the size of the TST.

The need to treat LTBI in pregnancy is controversial. There is some evidence that suggests that women in pregnancy and the early postpartum period may have a higher incidence of isoniazid-induced hepatitis, but not for progression of LTBI to disease. The risk of progression to active disease must be weighed against the risk of isoniazid-induced hepatitis. For women at high risk of hematogenous spread of the disease to the placenta or for progression to active disease (HIV-infected pregnant women or women who have been recently infected), treatment of latent infection should not be delayed owing to pregnancy. Isoniazid can even be used during the first trimester because it is not teratogenic. Clinical as well as laboratory monitoring for hepatitis should be done in pregnancy, while on isoniazid, and pyridoxine supplementation should be given. Breast-feeding is not contraindicated for women on isoniazid, although the infant should receive pyridoxine supplementation because it is not well secreted in breast milk. No efficacy data supports the use of other agents.

The risk for progression to active TB begins at 40% in untreated infants and decreases gradually throughout childhood. Infants and young children are more likely than others to develop life-threatening forms of TB, especially meningeal and disseminated disease. Isoniazid therapy for LTBI appears to be more effective for children than adults, with risk reduction of 70–90%. The risk of isoniazid hepatitis is minimal in children who tolerate the drug better than adults. The only published efficacy trials of the treatment of LTBI in children have studied isoniazid alone for 9 mo, studies in adults are not thought to be generalizable to children. Isoniazid has been given twice weekly to treat many children with LTBI. It appears safe when given twice a week, but its effectiveness has not been established. No studies have examined the treatment of LTBI in HIV-infected children. The American Academy of Pediatrics recommends a 9-mo course of isoniazid with routine monitoring of liver enzymes and pyridoxine supplementation.

If a person has contact with isoniazid-resistant, RIF-sensitive TB, RIF is recommended in combination with PZA for 2 mo. RIF alone should be used for 4 mo if the combination is not tolerated. Rifabutin can be substituted if RIF cannot be used. No definitive data exists on these treatments. An expert panel has recommended that susceptible contacts (e.g., those with HIV) exposed to this TB be treated with RIF alone. If the TB is resistant to multiple drugs the decision to treat and the selection of the drugs for a regime should be based on culture results in consultation with an expert. People suspected to be infected with multidrug resistant TB need followed for at least 2 yr whether or not they are treated.

SOURCES

1. Diagnostic Standards and Classification of Tuberculosis in Adults and Children (2000) Am J Respir Crit Care Med 161:1376–1395.
2. Targeted Tuberculin Testing and Treatment of Latent Tuberculosis Infection. Joint Statement of the American Thoracic Society and the Centers for Disease Control and Prevention (2000) Am J Respir Crit Care Med 161:S221–S247.
3. MMWR Aug. 31, 2001;50:733.
4. Guidelines for Using the QuantiFERON®-TB Gold Test for Detecting *Mycobacterium tuberculosis* Infection, United States. MM WR December 16, 2005;54:49.
5. MMWR 2001;50:733.

17

Sexually Transmitted Diseases Treatment Guidelines, 2006

Neil S. Skolnik, MD

CONTENTS

INTRODUCTION

In August 2006 the Centers for Disease Control (CDC) issued the Sexually Transmitted Diseases Treatment Guidelines, 2006. The guidelines contain and establish the standard of care for the treatment of sexually transmitted diseases (STDs) nationwide. This chapter summarizes the most important points and the treatment regimens recommended in the guidelines, and follows the organization of the guidelines. All treatment regimens, as well as selected text presented here, are taken verbatim from the guidelines. In addition to treatment, it is essential to understand that counseling patients routinely about prevention of STD acquisition is an important aspect of routine clinical care of adolescents and adults.

From: *Current Clinical Practice: Essential Practice Guidelines in Primary Care*
Edited by: N.S. Skolnik © Humana Press, Totowa, NJ

PARTNER MANAGEMENT

Treatment of the partners of patients who are treated is important because when partners are treated, the index patient has less chance of re-infection, and there is a decreased chance of the partners spreading the STD to other individuals. Clinicians should encourage patients treated for STDs to inform their sexual partners of the presence of an STD and encourage their partners to seek treatment. Another option for partner treatment is expedited partner therapy (EPT). In EPT, partners of infected patients are treated without medical evaluation or prevention counseling by giving the treated patient an extra prescription to be used for treatment of his or her partner. In the treatment of chlamydia and gonorrhea, EPT has been shown to prevent re-infection of the index case and is associated with a higher likelihood of partner notification, compared with recommending that a treated patient refer his or her partners. EPT should always be given with appropriate precautions and with the advise that it would be best for the partner to seek medical care. A potential problem with EPT is its unclear legal status.

SPECIAL POPULATIONS

Adolescents

Adolescents have one of the highest rates of STDs, therefore, emphasis on both preventing and treating STDs among adolescents is important. With rare exceptions, adolescents in the United States can legally consent to the confidential diagnosis and treatment of STDs. The guidelines state explicitly that, "in all 50 states and the District of Columbia, medical care for STDs can be provided to adolescents without parental consent or knowledge."

Men Who Have Sex With Men

Men who have sex with men (MSM) are at high risk for STDs. Routine screening is indicated for all sexually active MSM, and the following tests are recommended on an annual basis:

- HIV serology, if HIV negative or not tested within the previous year.
- Syphilis serology.
- A test for urethral infection with *Neisseria gonorrhoeae* and *Chlamydia trachomatis* in men who have had insertive intercourse during the preceding year.
- A test for rectal infection with *N. gonorrhoeae* and *C. trachomatis* in men who have had receptive anal intercourse during the preceding year.
- A test for pharyngeal infection with *N. gonorrhoeae* in men who have acknowledged participation in receptive oral intercourse during the preceding year; testing for *C. trachomatis* pharyngeal infection is not recommended.

In addition, clinicians can consider serological tests for herpes simplex virus (HSV)-2. Routine testing for anal cytological abnormalities or anal human papilloma virus (HPV) infection is not recommended.

More frequent screening at 3- to 6-mo intervals is indicated for MSM who have multiple or anonymous partners, have sex while using illicit drugs or methamphetamine, or whose sex partners participate in these activities. Vaccination against hepatitis A and B is recommended for all MSM.

DETECTION OF HIV INFECTION: SCREENING AND DIAGNOSTIC TESTING

All individuals who seek evaluation and treatment for STDs should be screened for HIV infection. The majority of HIV infections in the United States are caused by HIV-1; however, HIV-2 infection may be suspected in persons who have epidemiological risk factors linking infection to have possibly originated in West Africa.

Clinicians should be aware of acute retroviral syndrome, which may benefit from antiretroviral therapy, and which is characterized by fever, malaise, lymphadenopathy, and skin rash occuring in the first few weeks after HIV infection, before antibody test results become positive. It can be detected by checking an HIV nucleic acid (RNA) test.

DISEASES CHARACTERIZED BY GENITAL ULCERS

Management of Patients Who Have Genital Ulcers

The majority of young, sexually active patients who have genital ulcers in the United States have genital herpes, syphilis, or chancroid. Herpes is the most common of the three infections.

CHANCROID

Diagnosis

Chancroid typically has a combination of a painful genital ulcer and tender suppurative inguinal adenopathy. Culture testing is only positive in less than 80% of cases. A case can be considered probable if (a) the patient has one or more painful genital ulcers, (b) the patient has no evidence of *T. pallidum* infection by darkfield examination or by a serological testing at least 7 d after onset of ulcers, (c) the clinical presentation is typical for chancroid, and (d) HSV testing is negative. If the initial test results were negative, patients should be retested for syphilis and HIV 3 mo after the diagnosis.

Treatment

RECOMMENDED REGIMENS[1]

- Azithromycin 1 g orally in a single dose **OR**
- Ceftriaxone 250 mg intramuscularly (im) in a single dose **OR**

---

[1]Ciprofloxacin is contraindicated for pregnant and lactating women. Azithromycin and ceftriaxone offer the advantage of single-dose therapy. Worldwide, several isolates with intermediate resistance to either ciprofloxacin or erythromycin have been reported.

- Ciprofloxacin 500 mg orally twice a day for 3 d **OR**
- Erythromycin base 500 mg orally three times a day for 7 d

Genital ulcers should improve within 3–7 d of treatment. Improvement of adenopathy often takes longer and sometimes requires incision and drainage.

GENITAL HSV INFECTIONS

More than 50 million Americans have genital HSV infections. The majority of cases of recurrent genital herpes are caused by HSV-2 although HSV-1 can cause genital herpes. The majority of persons infected with HSV-2 have mild or rarely recurrent infection and are undiagnosed; therefore the majority of transmission occurs from individuals who shed virus intermittently and are often not aware that they are infected.

Diagnosis

The clinical diagnosis of HSV infection is imprecise. More than 50% of first episodes of genital herpes are HSV-1, although recurrence is less frequent for HSV-1 than HSV-2. Clinical diagnosis of genital herpes should be confirmed by laboratory testing.

Treatment

First Clinical Episode of Genital Herpes

Patients with an initial episode should be treated with oral antiviral medication.

RECOMMENDED REGIMENS[2]

- Acyclovir 400 mg orally three times a day for 7–10 d **OR**
- Acyclovir 200 mg orally five times a day for 7–10 d **OR**
- Famciclovir 250 mg orally three times a day for 7–10 d **OR**
- Valacyclovir 1 g orally twice a day for 7–10 d.

ESTABLISHED HSV-2 INFECTION

Intermittent asymptomatic shedding occurs with genital HSV-2 infection, even with longstanding or clinically silent infection. Antiviral therapy for established genital herpes can be given either episodically to diminish or shorten the duration of and outbreak or continuously as suppressive therapy to decrease the frequency of recurrences.

Suppressive Therapy for Recurrent Genital Herpes

Suppressive therapy reduces the frequency of genital herpes recurrences by 70–80% in patients with frequent recurrences, and often eliminates recurrences. The frequency of recurrent genital herpes outbreaks diminishes over time so it may be reasonable annually to consider a trial off suppressive therapy.

---

[2]Treatment might be extended if healing is incomplete after 10 d of therapy.

RECOMMENDED REGIMENS

- Acyclovir 400 mg orally twice a day **OR**
- Famciclovir 250 mg orally twice a day **OR**
- Valacyclovir 500 mg orally once a day **OR**
- Valacyclovir 1 g orally once a day.

Valacyclovir 500 mg once a day might be less effective than other valacyclovir or acyclovir dosing regimens in patients who have very frequent recurrences (i.e., >10 episodes per year).

Episodic Therapy for Recurrent Genital Herpes

When episodic treatment is chosen, it should be started within 1 d of lesion onset or during the prodrome before lesions are apparent.

RECOMMENDED REGIMENS

- Acyclovir 400 mg orally three times a day for 5 d **OR**
- Acyclovir 800 mg orally twice a day for 5 d **OR**
- Acyclovir 800 mg orally three times a day for 2 d **OR**
- Famciclovir 125 mg orally twice daily for 5 d **OR**
- Famciclovir 1000 mg orally twice daily for 1 d **OR**
- Valacyclovir 500 mg orally twice a day for 3 d **OR**
- Valacyclovir 1 g orally once a day for 5 d.

Severe Disease

Intravenous (iv) acyclovir therapy is recommended for severe HSV disease or complications that necessitate hospitalization (e.g., disseminated infection, pneumonitis, or hepatitis) or central nervous system (CNS) complications (e.g., meningitis or encephalitis). The recommended dose is acyclovir 5–10 mg/kg body weight iv every 8 h for 2–7 d, followed by oral antiviral therapy to complete at least 10 d of total therapy.

Special Situations

CO-INFECTION WITH HIV

Immunocompromised patients may have more severe outbreaks.

RECOMMENDED REGIMENS FOR DAILY SUPPRESSIVE THERAPY IN PERSONS INFECTED WITH HIV

- Acyclovir 400–800 mg orally twice to three times a day **OR**
- Famciclovir 500 mg orally twice a day **OR**
- Valacyclovir 500 mg orally twice a day.

RECOMMENDED REGIMENS FOR EPISODIC INFECTION IN PERSONS INFECTED WITH HIV

- Acyclovir 400 mg orally three times a day for 5–10 d **OR**
- Famciclovir 500 mg orally twice a day for 5–10 d **OR**
- Valacyclovir 1 g orally twice a day for 5–10 d.

Genital Herpes in Pregnancy

Most neonatal herpes infections occur in infants whose mothers lack a history of clinical herpes. The risk for transmission from an infected mother is 30–50% among women who acquire herpes near the time of delivery and is low (<1%) among women with histories of recurrent herpes at term or who acquire herpes earlier in pregnancy. *See* full guidelines for details of management.

Granuloma Inguinale (Donovanosis)

Granuloma inguinale is caused by the intracellular Gram-negative bacterium *Klebsiella granulomatis*. It is rare in the United States, and endemic in some tropical areas, including India; Papua, New Guinea; central Australia; and southern Africa. It causes painless, progressive ulcerative lesions without regional lymphadenopathy. The lesions have a beefy red appearance and bleed easily. Diagnosis is made by visualization of dark-staining Donovan bodies on tissue preparation or biopsy.

RECOMMENDED REGIMEN

• Doxycycline 100 mg orally twice a day for at least 3 wk and until all lesions have completely healed. Relapse can occur 6–18 mo after therapy.

ALTERNATIVE REGIMENS

• Azithromycin 1 g orally once a week for at least 3 wk and until all lesions have completely healed **OR**
• Ciprofloxacin 750 mg orally twice a day for at least 3 wk and until all lesions have completely healed **OR**
• Erythromycin base 500 mg orally four times a day for at least 3 wk and until all lesions have completely healed **OR**
• Trimethoprim–sulfamethoxazole one double-strength (160 mg/800 mg) tablet orally twice a day for at least 3 wk and until all lesions have completely healed

Some specialists recommend the addition of an aminoglycoside (e.g., gentamicin 1 mg/kg iv every 8 h) to these regimens if improvement is not evident within the first few days of therapy.

Special Considerations

PREGNANCY

Pregnant and lactating women should be treated with the erythromycin regimen, and consideration should be given to the addition of a parenteral aminoglycoside (e.g., gentamicin). Azithromycin might prove useful for treating granuloma inguinale during pregnancy, but published data are lacking.

HIV INFECTION

Individuals with both granuloma inguinale and HIV infection should receive the same regimens as those who are HIV-negative. Consideration should be given to the addition of a parenteral aminoglycoside (e.g., gentamicin).

Lymphogranuloma Venereum

Lymphogranuloma venereum (LGV) is caused by *C. trachomatis*. LGV manifests with tender inguinal and/or femoral lymphadenopathy that is typically unilateral. Rectal exposure in women or MSM can cause proctocolitis. If proctocolitis is not treated it can lead to chronic, colorectal fistulas and strictures. Genital and lymph node specimens (i.e., lesion swab or bubo aspirate) may be tested for *C. trachomatis* by culture, direct immunofluorescence, or nucleic acid detection. Chlamydia serology (complement fixation titers >1:64) can support the diagnosis. In the absence of specific LGV diagnostic testing, patients with a clinical syndrome consistent with LGV, including proctocolitis or genital ulcer disease with lymphadenopathy, should be treated for LGV.

Treatment

Treatment cures infection and prevents ongoing tissue damage, although tissue reaction to the injection can result in scarring. Buboes can require aspiration through intact skin or incision and drainage.

RECOMMENDED REGIMEN

- Doxycycline 100 mg orally twice a day for 21 d.

ALTERNATIVE REGIMEN

- Erythromycin base 500 mg orally four times a day for 21 d. Some STD specialists believe that azithromycin 1 g orally once a week for 3 wk is probably effective, although trial data is lacking.

Special Considerations

PREGNANCY

Pregnant and lactating women should be treated with erythromycin. Azithromycin might prove useful for treatment of LGV in pregnancy, but no published data are available regarding its safety and efficacy.

HIV INFECTION

Persons with both LGV and HIV infection should receive the same regimens as those who are HIV-negative. Prolonged therapy might be required, and delay in resolution of symptoms might occur.

Syphilis

GENERAL PRINCIPLES

Background

The clinical diagnosis of syphilis is divided into stages. Primary infection is characterized by an ulcer or chancre at the infection site. Secondary infection manifests with skin rash, mucocutaneous lesions, and lymphadenopathy. Tertiary infection can have cardiac and ophthalmic manifestations, auditory abnormalities, or gummatous lesions. Latent infection lacks clinical manifestations and is detected by serological testing. Latent syphilis acquired within the preceding year is referred to as early latent syphilis; all other cases of latent syphilis are either late latent syphilis or latent syphilis of unknown duration.

Serological Testing

Darkfield examinations and direct fluorescent antibody (DFA) tests of lesion exudate or tissue are used for diagnosing early syphilis. A presumptive diagnosis is possible with the use of two types of serological tests: (a) nontreponemal tests (e.g., Venereal Disease Research Laboratory [VDRL] and rapid plasma reagin) and (b) treponemal tests (e.g., fluorescent treponemal antibody absorbed [FTA-ABS] and *Treponema pallidum* particle agglutination [TP-PA]). The use of only one type of serological test is insufficient for diagnosis because false-positive nontreponemal test results are sometimes associated with various medical conditions unrelated to syphilis.

Nontreponemal test antibody titers usually correlate with disease activity. Nontreponemal tests usually become nonreactive with time after treatment; however they may persist at a low titer in some patients. Treponemal tests usually remain positive long-term, regardless of treatment or disease activity.

Treatment

The Jarisch-Herxheimer reaction is an acute febrile reaction frequently accompanied by headache, myalgia, and other symptoms that usually occurs within the first 24 h after any therapy for syphilis. It occurs most frequently among patients who have early syphilis.

Management of Sex Partners

Sexual transmission of *T. pallidum* occurs only when mucocutaneous syphilitic lesions are present. However, persons exposed sexually to a patient who has syphilis in any stage should be evaluated according to the following recommendations:

- Persons who were exposed within the 90 d preceding the diagnosis of primary, secondary, or early latent syphilis in a sex partner might be infected even if seronegative; therefore, such persons should be treated presumptively.
- Persons who were exposed more than 90 d before the diagnosis of primary, secondary, or early latent syphilis in a sex partner should be treated presumptively if serological test results are not available immediately and the opportunity for follow-up is uncertain.
- For purposes of partner notification and presumptive treatment of exposed sex partners, patients with syphilis of unknown duration who have high nontreponemal serological test titers (i.e., >1:32) can be assumed to have early syphilis.
- Long-term sex partners of patients who have latent syphilis should be evaluated clinically and serologically for syphilis and treated on the basis of the evaluation findings.

For identification of at-risk sexual partners, the periods before treatment are (a) 3 mo plus duration of symptoms for primary syphilis, (b) 6 mo plus duration of symptoms for secondary syphilis, and (c) 1 yr for early latent syphilis.

Primary and Secondary Syphilis

RECOMMENDED REGIMEN FOR ADULTS

• Benzathine penicillin G 2.4 million U im in a single dose.
• Serological follow-up is recommended at 6 and 12 mo after treatment.

Patients who have persistent or recurrent signs or symptoms or who have a sustained fourfold increase in nontreponemal test titer are likely to have failed treatment or have been re-infected. These patients should be retreated as well as evaluated for HIV infection and have a cerebrospinal fluid (CSF) analysis. Of patients with early syphilis treated with the recommended therapy, 15% will not achieve a two-dilution decline in nontreponemal titer used to define response at 1 yr after treatment.

For retreatment, weekly injections of benzathine penicillin G 2.4 million U im for 3 wk should be administered, unless CSF examination indicates that neurosyphilis is present.

SPECIAL CONSIDERATIONS

Penicillin Allergy

Doxycycline (100 mg orally twice daily for 14 d) and tetracycline (500 mg four times daily for 14 d) may be considered for treatment in penicillin-allergic patients. Although limited clinical studies, along with biological and pharmacological evidence, suggest that ceftriaxone is effective for treating early syphilis, the optimal dose and duration of ceftriaxone therapy have not been defined. Some specialists recommend 1 g daily either intramuscularly or intravenously for 8–10 d. Preliminary data suggest that azithromycin might be effective as a single oral dose of 2 g, although treatment failure with azithromycin has been reported. Patients with penicillin allergy whose compliance with therapy or follow-up cannot be ensured should be desensitized and treated with benzathine penicillin.

Pregnancy

Pregnant patients who are allergic to penicillin should be desensitized and treated with penicillin.

HIV Infection

See "Syphilis Among HIV-Infected Persons."

Latent Syphilis

Latent syphilis is defined as syphilis characterized by seroreactivity without other evidence of disease. Patients who have latent syphilis and who acquired syphilis within the preceding year are classified as having early latent syphilis.

TREATMENT

RECOMMENDED REGIMENS FOR ADULTS

- Early Latent Syphilis: Benzathine penicillin G 2.4 million U im in a single dose.
- Late Latent Syphilis or Latent Syphilis of Unknown Duration: Benzathine penicillin G 7.2 million U total, administered as three doses of 2.4 million U im each at 1-wk intervals.
- Other Management Considerations: All persons who have latent syphilis should be evaluated clinically for evidence of tertiary disease (e.g., aortitis and gumma) and syphilitic ocular disease (e.g., iritis and uveitis). Patients who have syphilis and who demonstrate any of the following criteria should have a CSF examination:
- Neurological or ophthalmic signs or symptoms,
- Evidence of active tertiary syphilis (e.g., aortitis and gumma),
- Treatment failure, **OR**
- HIV infection with late latent syphilis or syphilis of unknown duration.

A CSF examination may be performed for patients who do not meet these criteria. Some specialists recommend performing a CSF examination on all patients who have latent syphilis and a nontreponemal serological test of more than 1:32 or if the patient is HIV-infected with a serum CD4 count less than 350. However, the likelihood of neurosyphilis in this circumstance is unknown.

If a patient misses a dose of penicillin in a course of weekly therapy for late syphilis, the appropriate course of action is unclear. Pharmacological considerations suggest that an interval of 10–14 d between doses of benzathine penicillin for late syphilis or latent syphilis of unknown duration might be acceptable before restarting the sequence of injections. Missed doses are not acceptable for pregnant patients receiving therapy for late latent syphilis; pregnant women who miss any dose of therapy must repeat the full course of therapy.

FOLLOW-UP

Quantitative nontreponemal serological tests should be repeated at 6, 12, and 24 mo. Patients with a normal CSF examination should be re-treated for latent syphilis if (a) titers increase fourfold, (b) an initially high titer (>1:32) fails to decline at least fourfold (i.e., two dilutions) within 12–24 mo of therapy, or (b) signs or symptoms attributable to syphilis develop.

SPECIAL CONSIDERATIONS

Penicillin Allergy

Nonpregnant patients allergic to penicillin who have clearly defined early latent syphilis should respond to therapies recommended as alternatives to penicillin for the treatment of primary and secondary syphilis. The only acceptable alternatives for the treatment of late latent syphilis or latent syphilis of unknown duration are doxycycline (100 mg orally twice daily) or tetracycline

(500 mg orally four times daily), both for 28 d. Limited data suggests that ceftriaxone might be effective for treating late latent syphilis or syphilis of unknown duration.

Pregnancy

Pregnant patients who are allergic to penicillin should be desensitized and treated with penicillin (*see* the full guidelines for Management of Patients Who Have a History of Penicillin Allergy and Syphilis During Pregnancy).

HIV Infection

See "Syphilis Among HIV-Infected Persons."

Tertiary Syphilis

Tertiary syphilis refers to gumma and cardiovascular syphilis but not to all neurosyphilis. Patients who are not allergic to penicillin and have no evidence of neurosyphilis should be treated with the following regimens.

RECOMMENDED REGIMEN

- Benzathine penicillin G 7.2 million U total, administered as three doses of 2.4 million U im each at 1-wk intervals.

OTHER MANAGEMENT CONSIDERATIONS

- Patients who have symptomatic late syphilis should be treated in consultation with a specialist.

SPECIAL CONSIDERATIONS

Penicillin Allergy

Patients allergic to penicillin should be treated according to treatment regimens recommended for late latent syphilis.

Pregnancy

Pregnant patients who are allergic to penicillin should be desensitized, if necessary, and treated with penicillin.

HIV Infection

See "Syphilis Among HIV-Infected Persons."

Neurosyphilis

See the complete guidelines for treatment of neurosyphilis.

Syphilis Among HIV-Infected Persons

DIAGNOSTIC CONSIDERATIONS

Unusual serological responses have been observed among HIV-infected persons who have syphilis. Unusual serological responses are uncommon, and the majority of specialists believe that both treponemal and nontreponemal serological tests for syphilis can be interpreted in the usual manner for the majority of patients who are co-infected with *T. pallidum* and HIV.

Treatment

Compared with HIV-negative patients, HIV-positive patients who have early syphilis might be at increased risk for neurological complications and might have higher rates of treatment failure with currently recommended regimens. The magnitude of these risks is not defined precisely but is likely minimal.

Primary and Secondary Syphilis Among HIV-Infected Persons

TREATMENT

Treatment with benzathine penicillin G 2.4 million U im in a single dose is recommended. Some specialists recommend additional treatments (e.g., benzathine penicillin G administered at 1-wk intervals for 3 wk, as recommended for late syphilis) in addition to benzathine penicillin G 2.4 million U im.

Because CSF abnormalities (e.g., mononuclear pleocytosis and elevated protein levels) are common in patients with early syphilis and in persons with HIV infection, the clinical and prognostic significance of such CSF abnormalities in HIV-infected persons with primary or secondary syphilis is unknown. Although the majority of HIV-infected persons respond appropriately to standard benzathine penicillin therapy, some specialists recommend intensified therapy when CNS syphilis is suspected in these persons. Therefore, some specialists recommend CSF examination before treatment of HIV-infected persons with early syphilis, with follow-up CSF examination conducted after treatment in persons with initial abnormalities.

FOLLOW-UP

HIV-infected persons should be evaluated clinically and serologically for treatment failure at 3, 6, 9, 12, and 24 mo after therapy. Although of unproven benefit, some specialists recommend a CSF examination 6 mo after therapy.

HIV-infected persons who meet the criteria for treatment failure (i.e., signs or symptoms that persist or recur or persons who have fourfold increase in nontreponemal test titer) should be managed in the same manner as HIV-negative patients (i.e., a CSF examination and re-treatment). CSF examination and re-treatment also should be strongly considered for persons whose nontreponemal test titers do not decrease fourfold within 6–12 mo of therapy. The majority of specialists would re-treat patients with benzathine penicillin G administered as three doses of 2.4 million U im each at weekly intervals, if CSF examinations are normal.

SPECIAL CONSIDERATIONS

Penicillin Allergy

Penicillin-allergic patients who have primary or secondary syphilis and HIV infection should be managed according to the recommendations for penicillin-allergic, HIV-negative patients. The use of alternatives to penicillin has not been well studied in HIV-infected patients.

Latent Syphilis Among HIV-Infected Persons

DIAGNOSTIC CONSIDERATIONS

HIV-infected patients who have early latent syphilis should be managed and treated according to the recommendations for HIV-negative patients who have primary and secondary syphilis. HIV-infected patients who have either late latent syphilis or syphilis of unknown duration should have a CSF examination before treatment.

TREATMENT

Patients with late latent syphilis or syphilis of unknown duration and a normal CSF examination can be treated with benzathine penicillin G, at weekly doses of 2.4 million U for 3 wk. Patients who have CSF consistent with neurosyphilis should be treated and managed as patients who have neurosyphilis.

FOLLOW-UP

Patients should be evaluated clinically and serologically at 6, 12, 18, and 24 mo after therapy. If, at any time, clinical symptoms develop or nontreponemal titers rise fourfold, a repeat CSF examination should be performed and treatment administered accordingly. If during 12–24 mo the nontreponemal titer does not decline fourfold, the CSF examination should be repeated and treatment administered accordingly.

SPECIAL CONSIDERATIONS

Penicillin Allergy

The efficacy of alternative nonpenicillin regimens in HIV-infected persons has not been well studied.

Syphilis During Pregnancy

See complete guidelines for the details of treating syphilis in pregnancy. Note that no proven alternatives to penicillin exist. Pregnant women who have a history of penicillin allergy should be desensitized and treated with penicillin.

DISEASES CHARACTERIZED BY URETHRITIS AND CERVICITIS

Management of Male Patients Who Have Urethritis

Urethritis can result from infectious and noninfectious conditions. Patients can be symptomatic or asymptomatic. *N. gonorrhoeae* and *C. trachomatis* are clinically important infectious causes of urethritis. If Gram stain is not available, patients should be treated for both gonorrhea and chlamydia. Further testing to determine the specific etiology is recommended. Culture, nucleic acid hybridization tests, and nucleic acid amplification tests are available for the detection of both *N. gonorrhoeae* and *C. trachomatis*. Culture and hybridization tests require urethral swab specimens, whereas amplification tests can be performed on urine specimens. Because of their higher sensitivity, amplification tests are preferred for the detection of *C. trachomatis*.

Etiology

Several organisms can cause infectious urethritis. The presence of Gram-negative intracellular diplococci (GNID) on urethral smear is indicative of gonorrhea infection. Nongonoccocal urethritis (NGU) is diagnosed when microscopy indicates inflammation without GNID. *C. trachomatis* is a frequent cause of NGU (i.e., 15–55% of cases); however, the prevalence varies by age group, with lower prevalence among older men. The proportion of NGU cases caused by chlamydia has been declining gradually.

The etiology of the majority of cases of nonchlamydial NGU is unknown. *Ureaplasma urealyticum* and *Mycoplasma genitalium* have been implicated as etiological agents of NGU in some studies. *Trichomonas. vaginalis*, HSV, and adenovirus might also cause NGU. Diagnostic and treatment procedures for these organisms are reserved for situations in which these infections are suspected or when NGU is not responsive to therapy. Enteric bacteria have been identified as an uncommon cause of NGU and might be associated with insertive anal sex.

Confirmed Urethritis

Clinicians should document that urethritis is present. Urethritis can be documented on the basis of any of the following signs or laboratory tests:

- Mucopurulent or purulent discharge.
- Gram stain of urethral secretions demonstrating more than five white blood cells (WBC) per oil immersion field. The Gram stain is the preferred rapid diagnostic test for evaluating urethritis. It is highly sensitive and specific for documenting both urethritis and the presence or absence of gonococcal infection. Gonococcal infection is established by documenting the presence of WBC containing GNID.
- Positive leukocyte esterase test on first-void urine or microscopic examination of first-void urine sediment demonstrating more than 10 WBC per high-power field.

If none of these criteria are present, treatment should be deferred, and the patient should be tested for *N. gonorrhoeae* and *C. trachomatis*.

Management of Patients Who Have NGU Diagnosis

All patients who have confirmed or suspected urethritis should be tested for gonorrhea and chlamydia.

TREATMENT

Treatment should be initiated as soon as possible after diagnosis. Azithromycin and doxycycline are highly effective for chlamydial urethritis; however, infections with *Mycoplasma genitalium* may respond better to azithromycin.

RECOMMENDED REGIMENS

- Azithromycin 1 g orally in a single dose **OR**
- Doxycycline 100 mg orally twice a day for 7 d.

ALTERNATIVE REGIMENS

- Erythromycin base 500 mg orally four times a day for 7 d **OR**
- Erythromycin ethylsuccinate 800 mg orally four times a day for 7 d **OR**
- Ofloxacin 300 mg orally twice a day for 7 d **OR**
- Levofloxacin 500 mg orally once daily for 7 d.

FOLLOW-UP FOR PATIENTS WHO HAVE URETHRITIS

Patients should be instructed to abstain from sexual intercourse until 7 d after therapy is initiated.

Recurrent and Persistent Urethritis

Consider re-treatment if patient did not finish initial treatment or may have been re-exposed to infection. *T. vaginalis* culture should be performed using an intraurethral swab or a first-void urine specimen. Some cases of recurrent urethritis after doxycycline treatment might be caused by tetracycline-resistant *Ureaplasma urealyticum*. If the patient was compliant with the initial regimen and re-exposure can be excluded, the following regimen is recommended.

RECOMMENDED REGIMENS

- (Metronidazole 2 g orally in a single dose **OR**
- Tinidazole 2 g orally in a single dose) **PLUS**
- Azithromycin 1 g orally in a single dose (if not used for initial episode).

Management of Patients Who Have Cervicitis

Cervicitis frequently is asymptomatic, or can cause abnormal vaginal discharge and intermenstrual vaginal bleeding (e.g., after sexual intercourse). A finding of leukorrhea (>10 WBC per high-power field on microscopic examination of vaginal fluid) has been associated with chlamydial and gonococcal infection of the cervix. In the absence of inflammatory vaginitis, leukorrhea might be a sensitive indicator of cervical inflammation with a high negative-predictive value.

ETIOLOGY

When an etiological organism is isolated in the setting of cervicitis, it is typically *C. trachomatis* or *N. gonorrhoeae*. Cervicitis also can accompany trichomoniasis and genital herpes (especially primary HSV-2 infection). However, in the majority of cases of cervicitis, no organism is isolated, especially in women at relatively low risk for recent acquisition of these STDs (e.g., women aged >30 years). Limited data indicate that infection with *M. genitalium* and bacterial vaginosis (BV) as well as frequent douching might cause cervicitis.

DIAGNOSIS

Because cervicitis might be a sign of upper genital tract infection (endometritis), women who seek medical treatment for a new episode of cervicitis should be assessed for signs of pelvic inflammatory disease (PID) and should be tested for *C. trachomatis* and for *N. gonorrhoeae*. Women with cervicitis also should be evaluated for the presence of BV and trichomoniasis, and these conditions should be treated, if present. Because the sensitivity of microscopy to detect *T. vaginalis* is relatively low (approx 50%), symptomatic women with cervicitis and negative microscopy for trichomonads should receive further testing (i.e., culture or antigen-based detection). Although HSV-2 infection has been associated with cervicitis, the utility of specific testing (i.e., culture or serological testing) for HSV-2 in this setting is unclear. Standardized diagnostic tests for *M. genitalium* are not commercially available.

TREATMENT

RECOMMENDED REGIMENS FOR PRESUMPTIVE TREATMENT[1]

- Azithromycin 1 g orally in a single dose **OR**
- Doxycycline 100 mg orally twice a day for 7 d.

MANAGEMENT OF SEX PARTNERS

Sex partners of women treated for cervicitis should be treated. Patients and their sex partners should abstain from sexual intercourse until therapy is completed (i.e., 7 d after a single-dose regimen or after completion of a 7-d regimen).

Special Considerations

HIV INFECTION

Patients who have cervicitis and also are infected with HIV should receive the same treatment regimen as those who are HIV-negative.

Chlamydial Infections in Adolescents and Adults

In the United States, chlamydial genital infection is the most frequently reported infectious disease, and the prevalence is highest in persons younger than 25 yr. Asymptomatic infection is common among both men and women, and to detect chlamydial infections health care providers frequently rely on screening tests. Annual screening of all sexually active women aged younger than 25 yr is recommended, as is screening of older women with risk factors (e.g., those who have a new sex partner or multiple sex partners). Evidence is

---

[1]Consider concurrent treatment for gonococcal infection if prevalence of gonorrhea is high in the patient population under assessment.

insufficient to recommend routine screening for *C. trachomatis* in sexually active young men. However, screening of sexually active young men should be considered in clinical settings with a high prevalence of chlamydia (e.g., adolescent clinics, correctional facilities, and STD clinics).

TREATMENT

Treating infected patients prevents transmission to sex partners. In addition, treating pregnant women usually prevents transmission of *C. trachomatis* to infants during birth. Treatment of sex partners helps to prevent re-infection of the index patient and infection of other partners. Co-infection with *C. trachomatis* frequently occurs among patients who have gonococcal infection; therefore, presumptive treatment of such patients for chlamydia is appropriate.

RECOMMENDED REGIMENS

- Azithromycin 1 g orally in a single dose **OR**
- Doxycycline 100 mg orally twice a day for 7 d.

ALTERNATIVE REGIMENS

- Erythromycin base 500 mg orally four times a day for 7 d **OR**
- Erythromycin ethylsuccinate 800 mg orally four times a day for 7 d **OR**
- Ofloxacin 300 mg orally twice a day for 7 d **OR**
- Levofloxacin 500 mg orally once daily for 7 d.

FOLLOW-UP

Except in pregnant women, test-of-cure (repeat testing 3–4 wk after completing therapy) is *not* recommended. Repeat infections confer an elevated risk for re-infection; therefore, recently infected women are a major priority for repeat testing for *C. trachomatis*. Consider retesting approx 3 mo after treatment. Limited evidence is available on the benefit of retesting for chlamydia in men previously infected; however, some specialists suggest retesting men approx 3 months after treatment.

MANAGEMENT OF SEX PARTNERS

Sex partners should be evaluated, tested, and treated if they had sexual contact with the patient during the 60 d preceding onset of symptoms in the patient or diagnosis of chlamydia. The most recent sex partner should be evaluated and treated, even if the time of the last sexual contact was more than 60 days before symptom onset or diagnosis. If concerns exist that sex partners will not seek evaluation and treatment, then EPT should be considered (*see* "Partner Notification"). Patient-delivered partner therapy is not routinely recommended for MSM because of a high risk for coexisting infections, especially undiagnosed HIV infection, in their partners.

Patients should be instructed to abstain from sexual intercourse until they and their sex partners have completed treatment. Abstinence should be continued until 7 d after a single-dose regimen or after completion of a 7-d regimen.

SPECIAL CONSIDERATIONS

Pregnancy

Azithromycin is likely to be safe and effective. Repeat testing 3 wk after completion of therapy with the following regimens is recommended for all pregnant women to ensure therapeutic cure, considering the sequelae that might occur in the mother and neonate if the infection persists. The frequent gastrointestinal side effects associated with erythromycin might discourage patient compliance with the alternative regimens.

RECOMMENDED REGIMENS

- Azithromycin 1 g orally in a single dose **OR**
- Amoxicillin 500 mg orally three times a day for 7 d.

ALTERNATIVE REGIMENS

- Erythromycin base 500 mg orally four times a day for 7 d **OR**
- Erythromycin base 250 mg orally four times a day for 14 d **OR**
- Erythromycin ethylsuccinate 800 mg orally four times a day for 7 d **OR**
- Erythromycin ethylsuccinate 400 mg orally four times a day for 14 d.

Erythromycin estolate is contraindicated during pregnancy because of drug-related hepatotoxicity. The lower dose 14-d erythromycin regimens may be considered if gastrointestinal tolerance is a concern.

HIV Infection

Patients who have chlamydial infection and also are infected with HIV should receive the same treatment regimen as those who are HIV-negative.

Gonococcal Infections in Adolescents and Adults

Gonorrhea is the second most commonly reported bacterial STD. Because gonococcal infections among women frequently are asymptomatic, the US Preventive Services Task Force (USPSTF) recommends that clinicians screen all sexually active women, including those who are pregnant, for gonorrhea infection if they are at increased risk. Women younger than age 25 are at highest risk for gonorrhea infection. Other risk factors for gonorrhea include a previous gonorrhea infection, other sexually transmitted infections, new or multiple sex partners, inconsistent condom use, commercial sex work, and drug use. The prevalence of gonorrhea infection varies widely among communities and patient populations. The USPSTF does not recommend screening for gonorrhea in men and women who are at low risk for infection.

DIAGNOSTIC CONSIDERATIONS

A Gram stain of a male urethral specimen that demonstrates polymorphonuclear leukocytes with intracellular Gram-negative diplococci can be considered diagnostic for infection with *N. gonorrhoeae* in symptomatic men. A negative

Gram stain should not be considered sufficient for ruling out infection. Specific diagnosis of infection with *N. gonorrhoeae* may be performed by testing endocervical, vaginal, male urethral, or urine specimens.

Dual Therapy for Gonococcal and Chlamydial Infections

Patients treated for gonococcal infection should also be treated routinely with a regimen that is effective against uncomplicated genital *C. trachomatis* infection.

Quinolone-Resistant *N. gonorrhoeae*

Quinolone-resistant *N. gonorrhoeae* (QRNG) has continued to increase in prevalence. QRNG is common in parts of Europe, the Middle East, Asia, and the Pacific. In the United States, QRNG is becoming increasingly common. Previously, the CDC had advised that quinolones not be used in California and Hawaii because of the high prevalence of QRNG in these areas. The prevalence of QRNG has increased in other areas of the United States, which has resulted in changes in recommended treatment regimens by other states and local areas. QRNG prevalence will continue to increase, and quinolones will eventually not be advisable for the treatment of gonorrhea. The CDC website (http://www.cdc.gov/std/gisp) or state health departments can provide the most current information. QRNG was more common in 2004 among MSM than among heterosexual men (23.9 vs 2.9%). Quinolones should not be used for the treatment of gonorrhea among MSM or in areas with increased QRNG prevalence in the United States (e.g., California and Hawaii) or for infections acquired while traveling abroad.

Uncomplicated Gonococcal Infections of the Cervix, Urethra, and Rectum

RECOMMENDED REGIMENS

- (Ceftriaxone 125 mg im in a single dose **OR**
- Cefixime 400 mg orally in a single dose **OR**
- Ciprofloxacin 500 mg orally in a single dose **OR**
- Ofloxacin 400 mg orally in a single dose **OR**
- Levofloxacin 250 mg orally in a single dose) **PLUS**
- Treatment for chlamydia if chlamydial infection is not ruled out

(Note: quinolones should not be used for infections in MSM or in those with a history of recent foreign travel or partners' travel, infections acquired in California or Hawaii, or infections acquired in other areas with increased QRNG prevalence.)

RECOMMENDED REGIMENS FOR *MSM* OR HETEROSEXUALS WITH A HISTORY OF RECENT TRAVEL

- (Ceftriaxone 125 mg im in a single dose **OR**
- Cefixime 400 mg orally in a single dose) **PLUS**
- Treatment for chlamydia if chlamydial infection is not ruled out.

- Spectinomycin 2 g in a single im dose **OR**
- Single-dose cephalosporin regimens **OR**
- Single-dose quinolone regimens.

Uncomplicated Gonococcal Infections of the Pharynx

Gonococcal infections of the pharynx are more difficult to eradicate than infections at urogenital and anorectal sites. Although chlamydial coinfection of the pharynx is unusual, coinfection at genital sites sometimes occurs. Therefore, treatment for both gonorrhea and chlamydia is recommended.

RECOMMENDED REGIMENS

- (Ceftriaxone 125 mg im in a single dose **OR**
- Ciprofloxacin 500 mg orally in a single dose) **PLUS**
- Treatment for chlamydia if chlamydial infection is not ruled out.

Recommended regimens for MSM or heterosexuals with a history of recent travel include ceftriaxone 125 mg im in a single dose plus treatment for chlamydia if chlamydial infection is not ruled out.

FOLLOW-UP

There is no need to perform a test of cure if symptoms resolve. Patients who have symptoms that persist after treatment should be evaluated by culture for *N. gonorrhoeae*, and any gonococci isolated should be tested for antimicrobial susceptibility. Consider advising all patients with gonorrhea to be retested 3 mo after treatment.

MANAGEMENT OF SEX PARTNERS

Sex partners within 60 d of treatment, or the index patients last sexual partner, should be referred for evaluation and treatment. If it is felt to be unlikely that a partner will be referred or come in for treatment, delivery of antibiotic patient-delivered partner therapy is an option. Patient-delivered therapy for patients with gonorrhea should routinely include treatment for chlamydia. This approach should not be considered a routine partner management strategy in MSM because of the high risk of coexisting undiagnosed STDs or HIV infection.

SPECIAL CONSIDERATIONS

Allergy, Intolerance, and Adverse Reactions

Persons who cannot tolerate cephalosporins or quinolones should be treated with spectinomycin. Because spectinomycin is unreliable (52% effective) against pharyngeal infections, patients who have suspected or known pharyngeal infection should have a pharyngeal culture 3–5 d after treatment to verify eradication of infection.

Pregnancy

Pregnant women infected with *N. gonorrhoeae* should be treated with a recommended or alternate cephalosporin. Women who cannot tolerate a cephalosporin should be administered a single 2-g dose of spectinomycin intramuscularly. Either azithromycin or amoxicillin is recommended for treatment of presumptive or diagnosed *C. trachomatis* infection during pregnancy (*see* "Chlamydial Infections").

Administration of Quinolones to Adolescents

There has been caution around the use of Fluoroquinolones have in persons younger than 18 yr because based on studies showing damage to articular cartilage in young animals. No joint damage attributable to quinolone therapy has been observed in children treated with prolonged ciprofloxacin regimens. Therefore, children who weigh more than 45 kg can be treated with any regimen recommended for adults.

HIV Infection

Patients who have gonococcal infection and also are infected with HIV should receive the same treatment regimen as those who are HIV-negative.

DISEASES CHARACTERIZED BY VAGINAL DISCHARGE

Management of Patients Who Have Vaginal Infections

Vaginitis is usually characterized by a vaginal discharge and/ or vulvar itching and irritation, and a vaginal odor might be present. The three diseases most frequently associated with vaginal discharge are BV (replacement of the normal vaginal flora by an overgrowth of anaerobic microorganisms, mycoplasmas, and *Gardnerella vaginalis*), trichomoniasis (*T. vaginalis*), and candidiasis (usually caused by *Candida albicans*). Cervicitis can sometimes cause a vaginal discharge. Although vulvovaginal candidiasis (VVC) usually is not transmitted sexually, it is included in this section because it is frequently diagnosed in women being evaluated for STDs.

Bacterial Vaginosis

BV is a polymicrobial clinical syndrome resulting from replacement of the normal H_2O_2-producing *Lactobacillus* sp. in the vagina with high concentrations of anaerobic bacteria (e.g., *Prevotella* sp. and *Mobiluncus* sp.), *Gardnerella vaginalis*, and *Mycoplasma hominis*. BV is the most prevalent cause of vaginal discharge or malodor; however, more than 50% of women with BV are asymptomatic. It is not clear whether BV results from sexual transmission.

DIAGNOSTIC CONSIDERATIONS

BV can be diagnosed by the use of clinical criteria or Gram stain. Clinical criteria require three of the following symptoms or signs:

- Homogeneous, thin, white discharge that smoothly coats the vaginal walls.
- Presence of clue cells on microscopic examination.
- pH of vaginal fluid greater than 4.5.
- A fishy odor of vaginal discharge before or after addition of 10% KOH (i.e., the whiff test).

Culture of *G. vaginalis* is not recommended as a diagnostic tool because it is not specific. A DNA probe-based test for high concentrations of *G. vaginalis* (Affirm™ VP III, Becton Dickinson, Sparks, MD) might have clinical utility. Cervical Pap tests have no clinical utility for the diagnosis of BV because of low sensitivity. Other commercially available tests might be useful for the diagnosis of BV.

TREATMENT

Gardnerella

The established benefits of therapy for BV in nonpregnant women are to relieve vaginal symptoms and signs of infection and reduce the risk for infectious complications after abortion or hysterectomy.

The results of two randomized controlled trials have indicated that treatment of BV with metronidazole substantially reduced post-abortion PID. Because of the increased risk for postoperative infectious complications associated with BV, some specialists recommend that before performing surgical abortion or hysterectomy, providers should screen and treat women with BV in addition to providing routine prophylaxis. However, more information is needed before recommending treatment of asymptomatic BV before other invasive procedures.

RECOMMENDED REGIMENS FOR *BV*

- Metronidazole 500 mg orally twice a day for 7 d **OR**
- Metronidazole gel, 0.75%, one full applicator (5 g) intravaginally, once a day for 5 d **OR**
- Clindamycin cream, 2%, one full applicator (5 g) intravaginally at bedtime for 7 d.

Patients should be advised to avoid consuming alcohol during treatment with metronidazole and for 24 h thereafter. Clindamycin cream is oil-based and might weaken latex condoms and diaphragms for 5 d after use. Topical clindamycin preparations should not be used in the second half of pregnancy.

The recommended metronidazole regimens are equally efficacious. The recommended intravaginal clindamycin regimen might be less efficacious than the metronidazole regimens.

ALTERNATIVE REGIMENS

- Clindamycin 300 mg orally twice a day for 7 d **OR**
- Orclindamycin ovules 100 g intravaginally once at bedtime for 3 d.

Metronidazole 2 g single-dose therapy has the lowest efficacy for BV and is no longer a recommended or alternative regimen. The FDA has cleared metronidazole

750 mg extended-release tablets once daily for 7 d and a single dose of clindamycin intravaginal cream.

MANAGEMENT OF SEX PARTNERS

The results likelihood of relapse or recurrence are not affected by treatment of sex partner(s). Therefore, routine treatment of sex partners is not recommended.

SPECIAL CONSIDERATIONS

Allergy or Intolerance to the Recommended Therapy

Intravaginal clindamycin cream is preferred in case of allergy or intolerance to metronidazole. Intravaginal metronidazole gel can be considered for patients who do not tolerate systemic metronidazole, but patients allergic to oral metronidazole should not be administered intravaginal metronidazole.

Pregnancy

All pregnant women who have symptomatic disease require treatment. BV has been associated with adverse pregnancy outcomes (e.g., premature rupture of the membranes, chorioamnionitis, preterm labor, preterm birth, intraamniotic infection, postpartum endometritis, and postcesarean wound infection). Some specialists prefer using systemic therapy to treat possible subclinical upper genital tract infections.

Treatment of BV in asymptomatic pregnant women at high risk for preterm delivery (i.e., those who have previously delivered a premature infant) with a recommended oral regimen has reduced preterm delivery in three of four randomized controlled trials; some specialists recommend screening and oral treatment of these women. Screening (if conducted) and treatment should be performed during the first prenatal visit.

Multiple studies and meta-analyses have not demonstrated an association between metronidazole use during pregnancy and teratogenic or mutagenic effects in newborns.

RECOMMENDED REGIMENS

- Metronidazole 500 mg orally twice a day for 7 d **OR**
- Metronidazole 250 mg orally three times a day for 7 d **OR**
- Clindamycin 300 mg orally twice a day for 7 d

Whether treatment of asymptomatic pregnant women with BV who are at low risk for preterm delivery reduces adverse outcomes of pregnancy is unclear. In three trials, intravaginal clindamycin cream was administered at 16–32 wk gestation, and an increase in adverse events (e.g., low birthweight and neonatal infections) was observed in newborns. Therefore, intravaginal clindamycin cream should only be used during the first half of pregnancy.

Treatment of BV in asymptomatic pregnant women who are at high risk for preterm delivery might prevent adverse pregnancy outcomes. Therefore, a follow-up evaluation 1 mo after completion of treatment should be considered to evaluate whether therapy was effective.

HIV Infection

Patients who have BV and also are infected with HIV should receive the same treatment regimen as those who are HIV negative. BV appears to be more persistent in HIV-positive women.

Trichomoniasis

Trichomoniasis is caused by the protozoan *T. vaginalis*. Men may be asymptomatic or have symptoms of urethritis. Women can be asymptomatic or can have a diffuse, malodorous, yellow-green vaginal discharge with vulvar irritation. Microscopy of vaginal secretions has a sensitivity of 60–70%. In women in whom trichomoniasis is suspected but not confirmed by microscopy, vaginal secretions should be cultured for *T. vaginalis*.

RECOMMENDED REGIMENS

* Metronidazole 2 g orally in a single dose **OR**
* Tinidazole 2 g orally in a single dose.

ALTERNATIVE REGIMEN

* Metronidazole 500 mg orally twice a day for 7 d.

Metronidazole gel is considerably less efficacious for the treatment of trichomoniasis (<50%) than oral preparations of metronidazole.

If treatment failure occurs with metronidazole 2 g single dose and re-infection is excluded, the patient can be treated with metronidazole 500 mg orally twice daily for 7 d or tinidazole 2 g single dose. For patients failing either of these regimens, clinicians should consider treatment with tinidazole or metronidazole at 2 g orally for 5 d.

MANAGEMENT OF SEX PARTNERS

Sex partners of patients with *T. vaginalis* should be treated.

SPECIAL CONSIDERATIONS

Allergy, Intolerance, and Adverse Reactions

Metronidazole and tinidazole are both nitroimidazoles. Patients with an immediate-type allergy to a nitroimidazole can be managed by metronidazole desensitization in consultation with a specialist. Topical therapy with drugs other than nitroimidazoles can be attempted, but cure rates are low (<50%).

Pregnancy

Vaginal trichomoniasis has been associated with adverse pregnancy outcomes, particularly premature rupture of membranes, preterm delivery, and low birthweight. However, data do not suggest that metronidazole treatment results in a reduction in perinatal morbidity. Although some trials suggest the possibility of increased prematurity or low birthweight after metronidazole treatment, limitations of the studies prevent definitive conclusions regarding risks of treatment. Clinicians should counsel patients regarding the potential risks and benefits of treatment. Some specialists would defer therapy in asymptomatic pregnant women until after 37 wk gestation.

Women may be treated with 2 g of metronidazole in a single dose. Metronidazole is pregnancy category B. Multiple studies and meta-analyses have not demonstrated a consistent association between metronidazole use during pregnancy and teratogenic or mutagenic effects in infants. Tinidazole is pregnancy category C, and its safety in pregnant women has not been well evaluated.

In lactating women who are administered metronidazole, withholding breast-feeding during treatment and for 12–24 h after the last dose will reduce the exposure of metronidazole to the infant. While using tinidazole, interruption of breastfeeding is recommended during treatment and for 3 d after the last dose.

HIV Infection

Patients who have trichomoniasis and also are infected with HIV should receive the same treatment regimen as those who are HIV-negative.

Vulvovaginal Candidiasis

VVC usually is caused by *Candida albicans* but occasionally is caused by other *Candida* sp. or yeasts. VVC can be classified as either uncomplicated or complicated. Uncomplicated VVC is characterized by sporadic or infrequent VC which is mild-to-moderate in severity, is likely to be *C. albicans*, and occurs in a nonimmunocompromised woman. Complicated VVC is recurrent, severe, and is often nonalbicans candidiasis, occurring in women with uncontrolled diabetes, debilitation, or immunosuppression or pregnancy.

UNCOMPLICATED VVC

A diagnosis of *Candida* vaginitis is suggested clinically by history and physical exam. To treat uncomplicated VVC with a success rate of 80–90%, treatment should include short-course topical formulations (i.e., single dose and regimens of 1–3 d).

RECOMMENDED REGIMENS

- Butoconazole 2% cream 5 g intravaginally for 3 days* **OR**
- Butoconazole 2% cream 5 g (Butaconazole1-sustained release), single intrav-aginal application **OR**
- Clotrimazole 1% cream 5 g intravaginally for 7–14 d* **OR**
- Clotrimazole 100 mg vaginal tablet for 7 d **OR**
- Clotrimazole 100 mg vaginal tablet, two tablets for 3 d **OR**
- Miconazole 2% cream 5 g intravaginally for 7 d* **OR**

---

*Over-the-counter (OTC) preparations. The creams and suppositories in this regimen are oil-based and might weaken latex condoms and diaphragms. Intravaginal preparations of butaconazole, clotrimazole, miconazole, and tioconazole are available OTC.

- Miconazole 100 mg vaginal suppository, one suppository for 7 d* **OR**
- Miconazole 200 mg vaginal suppository, one suppository for 3 d* **OR**
- Miconazole 1,200 mg vaginal suppository, one suppository for 1 d* **OR**
- Nystatin 100,000-U vaginal tablet, one tablet for 14 d **OR**
- Tioconazole 6.5% ointment 5 g intravaginally in a single application* **OR**
- Terconazole 0.4% cream 5 g intravaginally for 7 d **OR**
- Terconazole 0.8% cream 5 g intravaginally for 3 d **OR**
- Terconazole 80 mg vaginal suppository, one suppository for 3 d

RECOMMENDED ORAL AGENT REGIMEN

- Fluconazole 150 mg oral tablet, one tablet in a single dose.

MANAGEMENT OF SEX PARTNERS

VVC is not usually acquired through sexual intercourse; treatment of sex partners is not recommended but may be considered in women who have recurrent infection. A minority of male sex partners might have balanitis, which may benefit from treatment with topical antifungal agents.

COMPLICATED VVC

Recurrent VVC (RVVC), usually defined as four or more episodes of symptomatic VVC in 1 yr, affects a small percentage of women (<5%). Vaginal cultures should be obtained from patients with RVVC to confirm the clinical diagnosis and to identify unusual species, including nonalbicans species, particularly *C. glabrata* (*C. glabrata* does not form pseudohyphae or hyphae and is not easily recognized on microscopy). *C. glabrata* and other nonalbicans *Candidia* species are observed in 10–20% of patients with RVVC. Conventional antimycotic therapies are not as effective against these species as against *C. albicans*.

Each individual episode of RVVC caused by *C. albicans* responds well to short duration oral or topical azole therapy. However, to maintain clinical and mycological control, some specialists recommend a longer duration of initial therapy (e.g., 7–14 d of topical therapy or a 100-, 150-, or 200-mg oral dose of fluconazole every third day for a total of three doses (days 1, 4, and 7) to attempt mycological remission before initiating a maintenance antifungal regimen.

A maintenance regimen should include oral fluconazole (i.e., 100-, 150-, or 200-mg dose) weekly for 6 mo as the first line of treatment. Suppressive maintenance antifungal therapies are effective in reducing RVVC.

SEVERE VVC

Severe vulvovaginitis (i.e., extensive vulvar erythema, edema, excoriation, and fissure formation) is associated with lower clinical response rates in

---

* Over-the-counter (OTC) preparations. The creams and suppositories in this regimen are oil-based and might weaken latex condoms and diaphragms. Intravaginal preparations of butaconazole, clotrimazole, miconazole, and tioconazole are available OTC.

patients treated with short courses of topical or oral therapy. Either 7–14 d of topical azole or 150 mg of fluconazole in two sequential doses (second dose 72 h after initial dose) is recommended.

Nonalbicans VVC

The optimal treatment of nonalbicans VVC remains unknown. Options include longer duration of therapy (7-14 d) with a nonfluconazole azole drug (oral or topical) as first-line therapy. If recurrence occurs, 600 mg of boric acid in a gelatin capsule is recommended, administered vaginally once daily for 2 wk. This regimen has clinical and mycological eradication rates of approx 70%. If symptoms recur, referral to a specialist is advised.

Compromised Host

Women with underlying debilitating medical conditions (e.g., those with uncontrolled diabetes or those receiving corticosteroid treatment) do not respond as well to short-term therapies. Efforts to correct modifiable conditions should be made, and more prolonged (i.e., 7–14 d) conventional antimycotic treatment is necessary.

Pregnancy

VVC frequently occurs during pregnancy. Only topical azole therapies, applied for 7 d, are recommended for use among pregnant women.

HIV Infection

The incidence of VVC in HIV-infected women is unknown. Vaginal *Candida* colonization rates among HIV-infected women are higher than among those for sero-negative women with similar demographic characteristics and high-risk behaviors, and the colonization rates correlate with increasing severity of immuno-suppression. Based on available data, therapy for VVC in HIV-infected women should not differ from that for sero-negative women.

PELVIC INFLAMMATORY DISEASE

Sexually transmitted organisms, especially *N. gonorrhoeae* and *C. tra-chomatis*, are implicated in many cases of PID; however, microorganisms that comprise the vaginal flora (e.g., anaerobes, *G. vaginalis*, *Haemophilus influenzae*, enteric Gram-negative rods, and *Streptococcus agalactiae*) also have been associated with PID. In addition, cytomegalovirus (CMV), *M. hominis*, *U. urealyticum*, and *M. genitalium* might be associated with some cases of PID. All women who are diagnosed with acute PID should be tested for *N. gonorrhoeae* and *C. trachomatis* and should be screened for HIV infection.

Diagnostic Considerations

The diagnosis of PID usually is based on clinical findings, which are imprecise. Data indicate that a clinical diagnosis of symptomatic PID has a positive predictive value (PPV) for salpingitis of 65–90% compared with laparoscopy.

Empiric treatment of PID should be initiated in sexually active young women and other women at risk for STDs if they are experiencing pelvic or lower abdominal pain, if no cause for the illness other than PID can be identified, and if one or more of the following minimum criteria are present on pelvic examination:

- Cervical motion tenderness or uterine tenderness or adnexal tenderness.

More elaborate diagnostic evaluation frequently is needed because incorrect diagnosis and management might cause unnecessary morbidity. These additional criteria may be used to enhance the specificity of the minimum criteria. The following additional criteria can be used to enhance the specificity of the minimum criteria and support a diagnosis of PID:

- Oral temperature greater than101°F (>38.3°C).
- Abnormal cervical or vaginal mucopurulent discharge.
- Presence of abundant numbers of WBC on saline microscopy of vaginal secretions.
- Elevated erythrocyte sedimentation rate.
- Elevated C-reactive protein.
- Laboratory documentation of cervical infection with *N. gonorrhoeaeor C. trachomatis.*

The majority of women with PID have either mucopurulent cervical discharge or evidence of WBC on a microscopic evaluation of a saline preparation of vaginal fluid.

Treatment

Treatment should be initiated as soon as the presumptive diagnosis has been made because prevention of long-term sequelae is dependent on immediate administration of appropriate antibiotics.

Some specialists have recommended that all patients with PID be hospitalized so that bed rest and supervised treatment with parenteral antibiotics can be initiated. However, in women with PID of mild or moderate clinical severity, outpatient therapy can provide short- and long-term clinical outcomes similar to inpatient therapy. Limited data support the use of outpatient therapy in women with more severe clinical presentations.

The following criteria for hospitalization are suggested:

- Surgical emergencies (e.g., appendicitis) cannot be excluded.
- The patient is pregnant.
- The patient does not respond clinically to oral antimicrobial therapy.
- The patient is unable to follow or tolerate an outpatient oral regimen.
- The patient has severe illness, nausea and vomiting, or high fever.
- The patient has a tubo-ovarian abscess.

Many practitioners have preferred to hospitalize adolescent girls whose condition is diagnosed as acute PID. No evidence is available suggesting that adolescents benefit from hospitalization for treatment of PID. Younger women with mild-to-moderate acute PID have similar outcomes with either outpatient or inpatient therapy. The decision to hospitalize adolescents with acute PID should be based on the same criteria used for older women.

Parenteral Treatment

For women with PID of mild or moderate severity, parenteral and oral therapy appears to have similar clinical efficacy. Transition to oral therapy can usually be initiated within 24 h of clinical improvement. The majority of clinicians recommend at least 24 h of direct inpatient observation for patients who have tubo-ovarian abscesses.

RECOMMENDED PARENTERAL REGIMEN A

- (Cefotetan 2 g iv every 12 h **OR**
- Cefoxitin 2 g iv every 6 h) **PLUS**
- Doxycycline 100 mg orally or iv every 12 h.

Because of the pain associated with infusion, doxycycline should be administered orally when possible, even when the patient is hospitalized. Oral and intravenous administration of doxycycline provide similar bioavailability.

Parenteral therapy may be discontinued 24 h after a patient improves clinically, and oral therapy with doxycycline (100 mg twice a day) should continue to complete 14 d of therapy. When tubo-ovarian abscess is present, many health care providers use clindamycin or metronidazole with doxycycline for continued therapy, rather than doxycycline alone, because it provides more effective anaerobic coverage.

Clinical data are limited regarding the use of other second- or third-generation cephalosporins (e.g., ceftizoxime, cefotaxime, and ceftriaxone), which also might be effective therapy for PID and may replace cefotetan or cefoxitin. However, these cephalosporins are less active than cefotetan or cefoxitin against anaerobic bacteria.

RECOMMENDED PARENTERAL REGIMEN B

- Clindamycin 900 mg iv every 8 h **PLUS**
- Gentamicin loading dose iv or im (2 mg/kg of body weight), followed by a maintenance dose (1.5 mg/kg) every 8 h. Single daily dosing may be substituted.

Although use of a single daily dose of gentamicin has not been evaluated for the treatment of PID, it is efficacious in analogous situations. Parenteral therapy can be discontinued 24 h after a patient improves clinically; continuing oral therapy should consist of doxycycline 100 mg orally twice a day or clindamycin 450 mg orally four times a day to complete a total of 14 d of therapy. When tubo-ovarian abscess is present, many health care providers use clindamycin for continued therapy, rather than doxycycline, because clindamycin provides more effective anaerobic coverage.

Limited data support the use of other parenteral regimens, but the following three regimens have been investigated in at least one clinical trial, and they have broad-spectrum coverage.

- Levofloxacin 500 mg iv once daily **WITH OR WITHOUT**
- (Metronidazole 500 mg IV every 8 h **OR**
- Ofloxacin 400 mg iv every 12 h) **WITH OR WITHOUT**
- (Metronidazole 500 mg IV every 8 h **OR**
- Ampicillin/Sulbactam 3 g iv every 6 h) **PLUS**
- Doxycycline 100 mg orally or iv every 12 h

(Note: quinolones should not be used in persons with a history of recent foreign travel or partners' travel, infections acquired in California or Hawaii, or infections acquired in other areas with increased QRNG prevalence.)

Intravenous ofloxacin has been investigated as a single agent; however, because of concerns regarding its spectum, metronidazole may be included in the regimen. Levofloxacin is as effective as ofloxacin and may be substituted; its single daily dosing makes it advantageous from a compliance perspective. One trial demonstrated high short-term clinical cure rates with azithromycin, either alone for 1 wk (at least one intravenous dose followed by oral therapy) or with a 12-d course of metronidazole. Ampicillin/sulbactam plus doxycycline is effective coverage against *C. trachomatis*, *N. gonorrhoeae*, and anaerobes and for patients who have tubo-ovarian abscess.

Oral Treatment

Oral therapy can be considered for women with mild-to-moderately severe acute PID, as the clinical outcomes among women treated with oral therapy are similar to those treated with parenteral therapy. The following regimens provide coverage against the frequent etiological agents of PID. Patients who do not respond to oral therapy within 72 h should be reevaluated to confirm the diagnosis and should be administered parenteral therapy on either an outpatient or inpatient basis.

- (Levofloxacin 500 mg orally once daily for 14 d **OR**
- Ofloxacin 400 mg orally once daily for 14 d) **WITH OR WITHOUT**
- Metronidazole 500 mg orally twice a day for 14 d.

(Note: quinolones should not be used in persons with a history of recent foreign travel or partners' travel, infections acquired in California or Hawaii, or infections acquired in other areas with increased QRNG prevalence.)

Azithromycin has been demonstrated in one randomized trial to be an effective regimen for acute PID. The addition of metronidazole should be considered, as anaerobic organisms are suspected in the etiology of the majority of PID cases. Metronidazole will also treat BV, which frequently is associated with PID.

RECOMMENDED REGIMEN *B*

- Ceftriaxone 250 mg im in a single dose **PLUS**
- Doxycycline 100 mg orally twice a day for 14 d **WITH OR WITHOUT**
- (Metronidazole 500 mg orally twice a day for 14 d **OR**
- Cefoxitin 2 g im in a single dose and Probenecid, 1 g orally administered concurrently in a single dose) **PLUS**
- Doxycycline 100 mg orally twice a day for 14 d **WITH OR WITHOUT**
- (Metronidazole 500 mg orally twice a day for 14 d **OR**
- Other parenteral third-generation cephalosporin [e.g., ceftizoxime or cefotaxime]) **PLUS**
- Doxycycline 100 mg orally twice a day for 14 d **WITH OR WITHOUT**
- Metronidazole 500 mg orally twice a day for 14 d.

The optimal choice of a cephalosporin for regimen B is unclear, although cefoxitin has better anaerobic coverage, ceftriaxone has better coverage against *N. gonorrhoeae.*

ALTERNATIVE ORAL REGIMENS

- Amoxicillin/clavulanic acid and doxycycline, which was effective in obtaining short-term clinical response in a single clinical trial; however, gastrointestinal symptoms might limit compliance.

Patients should demonstrate substantial clinical improvement within 3 d after initiation of therapy. If no clinical improvement has occurred within 72 h after outpatient oral or parenteral therapy an examination should be performed. Subsequent hospitalization, parenteral therapy, and diagnostic evaluation, including the consideration of diagnostic laparoscopy for alternative diagnoses, are recommended.

MANAGEMENT OF SEX PARTNERS

Male sex partners of women with PID should be examined and treated if they had sexual contact with the patient during the 60 d preceding the patient's onset of symptoms.

PREVENTION

Prevention of chlamydial infection by screening and treating high-risk women reduces the incidence of PID.

SPECIAL CONSIDERATIONS

Pregnancy

Because of the high risk for maternal morbidity and preterm delivery, pregnant women who have suspected PID should be hospitalized and treated with parenteral antibiotics.

HIV Infection

Differences in the clinical manifestations of PID between HIV-infected women and HIV-negative women have not been well delineated. HIV-infected women with PID have similar symptoms when compared with uninfected controls.

Intrauterine Device

The risk of PID associated with intrauterine device (IUD) use is primarily confined to the first 3 wk after insertion and is uncommon thereafter. No evidence suggests that IUDs should be removed in women diagnosed with acute PID. The rate of treatment failure and recurrent PID in women continuing to use an IUD is unknown.

Epididymitis

Acute epididymitis is a clinical syndrome consisting of pain, swelling, and inflammation of the epididymis of less than 6 wk. Chronic epididymitis is characterized by a 3-mo or longer history of symptoms of discomfort and/or pain in the scrotum, testicle, or epididymis that is localized on clinical examination. Among sexually active men younger than age 35, acute epididymitis is most frequently caused by *C. trachomatis* or *N. gonorrhoeae*. Acute epididymitis caused by sexually transmitted enteric organisms (e.g., Escherichia coli) also occurs among men who are the insertive partner during anal intercourse.

The evaluation of men for epididymitis should include either Gram stain of urethral secretions demonstrating more than 5 WBC per oil immersion field. or positive leukocyte esterase test on first-void urine or microscopic examination of first-void urine sediment demonstrating more than10 WBC per high-power field.

TREATMENT

As an adjunct to therapy, bed rest, scrotal elevation, and analgesics are recommended until fever and local inflammation have subsided.

RECOMMENDED REGIMENS FOR ACUTE EPIDIDYMITIS MOST LIKELY CAUSED BY GONOCOCCAL OR CHLAMYDIAL INFECTION

- Ceftriaxone 250 mg im in a single dose **PLUS**
- Doxycycline 100 mg orally twice a day for 10 d.

RECOMMENDED REGIMENS FOR ACUTE EPIDIDYMITIS MOST LIKELY CAUSED BY ENTERIC ORGANISMS OR FOR PATIENTS ALLERGIC TO CEPHALOSPORINS AND/OR TETRACYCLINES

- Ofloxacin 300 mg orally twice a day for 10 d **OR**
- Levofloxacin 500 mg orally once daily for 10 d.

MANAGEMENT OF SEX PARTNERS

Patients who have acute epididymitis, confirmed or suspected to be caused by *N. gonorrhoeae* or *C. trachomatis*, should be instructed to refer sex partners within the 60 d preceding onset of the patient's symptoms.

SPECIAL CONSIDERATIONS

HIV Infection

Patients who have uncomplicated acute epididymitis and also are infected with HIV should receive the same treatment regimen as those who are HIV-negative.

HPV Infection

Genital HPV infection can cause genital warts, usually associated with HPV types 6 or 11. Other HPV types that infect the anogenital region (e.g., high-risk HPV types 16, 18, 31, 33, and 35) are strongly associated with cervical neoplasia. Persistent infection with high-risk types of HPV is the most important risk factor for cervical neoplasia.

HPV TESTS

Screening women or men with the HPV test, outside of recommendations for use of the test with cervical cancer screening, is not recommended.

TREATMENT

In the absence of genital warts or cervical squamous intraepithelial lesion (SIL), treatment is not recommended for subclinical genital HPV infection. Genital HPV infection frequently goes away on its own, and no therapy has been identified that can eradicate infection.

If left untreated, visible genital warts might resolve on their own, remain unchanged, or increase in size or number. Treatment possibly reduces, but does not eliminate, HPV infection and impact on future transmission remains unclear.

Regimens

Treatment modality should be changed if a patient has not improved substantially. Treatment regimens are classified into patient-applied and provider-applied modalities.

RECOMMENDED PATIENT-APPLIED REGIMENS FOR EXTERNAL GENITAL WARTS

- Podofilox 0.5% solution or gel. Patients should apply podofilox solution with a cotton swab, or podofilox gel with a finger, to visible genital warts twice a day for 3 d, followed by 4 d of no therapy. This cycle may be repeated, as necessary, for up to four cycles. The total volume of podofilox should be limited to 0.5 mL/d. The safety of podofilox during pregnancy has not been established **OR**
- Imiquimod 5% cream. Patients should apply imiquimod cream once daily at bedtime, three times a week for up to 16 wk. The treatment area should be washed

with soap and water 6–10 h after the application. The safety of imiquimod during pregnancy has not been established.

RECOMMENDED PROVIDER-ADMINISTERED REGIMENS FOR EXTERNAL GENITAL WARTS

- Cryotherapy with liquid nitrogen or cryoprobe. Repeat applications every 1–2 wk **OR**
- Podophyllin resin 10–25% in a compound tincture of benzoin. A small amount should be applied to each wart and allowed to air dry. The treatment can be repeated weekly, if necessary. To avoid the possibility of complications associated with systemic absorption and toxicity, two important guidelines should be followed: (1) application should be limited to less than 0.5 mL of podophyllin or an area of less than 10 cm^2 of warts per session, and (2) no open lesions or wounds should exist in the area to which treatment is administered. Some specialists suggest that the preparation should be thoroughly washed off 1–4 h after application to reduce local irritation. The safety of podophyllin during pregnancy has not been established **OR**
- Trichloroacetic acid (TCA) or bichloroacetic acid (BCA) 80–90%. A small amount should be applied only to the warts and allowed to dry, at which time a white "frosting" develops. If an excess amount of acid is applied, the treated area should be powdered with talc, sodium bicarbonate (i.e., baking soda), or liquid soap preparations to remove unreacted acid. This treatment can be repeated weekly, if necessary **OR**
- Surgical removal either by tangential scissor excision, tangential shave excision, curettage, or electrosurgery.

ALTERNATIVE REGIMENS

- Intralesional interferon **OR**
- Laser surgery.

The efficacy and recurrence rates of intralesional interferon are comparable to other treatment modalities. Interferon therapy is not recommended as a primary modality because of inconvenient routes of administration, frequent office visits, and the association between its use and a high frequency of systemic adverse effects.

Because of the shortcomings associated with all available treatments, some clinics employ combination therapy (i.e., the simultaneous use of two or more modalities on the same wart at the same time).

RECOMMENDED REGIMENS FOR CERVICAL WARTS

- For women who have exophytic cervical warts, high-grade squamous intraepithelial lesion must be excluded before treatment is initiated. Management of exophytic cervical warts should include consultation with a specialist.

RECOMMENDED REGIMENS FOR VAGINAL WARTS

- Cryotherapy with liquid nitrogen. The use of a cryoprobe in the vagina is not recommended because of the risk for vaginal perforation and fistula formation **OR**

- TCA or BCA 80–90% applied to warts. A small amount should be applied only to warts and allowed to dry, at which time a white "frosting" develops. If an excess amount of acid is applied, the treated area should be powdered with talc, sodium bicarbonate, or liquid soap preparations to remove unreacted acid. This treatment can be repeated weekly, if necessary.

RECOMMENDED REGIMENS FOR URETHRAL MEATUS WARTS

- Cryotherapy with liquid nitrogen **OR**
- Podophyllin 10–25% in compound tincture of benzoin.

Some specialists recommend the use of podofilox and imiquimod for the treatment of distal meatal warts.

RECOMMENDED REGIMENS FOR ANAL WARTS

- Cryotherapy with liquid nitrogen **OR**
- TCA or BCA 80–90% applied to warts **OR**
- Surgical removal

Many persons with warts on the anal mucosa also have warts on the rectal mucosa, so patients with anal warts can benefit from an inspection of the rectal mucosa by digital examination or anoscopy.

COUNSELING GENITAL HPV INFECTION

Attempts should be made to convey the following key messages:

- Genital HPV infection is common among sexually active adults. The majority of sexually active adults will have it at some point in their lives.
- Genital HPV infection is usually sexually transmitted. The incubation period (i.e., the interval between initial exposure and established infection or disease) is variable, and determining the timing and source of infection is frequently difficult.
- No recommended uses of the HPV test to diagnose HPV infection in sex partners have been established. HPV infection is commonly transmitted to partners but usually goes away on its own.

MANAGEMENT OF SEX PARTNERS

Examination of sex partners is not necessary for the management of genital warts.

SPECIAL CONSIDERATIONS

Pregnancy

Imiquimod, podophyllin, and podofilox should not be used during pregnancy. However, because genital warts can proliferate and become friable during pregnancy, many specialists advocate their removal during pregnancy. HPV types 6 and 11 can cause respiratory papillomatosis in infants and children. The route of transmission (i.e., transplacental, perinatal, or postnatal) is not completely understood. Whether cesarean section prevents respiratory papillomatosis in infants and children is unclear; therefore, cesarean delivery should not be performed solely to prevent transmission of HPV infection to the newborn.

HIV Infection

No data suggest that treatment modalities for external genital warts should be different in the setting of HIV infection. Squamous cell carcinomas arising in or resembling genital warts might occur more frequently among immunosuppressed persons, therefore, requiring biopsy for confirmation of diagnosis.

Hepatitis A

PREVENTION

Two products are available for the prevention of hepatitis A viral (HAV) infection: hepatitis A vaccine and immunoglobulin (Ig) for intramuscular administration. When administered intramuscularly before or within 2 wk after exposure to HAV, Ig is more than 85% effective in preventing HAV infections.

PRE-EXPOSURE IMMUNIZATION

Persons in the following groups should be offered hepatitis A vaccine: all MSM; illegal drug users (both injecting and noninjecting drugs); and persons with chronic liver disease.

PREVACCINATION SEROLOGICAL TESTING FOR SUSCEPTIBILITY

Approximately one-third of the US population has serological evidence of previous HAV infection, which increases directly with age and reaches 75% among persons older than 70 yr of age. Screening for HAV infection might be cost-effective in populations where the prevalence of infection is likely to be high (e.g., persons over the age of 40 and persons born in areas of high HAV endemicity).

POSTEXPOSURE PROPHYLAXIS

Previously unvaccinated persons exposed to HAV (e.g., through household or sexual contact or by sharing illegal drugs with a person who has hepatitis A) should be administered a single intramuscular dose of Ig (0.02 mL/kg) as soon as possible but not more than 2 wk after exposure. Persons who have had one dose of hepatitis A vaccine at least 1 mo before exposure to HAV do not need Ig. If hepatitis A vaccine is recommended for a person receiving Ig, it can be administered simultaneously at a separate anatomic injection site.

Hepatitis B

All unvaccinated adults seeking services for STDs should be assumed to be at risk for hepatitis B and should receive hepatitis B vaccination.

Unvaccinated persons or persons known not to have responded to a complete hepatitis B vaccine series should receive both hepatitis B IG (HBIG) and hepatitis vaccine as soon as possible (preferably <24 h) after a discrete, identifiable exposure to blood or body fluids that contain blood from an hepatitis B surface antigen-positive source. *See* current recommendations for hepatitis B for details.

Hepatitis C

Hepatitis C virus (HCV) infection is the most common chronic blood-borne infection in the United States. Although HCV is not efficiently transmitted sexually, persons at risk for infection through injection-drug use might seek care in STD treatment facilities, HIV counseling and testing facilities, correctional facilities, drug treatment facilities, and other public health settings where STD and HIV prevention and control services are available. *See* hepatitis C guidelines for details.

Proctitis, Proctocolitis, and Enteritis

Sexually transmitted gastrointestinal syndromes include proctitis, proctocolitis, and enteritis. Proctitis occurs predominantly among persons who participate in receptive anal intercourse. When outbreaks of gastrointestinal illness occur among social or sexual networks of MSM, clinicians should consider sexual transmission as a mode of spread and provide counseling accordingly. Diagnostic and treatment recommendations for all enteric infections are beyond the scope of these guidelines.

TREATMENT

Acute proctitis of re◆nt onset among persons who have recently practiced receptive anal intercourse is usually sexually acquired. Such patients should be examined by anoscopy and should be evaluated for infection with HSV, *N. gonorrhoeae*, *C. trachomatis*, and *T. pallidum*. If an ano-rectal exudate is detected on examination or if polymorphonuclear leukocytes are detected on a Gram-stained smear of ano-rectal secretions, the following therapy may be prescribed while awaiting additional laboratory tests.

RECOMMENDED REGIMEN

- Ceftriaxone 125 mg im (or another agent effective against rectal and genital gonorrhea) **PLUS**
- Doxycycline 100 mg orally twice a day for 7 d. Patients with suspected or documented herpes proctitis should be managed in the same manner as those with genital herpes (see section on genital HSV infections).

Ectoparasitic Infections

PEDICULOSIS PUBIS

RECOMMENDED REGIMENS

- Permethrin 1% cream rinse applied to affected areas and washed off after 10 min **OR**
- Pyrethrins with piperonyl butoxide to the affected area and washed off after 10 min.

ALTERNATIVE REGIMENS

- Malathion 0.5% lotion applied for 8–12 h and washed off **OR**
- Ivermectin 250 mg/kg repeated in 2 wk.

Reported resistance to pediculcides has been increasing and is widespread. Malathion may be used when treatment failure is believed to have occurred because of resistance. Lindane is not recommended as first-line therapy because of toxicity.

The recommended regimens should not be applied to the eyes. Pediculosis of the eyelashes should be treated by applying occlusive ophthalmic ointment to the eyelid margins twice a day for 10 d. Bedding and clothing should be decontaminated (i.e., machine-washed, machine-dried using the heat cycle, or dry cleaned) or removed from body contact for at least 72 h. Fumigation of living areas is not necessary.

Follow-up should include an evaluation of the patient after 1 wk if symptoms persist. Re-treatment might be necessary if lice are found or if eggs are observed at the hair-skin junction. Patients who do not respond to one of the recommended regimens should be re-treated with an alternative regimen.

Special Considerations

Pregnancy

Pregnant and lactating women should be treated with either permethrin or pyrethrins with piperonyl butoxide; lindane is contraindicated in pregnancy.

SCABIES

RECOMMENDED REGIMEN

- Permethrin cream (5%) applied to all areas of the body from the neck down and washed off after 8–14 h **OR**
- Ivermectin 200 mg/kg orally, repeated in 2 wk.

ALTERNATIVE REGIMEN

- Lindane (1%) 1 oz of lotion or 30 g of cream applied in a thin layer to all areas of the body from the neck down and thoroughly washed off after 8 h.

Bedding and clothing should be decontaminated (i.e., either machine-washed, machine-dried using the hot cycle, or dry cleaned) or removed from body contact for at least 72 h. Fumigation of living areas is unnecessary.

CRUSTED SCABIES

Crusted scabies (i.e., Norwegian scabies) is an aggressive infestation that usually occurs in immunodeficient, debilitated, or malnourished individuals. Crusted scabies is associated with greater transmissibility than scabies. Substantial treatment failure might occur with a single topical scabicide or with oral ivermectin treatment. Some specialists recommend combined treatment with a topical scabicide and oral ivermectin or repeated treatments with ivermectin 200 µg/kg on days 1, 15, and 29.

Patients should be informed that the rash and pruritus of scabies might persist for up to 2 wk after treatment.

Management of Sex Partners and Household Contacts

Both sexual and close personal or household contacts within the preceding month should be examined and treated.

Management of Outbreaks in Communities, Nursing Homes, and Other Institutional Settings

Scabies epidemics frequently occur in nursing homes, hospitals, residential facilities, and other communities. Control of an epidemic can only be achieved by treatment of the entire population at risk. Ivermectin can be considered in this setting, especially if treatment with topical scabicides fails.

Special Considerations

Infants, Young Children, and Pregnant or Lactating Women

Infants, young children, and pregnant or lactating women should can be treated with permethrin. Ivermectin is not recommended for pregnant or lactating patients. The safety of ivermectin in children who weigh less than15 kg has not been determined.

SEXUAL ASSAULT AND STDs
Adults and Adolescents

The recommendations in this chapter are limited to the identification, prophylaxis, and treatment of sexually transmitted infections and conditions commonly identified in the management of such infections. The documentation of findings, collection of specimens for forensic purposes, and the management of potential pregnancy or physical and psychological trauma are beyond the scope of this chapter.

Trichomoniasis, BV, gonorrhea, and chlamydial infection are the most frequently diagnosed infections among women who have been sexually assaulted. Because the prevalence of these infections is high among sexually active women, their presence after an assault does not necessarily signify acquisition during the assault.

See the full guidelines for further information on sexual assault or abuse of children.

Evaluation for Sexually Transmitted Infections Initial Examination

An initial examination should include the following procedures:

- Testing for *N. gonorrhoeae* and *C. trachomatis* from specimens collected from any sites of penetration or attempted penetration.
- Culture or FDA-cleared nucleic acid amplification tests for either *N. gonorrhoeae* or *C. trachomatis*. Nucleic acid amplification testing offers the advantage of increased sensitivity in detection of *C. trachomatis*.
- Wet mount and culture of a vaginal swab specimen for *T. vaginalis* infection. If vaginal discharge, malodor, or itching is evident, the wet mount also should be examined for evidence of BV and candidiasis.
- Collection of a serum sample for immediate evaluation for HIV, hepatitis B, and syphilis.

Follow-Up Examinations

After the initial post-assault examination, follow-up examinations provide an opportunity to (a) detect new infections acquired during or after the assault; (b) complete hepatitis B immunization, if indicated; (c) complete counseling and treatment for other STDs; and (d) monitor side effects and adherence to postexposure prophylactic medication, if prescribed.

Examination for STDs should be repeated within 1–2 wk of the assault. Because infectious agents acquired through assault might not have produced sufficient concentrations of organisms to result in positive test results at the initial examination, testing should be repeated during the follow-up visit, unless prophylactic treatment was provided. Serological tests for syphilis and HIV infection should be repeated 6 wk, 3 mo, and 6 mo after the assault if initial test results were negative.

Prophylaxis

Many specialists recommend routine preventive therapy after a sexual assault because follow-up of survivors of sexual assault can be difficult. The following prophylactic regimen is suggested as preventive therapy:

- Postexposure hepatitis B vaccination, without HBIG. Hepatitis B vaccination should be administered to sexual assault victims at the time of the initial examination if they have not been previously vaccinated. Follow-up doses of vaccine should be administered 1–2 and 4–6 mo after the first dose.
- An empiric antimicrobial regimen for chlamydia, gonorrhea, trichomonas, and BV.
- Emergency contraception should be offered if the post-assault could result in pregnancy in the survivor.

RECOMMENDED REGIMENS

- Ceftriaxone 125 mg im in a single dose **PLUS**
- Metronidazole 2 g orally in a single dose **PLUS**
- Azithromycin 1 g orally in a single dose **OR**
- Doxycycline 100 mg orally twice a day for 7 d.

For patients requiring alternative treatments, refer to the sections in this chapter relevant to the specific agent. Providers might also consider anti-emetic medications, particularly if emergency contraception also is provided.

Risk for Acquiring HIV Infection

HIV sero-conversion has occurred in persons whose only known risk factor was sexual assault or sexual abuse, but the frequency of this occurrence is probably low. In consensual sex, the risk for HIV transmission from vaginal intercourse is 0.1–0.2% and for receptive rectal intercourse, 0.5–3%. The risk for HIV transmission from oral sex is substantially lower. Specific circumstances of an assault might increase risk for HIV transmission.

Although a definitive statement of benefit cannot be made regarding post-exposure prevention after sexual assault, the possibility of HIV exposure from the assault should be assessed at the time of the post-assault examination and a risk-benefit discussion made. Specialist consultation on postexposure prevention regimens is recommended if HIV exposure during the assault was possible and if postexposure prevention is being considered. (For more details *see* CDC-Antiretroviral postexposure prophylaxis after sexual, injection-drug use, or other nonoccupational exposure to HIV in the United States. Recommendations from the U.S. Department of Health and Human Services. MMWR 2005; 54[No. RR-2]).

SOURCES

Workowski KA, Berman SM. Sexually Transmitted Diseases Treatment Guidelines, 2006; MMWR Recommendations and Reports Vol 55, RR-11, August 4, 2006.

18

Updated US Public Health Service Guidelines for the Management of Occupational Exposure to HBV, HCV, and HIV and Recommendations for Postexposure Prophylaxis

David Gary Smith, MD, FACP

CONTENTS

INTRODUCTION

Occupational exposure to potentially infectious agents has received great attention because of the advent of HIV and the growing awareness of the possible serious clinical ramifications of hepatitis C. However, there are more than 20 diseases that have been linked to needle-stick injury. The latter group of illnesses are beyond the scope of this chapter but should be considered when developing institutional policies or when providing care for exposed health care personnel (HCP). The following guidelines apply to any health care worker (HCW; e.g., employees, students, contractors, attending clinicians, public safety workers, volunteers).

From: *Current Clinical Practice: Essential Practice Guidelines in Primary Care*
Edited by: N. S. Skolnik © Humana Press, Totowa, NJ

The definition of an exposure is any incident involving a percutaneous injury (e.g., needle stick or sharp object) or contact of mucous membrane or non-intact skin (e.g., exposed skin that is chapped, abraded, or afflicted with dermatitis) with blood, tissue, or other body fluids that are potentially infectious. In addition to blood and body fluids containing visible blood, semen and vaginal secretions are also considered potentially infectious. Although semen and vaginal secretions have been implicated in the sexual transmission of hepatitis B virus (HBV), hepatitis C virus (HCV) and HIV, they have not been implicated in occupational transmission from patients to HCP. The following fluids are also considered to be potentially infectious: cerebrospinal fluid (CSF), synovial, pleural, peritoneal, pericardial and amniotic. The risk of transmission from these fluids is unknown because the potential risk to HCP from occupational exposures has not been assessed by epidemiological studies in health care settings. Feces, nasal secretions, saliva, sputum, sweat, tears, urine, and vomitus are not considered potentially infectious unless they contain blood.

Occupational exposure still occurs despite HCW educational programs, strict policies, and innovations in available equipment. The most recent data suggest that the overall rate for sharp object injuries was 34 per 100 occupied beds per year for non-teaching hospitals and 40 injuries per 100 occupied beds per year in teaching hospitals. Most exposures occurred in patient rooms (30%), the operating room (25%), critical care units (8%), the emergency department (7%), and outpatient offices (6%). Nurses report the most frequent exposure (40%), followed by physicians who are residents or fellows (14%), attending physicians (8%), surgery attendings (5%), and non-laboratory technologists (6%). Disposable syringes (26%) and suture needles (16%) were the most common devices involved in the injury.

BASIC PRINCIPLES

All HCWs should receive education on the issues involved in occupational exposures and the methods used to prevent these injuries. They should be provided with the most up-to-date protective gear available in the community. The types of equipment are beyond the scope of this chapter but information is readily available.

All HCP should receive hepatitis B vaccination. Every clinical contact should have the available resources to comply with the standard precautions (preciously known as universal precautions). Protocols for management of exposure within particular clinical settings should be publicized widely and should include 24/7 access to care and educational resources for the HCP and the treating clinicians. Individuals with significant questions, should call the National Clinicians' Postexposure Prophylaxis Hotline (PEPline) at 1-888-448-4911. Local experts within the clinical setting should also be easily accessed.

Details of the initial management of an exposure should be provided as a checklist within each clinical setting and should include the following:

- Date and time of exposure.
- Nature of procedure.
- Details of exposure including type of injury, type of bodily fluid, and severity.
- Details of exposure source (e.g., was there known presence of HBV, HCV, HIV?).
- Details of exposed person (e.g., HBV vaccination status and vaccination response status).
- Provision of counseling, postexposure prophylaxis (PEP) management, and follow-up.

The evaluation of occupational exposure sources should consider the following:

- Testing known sources for hepatitis B surface antigen (HbsAg), anti-HCV and HIV antibodies.
- Direct virus assays for routine screening of source patients are not recommended.
- If the source person is not infected with a blood-borne pathogen, baseline testing or further follow-up of the exposed person is not necessary.
- For sources whose infection status remains unknown (e.g., the source person refused testing and local legal resource do not provide for this contingency), medical diagnoses, clinical symptoms, and history of risk behaviors should be considered.

The definition of exposure is a critical step in the initial evaluation and should be restricted to the following:

- Any percutaneous injury with a needle or sharp object that involves bodily fluids or exposure with mucous membranes or non-intact skin with bodily fluids.
- Any direct contact with materials involving high concentrations of infectious agents.

The following sections deal with the details of the policy concerning exposure to HBV, HCV, and HIV.

HBV EXPOSURE

Prior to widespread HBV vaccination of HCP, the prevalence of HBV was extremely high. The mandatory vaccination with HBV has reduced the number of serologically positive infected HCP by 95%. The risk of transmitting HBV through percutaneous exposure depends on the nature of the exposure, the serological and viral state of the sources, and the immunological status of the HCP. The risk of clinical hepatitis is as follows:

1. Risk of clinical hepatitis
   a. Source is HBsAg-positive and hepatitis "e" antigen (HBeAg)-positive: 22–31%
   b. Source is HBsAg-positive and HBeAg-negative: 1–6%
2. Risk of serological conversion
   a. Source is HBsAg-positive and HBeAg-positive: 37–62%
   b. Source is HBsAg-positive and HBeAg-negative: 23–37%

PEP for HCP-negative and source-positive situations include the use of HB immunoblobulin (HBIG) and the initiation of the HBV vaccination program (*see* Table 1). Use of HBIG should occur as soon as possible (preferably within 24 h). Regimens involving multiple doses of HBIG within 1 wk of exposure or the hepatitis B vaccine series are 70–75% effective in preventing the infection in HCP. Although not studied in HCP exposure incidents, the data from perinatal transmission provide the basis for the recommendations for the combination of HBIG and HBV treatments.

The safety of HBV PEP is excellent with the incidence of anaphylaxis being 1 in 600,000 and significant reactions to HBIG being even rarer.

The recommended regimen is as follows:

- Source is HBsAg-positive: HBIG and HBV vaccination if exposed individual has not been vaccinated or has had an inadequate response.
- Source is HBsAg-negative: HBV vaccination in the event that the exposed individual has not been vaccinated.
- Wounds and skin sites that have been in contact with blood or body fluids should be washed with soap and water. Mucous membranes should be flushed with water.

HCV EXPOSURE

HCV is not transmitted efficiently through occupational exposures to blood. The average risk of infection given percutaneous exposure is approx 1.8%. Transmission rarely occurs from mucous membrane exposures to blood and no transmission in HCP has been documented from intact or non-intact skin exposures to blood. Its relative importance stems from the successes in preventing HBV infection (and thus the marked reduction of HBV in the occupational setting) and the real clinical complications following infection. The unfortunate consideration is that there is no known PEP for HCV exposure and no existing vaccination for HCP. The only requirements for postexposure programs is serological surveillance and for treatment of established infections. Some of the observations from experimental studies included the data suggestion that there was no protection from immunoglobulin therapy.

The serological surveillance should include testing of the source to establish the risk of exposure and the testing of the HCP for anti-HCV antibodies, HCV RNA quantitative assay, and liver function tests at the time of exposure. Referral to HCV specialists should occur when an HCP shows any sign of infection.

HIV EXPOSURE

The occupational exposure to HIV has probably done the most to sensitize HCP to all the risks of infection in the workplace. The risk of infection is far less than HBV but the implications of the infection are far greater. The risk of infection

Table 1

Vaccination and antibody response status of exposed HCP	Treatment: source HBsAg-positive	Treatment: source HBsAg-negative	Treatment: source unknown or not available for testing
Unvaccinated	HBIG × 1 and initiate HB vaccine series	Initiate HB vaccine series	Initiate HB vaccine series
Previously vaccinated			
Known responder	No treatment	No treatment	No treatment
Known nonresponder	HBIG × 1 and initiate revaccination or HBIG × 2HB vaccine series	No treatment	If known high-risk source reat as if source were HBsAg-positive
Antibody response unknown	Test exposed person for anti-HBs. If adequate, no treatment. If inadequate give HBIG × 1 and vaccine booster	No treatment	Test exposed person for anti-HBs. If adequate, no treatment. If inadequate give vaccine booster and recheck titer in 1–2 mo

HCP, health care personnel; HBsAg, hepatitis B surface antigen; HBIG, hepatitis B immunoglobulin; HB, hepatitis B.

given percutaneous exposure is approx 0.3%. The risk of infection given mucous membrane exposure is 0.09%. As with many viral illnesses, the transmission to HCP depends on the serological and viral status of the source. The HIV viral load in the source patient does correlate with the risk of transmission to the exposed HCP. The potential for transmission and the impact on the HCP require the availability of specialized caregivers to manage such exposures. Important considerations include the data from the source patient, the status of the HCP, and the need for the HCP to follow strict guidelines until a clinical judgement can be made about the HCP's subsequent infection status.

The use of PEP in HCP has been supported with the early studies using zidovudine (AZT) that demonstrated an efficacy of 81%. Some of the efficacy estimates should be interpreted with caution given the lack of widespread resistant virus in the source populations and the low likelihood of transmission of exposures. Given the current highly active anti-retroviral therapy era, the possibility of exposure to resistant virus is a real consideration. PEP in HCP given known exposure is recommended with drugs believed to be active against source patient's virus and based on the nature of the exposure. Individuals with questions should consult their local experts or call the National Clinicians Postexposure Prophylaxis Hotline (PEPline)–1-888-448-4911. Some additional reasons to consult an expert include the following:

- Delayed reporting of exposure.
- Unknown source (e.g., needle in sharps disposal container or laundry).
- Known or suspected pregnancy in exposed individual.
- Resistance of source virus to anti-retroviral agents.
- Toxicity of the initial PEP regimen.

The choice of the initial regimen should be based on clinical assessment of the source exposure viral history and treatment status and should include multiple agents likely to be effective. The initial treatment may be the best chance of preventing the establishment of a chronic infection.

Initial testing of the source and HCP should include anti-HIV antibodies and review of the sources treatment history and current status (viral load, available genotypic profiles). Surveillance of the HCP should include regular testing for HIV antibodies at 0, 3, 6, and 12 mo. If the HCP develops any clinical symptoms of sero-conversion, immediate testing should be done for antibodies to HIV and a qualitative HIV viral assessment (local experts or the national hotline listed above should be consulted for the specific tests used in particular clinical settings).

For current recommended PEP regimens, *see* the Updated US Public Health Service Guidelines for the Management of Occupational Exposures to HIV and Recommendations for Postexposure Prophylaxis. MMWR Recommendations and Reports September 30, 2005/54(RRO9); 1-17. (located at http://www.cdc.gov/mmwr/preview/mmwrhtml/rr5409a1.htm)

SUMMARY

The best management of occupational exposure is through an effective prevention program of HCP via education and the provision of resources to protect HCP. Despite best efforts, however, exposures will still occur albeit at a much lower level. All health care settings should have an effective management team to provide the above protocols in the management of their HCPs.

SOURCES

1. Updated U.S. Public Health Service Guidelines for the Management of Occupational Exposures to HBV, HCV, and HIV and Recommendations for Postexposure Prophylaxis. MMWR June 29, 2001; 50 (RR11):1–42.

IV   ENDOCRINOLOGY

19

Screening for Osteoporosis in Postmenopausal Women

Richard Neill, MD

CONTENTS

INTRODUCTION

The US Preventive Services Task Force recommends screening all women age 65 and over for osteoporosis using dual-energy X-ray absorptiometry (DXA) of the femoral neck. Neither the frequency of screening nor the age at which screening may stop are specified. Women at high risk should begin screening at age 60; however, the criteria for determining which women are at high risk are controversial. There is insufficient evidence to recommend for or against screening women younger than 60 or low-risk women aged 60–64. In making their recommendation, the US Preventive Services Task Force reviewed evidence related to five key questions, each of which is summarized next *(1)*.

From: *Current Clinical Practice: Essential Practice Guidelines in Primary Care*
Edited by: N. S. Skolnik © Humana Press, Totowa, NJ

DOES RISK FACTOR ASSESSMENT ACCURATELY IDENTIFY WOMEN WHO MAY BENEFIT FROM BONE DENSITY TESTING?

Multiple risk assessment tools were reviewed by the panel. The tools included varyingly complex scoring systems. Thus includes combination of the many risk factors with most including combinations of age, weight, estrogen use, ethnicity history of fractures, and presence of rheumatoid arthritis. Age is the strongest predictor of osteoporosis risk, followed by weight of 70 kg or less. The osteoporosis risk assessment instrument is a simple three-item scoring system that combines age, estrogen use status, and weight. A total osteoporosis risk assessment instrument score of 9 or more has 95% sensitivity for identifying women at high risk of osteoporosis (*see* Table 1).

DO BONE DENSITY MEASUREMENTS ACCURATELY IDENTIFY WOMEN WHO MAY BENEFIT FROM TREATMENT?

There are several methods for measuring bone density, including computed tomography, ultrasound, and DXA. Each of these methods yields varying results depending on the skeletal site selected for study and the criteria used for establishing a diagnosis of osteoporosis. DXA scan of the femoral neck is the best predictor of hip fracture and is comparable to forearm measurements for predicting fractures at other sites. Osteoporosis risk assessment that relies on ultrasound or X-ray absorptiometry of peripheral skeletal sites (heel, forearm, or finger) predicts 1-yr risk of fracture, but these measurements have not been correlated with traditional DXA measurements.

WHAT ARE THE HARMS OF SCREENING?

Potentially unwarranted anxiety and perceived vulnerability are associated with positive screening tests. Because various screening methods yield results that cannot be compared directly, women undergoing testing using multiple methods overtime risk misclassification as normal or at risk. The time, effort, expense, and radiation exposure risk of repeated scans over a lifetime have not been determined.

WHAT ARE THE HARMS OF TREATMENT?

The harms of treatment depend on the treatment used. Medication use, specifically with selective estrogen receptor modulators, is associated with gastrointestinal side effects in a significant number of patients. Increased weight is associated with lower risk of osteoporosis but higher risk of cardiovascular disease and diabetes.

Table 1
Osteoporosis Risk Assessment Instrument

Risk factor	Value	Score
Age (yr)	≥75	15
	65–74	9
	55–64	5
	≤54	0
Weight (kg)	<60	9
	60–69.9	3
	≥70	0
Current estrogen use	Yes	2
	No	0

Total score ≥9 is high risk of osteoporosis.

DOES TREATMENT REDUCE THE RISK OF FRACTURES IN WOMEN IDENTIFIED BY SCREENING?

There are no published trials of the effectiveness of screening in reducing osteoporotic fractures. There are many studies that demonstrate the benefits of treatment in reducing fracture incidence, primarily using estrogen, bisphosphonates, or selective estrogen receptor modulators. The benefits of exercise, smoking cessation, and adequate dietary calcium and vitamin D have also been demonstrated.

SOURCES

1. US Preventive Services Task Force (2002) Screening for osteoporosis in postmenopausal women: Recommendations and rationale. Ann Intern Med 137:526–528.

V   GYNECOLOGY

20

Managing Abnormal Cervical Cytology and Cervical Intraepithelial Neoplasia

2001 Consensus Guidelines

Amy Clouse, MD

CONTENTS

INTRODUCTION

About 70% of the nearly 60 million women who undergo Papanicolaou (Pap) testing each year in the United States will be told they have abnormal results. In the past, deciding who gets a colposcopy, when to repeat the Pap test, and which patients should be treated has been both confusing and controversial. The publication of two sets of guidelines from the American Society for Colposcopy and Cervical Pathology (ASCCP) has greatly clarified these issues. These new evidence-supported consensus-based guidelines provide algorithms for managing cervical cytological abnormalities and histologically confirmed cervical intraepithelial neoplasia (CIN). They were developed out of a consensus workshop convened by ASCCP in 2001 and subsequently published in *JAMA* and the *American Journal of Obstetrics and Gynecology*. These new guidelines were preceded by revisions to the Bethesda System of nomenclature for cervical cytology. This updated terminology, as well as advances in the

From: *Current Clinical Practice: Essential Practice Guidelines in Primary Care*
Edited by: N. S. Skolnik © Humana Press, Totowa, NJ

understanding of human papillomavirus (HPV) as a cervical cancer precursor and the increased use of advanced technologies like liquid-based cervical cytology and HPV-DNA typing, were key in developing these guidelines.

THE 2001 BETHESDA SYSTEM

The National Cancer Institute organized a workshop in 2001 to update the 1991 Bethesda System used by pathologists to report cervical cytology results. There are three components of a Pap test result as reported under the new Bethesda System: specimen adequacy, a general categorization, and the interpretation or result.

Specimens are categorized as either "satisfactory" or "unsatisfactory." The once potentially confusing designation of "satisfactory but limited by…" has been eliminated. A specimen is considered adequate if it contains at least 8000–12,000 well-visualized squamous cells for conventional smears and at least 5000 cells with newer liquid-based technologies. The presence or absence of the endocervical/transformation zone component is noted here.

The general categorization section is considered an optional part of the interpretation, designed to offer rapid triage of abnormal results. Here, a single category, "negative for intraepithelial lesion or malignancy" replaces the previous two designations "within normal limits" and "benign cellular changes." This was changed to more clearly indicate that reactive changes are considered negative. Any abnormal cellular findings will be categorized as an "epithelial cell abnormality." An additional category of "other" has also been added here to indicate findings that, although benign, may impart some increased risk to the patient, such as benign-appearing endometrial cells in a woman over the age of 40.

The third section of the revised Bethesda System is the actual interpretation or result section. This has been renamed from the diagnosis section to reflect the concept that a Pap test is a screening test and should be interpreted in its full clinical context. Specimens that are without any epithelial abnormalities are designated "negative for intraepithelial lesion or malignancy." Other findings, such as *Trichomonas vaginalis*, fungal organisms, or atrophy, may also be reported under this heading.

Abnormal specimens are reported as "epithelial cell abnormalities" and are further categorized as either involving squamous cells or glandular cells. Of the squamous abnormalities, the old term "atypical squamous cells of undetermined significance" has undergone the most change. Atypical squamous cells can now be reported as either "of undetermined significance" (ASC-US) or as "cannot exclude high-grade squamous intraepithelial lesions" (ASC-H). The previous term "atypical squamous cells favor reactive" has been eliminated.

The designations "low-grade squamous intraepithelial lesion" (LSIL) and "high-grade squamous intraepithelial lesion" (HSIL) have remained unchanged in the new Bethesda System. LSIL continues to include HPV/mild dysplasia and cervical intraepithelial neoplasia grade 1 (CIN-1). Moderate and severe dysplasia, carcinoma *in situ*, CIN-2, and CIN-3 are clustered under the HSIL category.

The other type of epithelial cell abnormality that can be reported is glandular cell. These are now designated as "atypical glandular cells" (AGC) instead of the previous "atypical glandular cells of undetermined significance" (AGUS), which could have been confused with ASC-US. The category is further qualified as AGC either endocervical, endometrial, or not otherwise specified (AGC-NOS); AGC favor neoplasia; and endocervical adenocarcinoma *in situ* (AIS).

MANAGING WOMEN WITH CERVICAL CYTOLOGICAL ABNORMALITIES

Using this new terminology and incorporating information from the large, randomized ASCUS/LSIL Triage Study (ALTS), the ASCCP published consensus-based guidelines for managing cervical cytological abnormalities *(1)*.

Atypical Squamous Cells

There is a 5–17% chance that a cytology result of ASC will turn out to be CIN-2,3 on biopsy. This risk increases to 24–94% in those with ASC-H. However, the risk for invasive cervical cancer after an ASC Pap test is as low as 0.1%. The guidelines recommend follow-up for these ASC results but caution that unnecessary inconvenience, anxiety, cost, and potential patient discomfort should be avoided.

Atypical Squamous Cells of Undetermined Significance

According to the guidelines, clinicians may choose one of three options for managing an initial Pap result of ASC-US: repeat cytology, immediate colposcopy, and HPV-DNA testing for high-risk DNA types. The HPV-DNA testing route is the preferred approach when both liquid-based cytology system and reflex HPV-DNA typing are available. This approach has the advantages of a higher sensitivity than a single-repeat Pap test as well as the potential to avoid an unnecessary procedure.

If the HPV-DNA testing is negative for high-risk types; those women can be followed with repeat Pap testing at 12 mo. Those with high-risk types of HPV-DNA should be triaged to colposcopy. Any CIN discovered after colposcopy should be managed according to the ASCCP guidelines as outlined below. However, if CIN is not identified during this colposcopy, either cytology testing at 6 and 12 mo or HPV-DNA testing at 12 mo should be performed. If any Pap reveals ASC or greater or if the HPV test is positive for high-risk types, repeating the colposcopy is recommended. Otherwise, a return to routine screening is appropriate.

If the clinician chooses to repeat the cervical cytology at 4- to 6-mo intervals with an initial Pap of ASC-US, another Pap of ASC or greater warrants a colposcopy. When two consecutive "negative for intraepithelial lesion or malignancy" results are confirmed, the guidelines recommend resuming routine screening.

Immediate colposcopy is the third option for management of ASC-US. CIN found on colposcopic biopsies should be treated according to the ASCCP guidelines. Without evidence of CIN, women may have the Pap test repeated at 12 mo. More aggressive management of an ASC-US Pap with a diagnostic excisional procedure such as loop electrosurgical excision procedure (LEEP) is not appropriate without evidence of biopsy-confirmed CIN.

ASC-US in Special Circumstances

Postmenopausal women are at lower risk for CIN-2,3 than their premenopausal counterparts, whereas immunosuppressed women are more likely to have both CIN-2,3 and high-risk HPV-DNA types. Pregnant women with ASC-US should be managed the same way as nonpregnant women.

For postmenopausal women with ASC-US, the guidelines suggest a course of intravaginal estrogen followed by a repeat Pap test approx 1 wk later. This is considered an acceptable alternative in those women with evidence of atrophy and no contraindication for estrogen therapy. If this test is negative and a follow-up Pap in 4–6 mo is also negative, the patient can return to routine screening. A colposcopy is indicated if either repeat Pap test shows ASC or greater. Immunosuppressed women with ASC, including those with HIV regardless of CD4 count or viral load, should be triaged to a colposcopy.

Atypical Squamous Cells, That Cannot Exclude HSIL

A colposcopy is the only recommended approach for managing women with ASC-H. Biopsy-confirmed CIN should be managed according to the ASCCP guideline for managing CIN. If a lesion is not identified at the time of colposcopy, then the cytology and histology results should be reviewed to determine if there is a change in the interpretation. If this review changes the diagnosis to include identified CIN, this would be managed per the CIN guidelines. If no change in the original interpretation can be confirmed, cytology should be repeated in 6 and 12 mo or HPV-DNA testing can be performed at 12 mo. Another colposcopy is suggested when results of ASC or greater is found during cytology follow-up or if high-risk HPV-DNA is identified at the 1 yr mark.

Low-Grade Squamous Intraepithelial Lesion

Of those women with LSIL on cervical cytology, approx 15–30% will subsequently have CIN-2,3 found on biopsy. This higher risk of more significant disease, in addition to the risk of losing a patient to follow-up, has prompted ASCCP to recommend immediate colposcopy for women with LSIL. Further management is dictated based on the adequacy of the colposcopical examination and whether or not a lesion is identified. Diagnostic excisional procedures and ablative procedures are unacceptable as the initial management of LSIL.

With a satisfactory colposcopy and an identified lesion, endocervical sampling is considered an accepted approach in nonpregnant women. Even when there is no a lesion identified or the colposcopy is not satisfactory, endocervical sampling is still preferred in the management of LSIL. Any biopsy-proven CIN should be treated according the ASCCP guidelines. If biopsy and/or endocervical sampling does not identify CIN, either cytology at 6 and 12 mo or HPV-DNA testing at 12 mo is the appropriate next step. If both Pap tests are negative or no high-risk HPV types are found, it is safe to return to routing screening. Otherwise, a repeat colposcopy is recommended.

LSIL in Special Circumstances

Postmenopausal women with LSIL can be managed with conservative follow-up instead of an immediate colposcopy. Repeat cytological testing at 6 and 12 mo or HPV-DNA typing at 12 mo are both acceptable alternatives. A colposcopy should be recommended if either of the Pap tests reveal ASC or greater or if high-risk types of HPV-DNA are identified. Similar to the approach to ASC-US in the postmenopausal woman, a course of vaginal estrogen may also be offered, provided there are no contraindications to estrogen therapy and there is atrophy present. Another Pap test should follow this after 1 wk of estrogen completion. Colposcopy is recommended if this repeat Pap shows ASC or greater. Cytology should be repeated again in 4–6 mo.

Adolescents with LSIL may also be followed with repeat Pap testing at 6 and 12 mo or with HPV-DNA testing at 12 mo. Again, triage to colposcopy is appropriate if either the cytology tests show ASC or greater or if testing reveals high-risk types of HPV-DNA. For pregnant women with LSIL, *see* section on HSIL in special circumstances.

High-Grade Squamous Intraepithelial Lesion

Although relatively uncommon, women with HSIL cytology results have up to a 75% chance of having biopsy-confirmed CIN-2,3 and a 1–2% chance of invasive cervical cancer. The ASCCP continues to recommend colposcopy coupled with endocervical sampling for these women. Immediate treatment of the transformation zone with a LEEP is an acceptable option, especially in those whom may be lost to follow-up or if fertility is not an issue.

With a satisfactory colposcopy, biopsy-confirmed CIN-2,3 should be treated according to the CIN management guidelines. However, when no lesion or only CIN-1 is identified on a satisfactory colposcopy, there remains a considerable risk of missing more significant disease. In these cases, a thorough review of the material, including the cytology, colposcopic findings, and all biopsies, is recommended. If this review results in an upgrade of the diagnosis to CIN-2,3, the patient should be managed in accordance with the revised diagnosis. If still no lesion or only CIN-1 is identified after the review, a diagnostic excisional procedure is recommended to ensure there is no higher-grade dysplasia.

With an unsatisfactory colposcopy, review is again appropriate when no lesion is identified. If review is not possible or the original diagnosis is upheld, a diagnostic excisional procedure is recommended. Any biopsy-confirmed CIN should be managed according to the ASCCP guidelines.

HSIL in Special Circumstances

Pregnant women with HSIL (and also those with LSIL) on initial cytology should undergo a colposcopy performed by an experienced clinician. Lesions suspicious for high-grade disease can be biopsied, however, endocervical sampling is not recommended. If the colposcopy is unsatisfactory, it should be repeated in 6–12 wk because the transformation zone may become more easily visualized as pregnancy progresses. Neither treatment of the transformation zone nor a diagnostic excisional procedure is acceptable during pregnancy unless invasive disease is identified.

In adolescents with HSIL cytology results and no CIN-2,3 identified on colposcopy, observation with cytology and colposcopy at 4- to 6-mo intervals for 1 yr instead of a diagnostic excisional procedure is acceptable. This more conservative approach may only be followed if the initial colposcopy was satisfactory, endocervical sampling was negative, and the patient understands the risk of occult disease. The diagnostic excisional procedure should eventually be performed if there is any evidence of disease progression or if the HSIL cytology persists.

ATYPICAL GLANDULAR CELLS AND ADENOCARCINOMA *IN SITU*

AGC abnormalities have a greater risk for cervical neoplasia than the ASC or LSIL categories. Studies have found that women with AGC have up to a 54% chance of having biopsy-confirmed CIN, an 8% chance of having AIS, and a 1–9% chance of invasive carcinoma.

The three methods used to evaluate AGC—repeat cytology, colposcopy, and endocervical sampling—have low sensitivity for detecting glandular abnormalities. Those women in whom cervical neoplasia is not found during the initial workup may continue to be at risk for cancer and its precursors.

Women with all the subcategories of AGC or AIS, except atypical endometrial cells, should undergo colposcopy with endocervical sampling. The guidelines recommend endometrial sampling for those with atypical endometrial cells. Furthermore, endometrial sampling should accompany colposcopy in women aged 35 and older with AGC and in those with unexplained vaginal bleeding. It is not acceptable to use repeat Pap testing for AGC or AIS results and there is not a role for HPV-DNA typing in the management of these lesions.

If the initial Pap test showed AGC "favor neoplasia" or AIS and invasive disease is not identified with the initial colposcopy and biopsies, further evaluation with a diagnostic excisional procedure is recommended, preferably with a cold knife conization. Invasive disease requires referral to an appropriate specialist. If the initial Pap showed AGC-NOS, biopsy-confirmed CIN should be managed according to the ASCCP guidelines. If no CIN is identified in these women, they should be followed with repeat cytology at 4- to 6-mo intervals until four consecutive "negative for intraepithelial lesion or malignancy" results. At this point, results of ASC or LSIL warrant another colposcopy and results of HSIL or AGC warrant a diagnostic excisional procedure.

MANAGING WOMEN WITH CIN

The prevention of cervical cancer not only involves performing Pap tests and following up on abnormal cytology results, but also in the destruction or removal of cervical cancer precursors. Using information from the same consensus conference, the ASCCP published further guidelines to help clarify management options for biopsy-confirmed intraepithelial neoplasia *(2)*.

Cervical Intraepithelial Neoplasia Grade 1

Most untreated CIN-1 spontaneously regresses without treatment. Research indicates that CIN-1 lesions may regress in up to 57% of women but advance to CIN-2,3 or cancer in only 11%. Overall, there is a 0.3% chance of progression to invasive cancer and most of these cancers are in those lost to follow-up. The management guidelines, therefore, recommend a conservative follow-up strategy for CIN-1. However, when the colposcopy is not satisfactory, there is still the risk that higher-grade dysplasia could be missed so the guidelines suggest managing these women more aggressively *(3)*.

With a satisfactory colposcopy, follow-up without treatment using either repeat cytology at 6 and 12 mo or HPV-DNA testing at 12 mo is the preferred approach. After two consecutive negative Pap tests or no high-risk HPV at the 1-yr mark, a return to annual screening is appropriate. If either Pap reveals ASC or greater or if high-risk types of HPV are found, the colposcopy should be repeated. An acceptable alternate follow-up strategy is to perform both colposcopy and Pap testing at 12 mo after the initial CIN-1 diagnosis. If colposcopic and cytological regression is demonstrated, annual cytological screening may be resumed. Otherwise, any CIN found should be treated according to these guidelines. Persistent CIN-1 can also be treated depending on provider and patient preferences.

Treating biopsy-confirmed CIN-1 is also an acceptable management option if the colposcopy was satisfactory. Cryotherapy, electrofulguration, laser ablation, cold coagulation, and LEEP are all acceptable treatment modalities. Although the choice of method is based on provider experience and available resources, endocervical sampling should precede any ablative method. Excisional methods are preferred in the setting of recurrent CIN-1 after previous ablative therapy. Hysterectomy is not an appropriate treatment for CIN-1.

When the colposcopy is not satisfactory, a diagnostic excisional procedure is preferred to manage biopsy-confirmed CIN-1. However, one of the conservative follow-up protocols above may be used for immunosuppressd or pregnant women (*see* section on CIN-2,3 in special circumstances). Adolescents with CIN-1 and an unsatisfactory colposcopy may also be treated conservatively as higher-grade disease is unlikely in this population.

Cervical Intraepithelial Neoplasia Grades 2 and 3 (CIN-2,3)

Unlike CIN-1, untreated moderate dysplasia, severe dysplasia, and carcinoma *in situ* are all more likely to persist or progress rather than regress. Of CIN-2 lesions, 43% will regress spontaneously, whereas 35% will persist and 22% will progress to carcinoma *in situ* or cancer when left untreated. Likewise, 32% of untreated CIN-3 lesions will regress; 56% will persist, and 14% will progress. The similarities in the behavior of these two lesions have led the ASCCP to combine their management in the 2001 consensus guidelines.

With a satisfactory colposcopy and biopsy-confirmed CIN-2,3, the guidelines recommend treatment with either excision or ablation of the transformation zone. Excisional methods are preferred in the case of recurrent CIN-2,3. When the colposcopy is unsatisfactory, a diagnostic excisional procedure is recommended as initial management of CIN-2,3. Following these lesions without treatment is generally unacceptable. This would only be appropriate in pregnancy or with adolescents (*see* the section on special circumstances). Hysterectomy is also not acceptable as initial management for CIN-2,3 but could be considered for recurrent or persistent lesions.

Follow-Up Posttreatment for CIN-2,3

Recommendations for follow-up after the initial treatment for CIN-2,3 include either cervical cytology and colposcopy or cytology alone at 4- to 6-mo intervals. Once three consecutive "negative for squamous intraepithelial lesion or malignancy" results are obtained, the patient may return to annual screening. However, if any of the Pap tests during this follow-up period reveals ASC or greater, another colposcopy is warranted.

Another option for follow-up posttreatment of CIN-2,3 is HPV-DNA testing at least 6 mo after treatment. If high-risk types are identified at this point, another colposcopy should be performed. Annual cytological screening can be resumed if this testing is negative for high-risk HPV-DNA types.

If the margins of a diagnostic excisional procedure or a postprocedure endocervical sampling contain CIN, the 4- to 6-mo follow-up visit should include colposcopy as well as another endocervical sampling. When CIN-2,3 is identified at the margins or in the endocervical sampling, it is also acceptable to repeat the diagnostic excisional procedure. If this is not possible, an acceptable alternative is a hysterectomy. A hysterectomy is also acceptable for treatment of recurrent or persistent biopsy-confirmed CIN-2,3.

CIN-2,3 in Special Circumstances

Because of the minimal risk of progression of CIN-2,3 to invasive cervical cancer during pregnancy and a reported 69% spontaneous regression rate after delivery, pregnant women with CIN-2,3 can be treated conservatively. The guidelines suggest shifting management goals to identifying invasive cervical cancers only and avoiding diagnostic excisional procedures unless invasive cancer cannot be ruled out.

Likewise, some adolescents can also be treated more conservatively. Invasive cervical cancer is rare in adolescents and there is a relatively higher rate of spontaneous regression with CIN-2 compared with CIN-3. Follow-up with Pap tests and colposcopy at 4- to 6-mo intervals for 1 yr is an appropriate alternative in adolescents with CIN-2 assuming the following conditions are met: the initial colposcopy was satisfactory, endocervical sampling results were negative, and the patient understands the risk of occult disease. Treatment with either ablation or excision is the only acceptable option for biopsy-proven CIN-3 in this population.

In immunosuppressed women with HIV, there is a high rate of recurrence and persistence of CIN-2,3 even after appropriate treatment. However, treatment does appear to be effective in preventing the progression of CIN-2,3 to invasive cervical cancer.

SOURCES

1. Wright TC, Cox JT, Massad LS, et al. (2002) *2001 Consensus Guidelines for the Management of Women with Cervical Cytological Abnormalities.* JAMA 287:2120–2129.
2. Wright TC, Cox JT, Massad LS, et al. (2003) *2001 Consensus Guidelines for the Management of Women with Cervical Intraepithelial Neoplasia.* Am J Obstet 189:295–304.
3. Solomon D, Davey D, Kurman R, et al. (2002) *The 2001 Bethesda System. Terminology for Reporting Results of Cervical Cytology.* JAMA 287:2114–2119.

VI NEUROLOGY

21 Dementia

William McCarberg, MD

Contents

INTRODUCTION

As the US population ages, the incidence and prevalence of various dementias will increase in the absence of new methods for preventing or reversing dementia. With 4 million individuals with Alzheimer's disease (AD) in 1990, the National Institutes of Health estimates that there will be 8.5 million Americans with this disease by the year 2030, and an unknown number of people with other dementias. In 1998, the annual cost for the care of patients with AD in the Unites States was approx $40,000 per patient. If one were able to successfully identify and treat mild cognitive impairment (MCI) such that the progression of these individuals to AD could be delayed by 1 yr, there would be significant savings.

In 1994, the Quality Standards Subcommittee of the American Academy of Neurology (AAN) published the Diagnosis and Evaluation of Dementias. This practice parameter was designed for use by neurologists in the evaluation of patients with possible dementia and was based on evidence. Since 1994, considerable progress has been made prompting an updated report from the Quality Standards Subcommittee. The 2001 guideline was published in three parts: early detection of dementia: MCI; diagnosis of dementia; and management of dementia *(1–3)*.

From: *Current Clinical Practice: Essential Practice Guidelines in Primary Care*
Edited by: N. S. Skolnik © Humana Press, Totowa, NJ

Table 1
Classification of the Evidence

Class	Description
I	Highest quality, well-designed prospective study in broad group of patients
II	Well-designed prospective study of a narrow spectrum of patients with the condition, or a well-performed retrospective study of a broad group of patients
III	Evidence from a retrospective study in which a narrow spectrum of patients are studied, and in which tests were applied in a blinded fashion
IV	Evidence from studies that were not blinded or recommendation provided by expert opinion

All three reports follow a similar format:

- *Clinical question statement:* strategic questions are asked about each topic.
- *Analysis of evidence:* the clinical questions are analyzed presenting the quality of available evidence.
- *Practice recommendations:* grouped into three categories of patient management recommendations based on the quality of the evidence: (a) standard—high degree of clinical certainty; (b) guidelines—moderate clinical certainty; (c) option—clinical utility is uncertain.

The databases searched for the analysis of evidence comprised of MEDLINE, EMBASE, Excerpta Medica, BIOSIS, Current Contents, Psychological Abstract, Psycho Info, Cochrane Database and CINAHL. Each identified article was classified on the quality of evidence (classes I–IV; Table 1). When available, data on specificity and sensitivity were used. Inclusion of articles was dependent on a consensus of the Quality Standards Subcommittee and the Practice Committee of the AAN.

EARLY DETECTION OF DEMENTIA: MCI

Epidemiological studies of aging and dementia have demonstrated three groups of subjects—those who are demented, those who are not demented, and individuals who cannot be classified because of cognitive (memory) impairment but do not meet criteria for dementia. MCI (Table 2) refers to the state of cognitive and functional ability between normal aging and very mild AD. It is characterized by a memory complaint corroborated by a close friend or partner, objective memory impairment, and generally normal cognitive function with intact activities of daily living.

Clinical Question Statement

1. Does the presence of MCI predict the development of dementia?

   Four class II studies, three in the United States and one in Canada, showed conversion from MCI to AD of 6 to 15% per year. Taken together, these studies indicate that individual as being cognitively impaired but not meeting the clinical criteria for dementia and has a high risk of progressing to dementia or AD.

2. Does screening at-risk subjects lead to the diagnosis of dementia?

   The Mini-Mental Status Examination (MMSE) is a widely recognized instrument for the detection of cognitive impairment. Two large class I and several class II studies provide data on this instrument. The MMSE, originally designed as a bedside screening tool, appears to have limitations as a general population screening tool. It is still useful in examining patients with MCI. Other less-studied tools including Kokmen Short Test of Mental Status, 7-min screen, and memory impairment screen are useful for the detection of dementia when used in patient populations with elevated prevalence. Brief focused screening instruments such as drawing the face of a clock with a designated time, the subject's ability to tell time, and ability to make change are less useful.

Neuropsychological batteries include nonverbal memory, confrontational naming, recall of prose passages, calculation, visuomotor function, construction memory, attention, and other tests. Class II and III studies showed good predictive value. A close observer such as a significant other often is the first to complain of the patient's cognitive decline. Several tools (informant-based instruments) emphasize the history from such observers. Not enough work has been done to recommend these tools.

Practice Recommendations

- There were sufficient data to recommend the evaluation and clinical monitoring of person with MCI because of the person's increased risk for developing dementia (guideline).
- Screening instruments such as the MMSE were found to be useful to the clinician for assessing the degree of cognitive impairment (guideline), as were neuropsychological batteries (guideline).
- Brief focused cognitive instruments and structured informant interviews were not thought to be as helpful (option).

DIAGNOSIS OF DEMENTIA

Dementia describes a variety of diseases with resultant loss of cognitive functioning. These include AD, vascular dementia (VAD), dementia with Lewy bodies (DLB), frontotemporal dementia (FTD), prion diseases, and others.

Clinical Question Statement

1. Are the current criteria for the diagnosis of dementia reliable?

   The diagnostic criteria most widely used in the United States are based on definitions contained in the *Diagnostic and Statistical Manual,* 3rd edition, revised (DSM-IIIR). DSM-IIIR states:

   The essential feature of Dementia is impairment in short- and long-term memory, associated with impairment in abstract thinking, impaired judgment, other disturbances of higher cortical function, or personality change. The disturbance is severe enough to interfere significantly with work or usual social activities and relationship with others. The diagnosis of Dementia is not made if these symptoms occur in Delirium.

   The DSM-IIIR definition of dementia has good to very good reliability. The DSM-IV definition, which is identical to DSM-IIIR, has not been subjected to assessment but presumably would have similar reliability.

2. Are current diagnostic criteria sufficiently accurate to establish a diagnosis for the prevalent dementias in the elderly?

   AD: Three class I and 10 class II studies addressed the diagnostic accuracy of AD using neuropathological confirmation. DSM-IIIR of "probable" AD achieved good sensitivity (81%) and average specificity (70%) across studies.

   VAD: The diagnosis of VAD is difficult using current criteria. Recent studies distinguished between "some or any" vascular lesions against "pure" vascular pathology (the circumstance in which vascular pathology was both sufficient to account for cognitive symptoms and unaccompanied by other pathology). Some vascular pathology existed in 29–41% of dementia cases coming to autopsy with pure vascular pathology accounting for about only 10%. The Hachinski ischemic score is the most suitable for identifying the majority of patients with VAD.

   DLB: DLB has been defined clinically by the presence of dementia, gait/balance disorder, prominent hallucinations and delusions, sensitivity to traditional antipyschotics, and fluctuations in alertness. Multiple class I and II studies have investigated the diagnostic criteria for DLB and all either demonstrate low sensitivity and/or specificity. Current neuropsychological tests do not reliably differentiate DLB from either AD or VAD. Neuroimaging is also unsuccessful in differentiating DLB from AD despite reported less atrophy of the temporal lobe in AD.

   FTD: Early loss of social awareness, hyperorality, and stereotyped, perseverative behavior were somewhat sensitive (63–73%) and highly specific (>96%) in diagnosing FTD. Neuropsychological test profiles of patients with FTD typically reveal deficits in verbal fluency, abstraction, and executive function; however, patients with AD demonstrate substantial impairment in all of these functions as well. Neither the clinical nor neuropsychological profile of the frontotemporal syndrome is specific for FTD.

   Prion disease: The diagnostic criteria of Masters were used in a class I study of 188 patients with Creutzfeldt-Jakob disease (CJD). Autopsy-proven disease was found in 97% of the "probable" and 44% of the "possible" cases.

3. Do laboratory tests improve the accuracy of the clinical diagnosis of dementing illness?

Given the goal of minimal undetected structural lesions, the data supports the use of a neuroimaging examination—either a noncontrast computed tomography (CT) or magnetic resonance imaging (MRI) scan—usually at the time of the initial dementia assessment to identify pathology such as brain neoplasms or subdural hematomas. Normal pressure hydrocephalus, which might be detected by CT or MRI and might be responsive to treatment, is very rare.

Genetic biomarkers—the genetics of dementing illness is a maturing field. Although autosomal-dominant transmission is not evident, advances in the identification of genetic markers for dementia of the familial nature increases awareness of these disorders. One large pathologically confirmed class II study using apolipoprotien (APO) E4 found only a slight increase in positive-predictive value. In patients with a clinical diagnosis of AD, APO E testing increased predictive value by only 4% with the presence of APO E4. No genetic testing is recommended for AD, DLB, or CJD. The CSF 14-3-3 protein is recommended in the diagnosis of CJD.

4. What comorbidities should be evaluated in elderly patients undergoing an initial assessment for dementia?

Up to 12% of demented patients were also depressed. Screening with the appropriate office-based tool is recommended.

Vitamin B_{12} deficiency is common in elderly patients; however, improved cognition with treatment is uncertain. As a cause of dementia, vitamin B_{12} deficiency is unusual, but ease of screening and treatment warrant monitoring for this disorder.

Hypothyroidism is also common in the elderly. The link between decreased thyroid function and cognition is unclear, with variable results from several studies. In population-based studies, increased thyroid-stimulation hormone carried an increased risk of dementia; however, this risk is small and often not reversible with treatment. However, screening is recommended for this comorbidity.

No other testing, including testing for syphilis, hypoparathyroidism, or hepatic encephalopathy, is recommended by current evidence.

Practice Recommendations

- DSM-IIIR definition of dementia is reliable and should be used in diagnosis of AD and CJD (guideline).
- Diagnostic criteria for VAD, DLB, FTD is imprecise with current evidence (option).
- Structural neuroimaging with noncontrast CT or MRI is appropriate (guideline).
- No genetic markers are recommended for routine diagnostic purposes. CSF 14-3-3 protein is useful for confirming the diagnosis of CJD (guideline).
- Depression, vitamin B_{12}, and hypothyroidism, but not syphilis, should be screened (guideline).

MANAGEMENT OF DEMENTIA

The previously identified databases were searched and revealed 2548 articles identified with 380 meeting predefined inclusion criteria to help answer the following questions. Drugs that were reviewed are shown in Table 3.

Clinical Question Statement

1. Does pharmacotherapy improve outcomes in patient with dementia compared with no therapy?

   AD—multiple drugs were identified in the cholinesterase inhibitors category for the 2001 study. All were approved for use in AD: tacrine, donepezil, rivastigmine, and galantamine (Note: since issue of the guideline: Memantine, an *N*-methyl-D-aspartate receptor antagonist [a newer drug], was not reviewed but has been approved by the Food and Drug Administration).

   Cholinesterase inhibitors as a class are consistently better than placebo. However, the disease eventually continues to progress and the average treatment effect is modest. The main difference between the multiple agents is in side-effect profile and ease of administration.

   One study of vitamin E or selegiline showed a possible benefit. These agents should not be combined.

   A wide group of agents with diverse mechanisms of action have been tested in at least one class I trial but there is incomplete or conflicting evidence for these agents. Nonsteroidal anti-inflammatory agents show a slight decline with high drop-out rates. Two well-designed trials failed to show that Premarin® slowed decline in AD.

2. Does pharmacotherapy for noncognitive symptoms improve outcomes in patients with dementia compared with no therapy?

   Behavioral disturbances including agitation, psychosis, anxiety, disinhibition, sleep disturbances, wandering, shadowing, compulsive behaviors, apathy, and others are common in dementia. Pain or environmental triggers may be associated with these disturbances. Treatment of these behaviors can improve quality of life for patients and caregivers. When nonpharmacological strategies for environmental triggers are not apparent, class I evidence supports the use of both traditional and atypical antipyschotics in the treatment of both agitation and psychosis. Atypical agents are better tolerated. Anticonvulsants, benzodiazepines, antihistamines, monoamine oxidase (MOA) inhibitors, and selective serotonin reuptake inhibitors (SSRI) lack evidence of efficacy. Other behavioral disturbances also lack convincing evidence in any drug trials. Depression is also commonly found in the patient with dementia. Selected tricyclics, SSRIs, and MAO-B inhibitors offer benefit in treatment of depression in the demented patient.

3. Do educational interventions improve outcomes in patient and/or caregivers of patients with dementia compared with no such interventions?

Trials comparing educational programs to no program or a support group, showed impact only on patients and caregivers without effect on disease severity or patient outcome. Short-term improvement in caregivers' disease knowledge and ability to cope occurs, but decision-making skills and perceived burden did not improve. Intensive long-term education and support delayed time to nursing home placement by 12–24 mo.

4. Do nonpharmacological interventions other than education improve outcomes in patients and/or caregivers of patients with dementia compared with no such interventions?

Interventions to improve functional performance: Two class I studies show that behavior modification, scheduled toileting, and prompted voiding can reduce urinary incontinence. Graded assistance, skills practice, and positive reinforcement can increase functional independence.

Nonpharmacological interventions for problem behaviors: Sensory stimulation of various types (music, bright lights, verbal cues, walking, light, exercise) are usually studied in a multifaceted approach to treatment of patients with dementia and make it difficult to judge any one treatment; however, they may have a beneficial impact on agitation.

Psychosocial interventions for caregivers: Psychosocial interventions directed toward caregivers, which may include education, support, and respite care, may improve caregivers' emotional well-being and quality of life as well as delay nursing home placement.

Practice Recommendations

- Cholinesterase inhibitors (and memantine) benefit patients with AD, although the benefit appears small (standard). Vitamin E delays the time to clinical worsening (guideline). Selegiline, other antioxidants, anti-inflammatories, and estrogen are not supported by current evidence.

- Antipyschotics are effective for agitation and psychosis in which environmental manipulation fails (standard). Antidepressants are effective in depressed patients (guideline).

- Staff at long-term care facilities should be educated about AD to minimize the unnecessary use of antipsychotic medications (guideline).

- Behavior modification, scheduled toileting, and prompted voiding reduce urinary incontinence (standard). Functional independence can be increased by graded assistance, skills practice, and positive reinforcement (guideline).

More evidence-based studies must explore the early detection of dementia, better methods of diagnosis including biogenetic markers and earlier treatments that include preventative strategies. These should include prospective studies of elderly at-risk individuals prior to the development of dementia.

Studies must be designed to guide routine clinical care and research involving patient with dementia. Guidance in these areas is critical for therapeutic research to continue effectively.

SOURCES

1. Early Detection of Dementia: Mild Cognitive Impairment (2001) Neurology 56:113.
2. Diagnosis of Dementia (2001) Neurology 56:1143.
3. Management of Dementia (2001) Neurology 56:1154.

22

Diagnosis and Treatment of Migraine Headaches

Richard Neill, MD

DIAGNOSIS AND TREATMENT OF MIGRAINE HEADACHES

Migraine headache is a common disorder affecting nearly 18% of women and 6% of men in the United States. The American Academy of Neurology, in conjunction with the seven participating specialty societies of the US Headache Consortium, performed an evidence-based review of available treatments for migraine headache in both acute and preventive settings, as well as assessing the role of diagnostic imaging in evaluation and treatment of headache *(1,2)*.

DIAGNOSIS OF MIGRAINE

The current classification system for headache is based on the 1988 International Headache Society system and updated in 2004, characterizes migraine as a chronic condition with recurrent episodic attacks. Its characteristics vary among patients and often among attacks in a single patient. Migraine types include migraine with and without aura and chronic migraine (lasting more than 15 d). Migraine diagnosis requires consideration of secondary causes of headache and also whether the patient has any coexisting primary headache type such as tension headache or trigeminal neuralgia.

From: *Current Clinical Practice: Essential Practice Guidelines in Primary Care*
Edited by: N. S. Skolnik © Humana Press, Totowa, NJ

Migraine symptoms typically start in the morning with gradual onset of moderate to severe pain described as throbbing and often accompanied by nausea, anorexia, and vomiting. Physical activity, light, or sound often exacerbates symptoms, which without treatment slowly subside in 4–72 h in most adults. The majority of migraneurs have attacks infrequently, although nearly 30% have attacks monthly or more frequently.

The diagnosis is made on the basis of history suggestive of migraine and a normal neurological examination. Neurodiagnostic imaging should be reserved for patients with an unexplained abnormal finding on neurological examination (grade B recommendation) or with atypical headache features or headaches that do not fulfill the strict definition of migraine or other primary headache disorder (or have some additional risk factors such as immune deficiency), when a lower threshold for neuroimaging may be applied (grade C recommendation). There is insufficient evidence to support evidence-based guidelines for any other diagnostic testing other than neuroimaging (grade C recommendation).

TREATMENT OF MIGRAINE

Nonpharmacological and pharmacological treatment goals include the following:

1. Reduction in attack frequency, severity, and disability.
2. Reduce reliance on poorly tolerated, ineffective, or unwanted acute pharmacotherapies.
3. Improve quality of life.
4. Avoid acute headache medication escalation.
5. Educate and enable patients to manage their disease to enhance personal control of their migraine.
6. Reduce headache-related distress and psychological symptoms.

Although nonpharmacological treatments are helpful in the prevention of migraine recurrence, they are typically used in conjunction with pharmacotherapy in the acute setting.

Cognitive and Behavioral Treatment Recommendations

Relaxation training, thermal biofeedback combined with relaxation training, electromyographic biofeedback, and cognitive-behavioral therapy may be considered as treatment options for prevention of migraine (grade A). Specific recommendations regarding which of these to use for specific patients cannot be made. Behavioral therapy may be combined with preventive drug therapy to achieve additional clinical improvement for migraine relief (grade B). Evidence-based treatment recommendations regarding the use of hypnosis, acupuncture, transcutaneous electrical nerve stimulation, chiropractic or osteopathic cervical manipulation, occlusal adjustment, and hyperbaric oxygen as preventive or acute therapy for migraine are not yet possible.

Nonpharmacological interventions should be considered in the following circumstances:

1. Patient preference for nonpharmacological interventions.
2. Poor tolerance to specific pharmacological treatments.
3. Medical contraindications for specific pharmacological treatments.
4. Insufficient or no response to pharmacological treatment.
5. Pregnancy, planned pregnancy, or nursing.
6. History of long-term, frequent, or excessive use of analgesic or acute medications that can aggravate headache problems (or lead to decreased responsiveness to other pharmacotherapies).
7. Significant stress or deficient stress-coping skills.

Goals of acute migraine treatment are as follows:

1. Treat attacks rapidly and consistently without recurrence.
2. Restore the patient's ability to function.
3. Minimize the use of back-up and rescue medications. (A rescue medication is used at home when other treatments fail and permits the patient to achieve relief without the discomfort and expense of a visit to the physician's office or emergency department.)
4. Optimize self-care and reduce subsequent use of resources.
5. Be cost-effective for overall management.
6. Have minimal or no adverse events.

To meet these goals:

1. Use migraine-specific agents (triptans, dihydroergotamine [DHE]) in patients with moderate or severe migraine or whose mild to moderate headaches respond poorly to nonsteroidal anti-inflammatory drugs (NSAIDs) or combinations such as aspirin plus acetaminophen plus caffeine. Failure to use an effective treatment promptly may increase pain, disability, and the impact of the headache.
2. Select a non-oral route of administration for patients with migraine associated with severe nausea or vomiting.
3. Antiemetics should not be restricted to patients who are vomiting or likely to vomit. Nausea itself is one of the most aversive and disabling symptoms of a migraine attack and should be treated appropriately.
4. Consider a self-administered rescue medication for patients with severe migraine who do not respond to (or fail) other treatments.
5. Guard against medication-overuse headache (rebound headache or drug-induced headache). Frequent use of acute medications (ergotamine [not DHE], opiates, triptans, simple analgesics, and mixed analgesics containing butalbital, caffeine, or isometheptene) is generally thought to cause medication-overuse headache. Many experts limit acute therapy to 2 d of headache per week on a regular basis. Patients with medication overuse should use preventive therapy.

PHARMACOTHERAPY OF ACUTE MIGRAINE

Triptans and DHE are specific treatments for migraine that should be considered as first-line therapy. Triptans are effective and relatively safe for the acute treatment of migraine headaches and are an appropriate initial treatment choice in patients with moderate to severe migraine who have no contraindications for its use (grade A). Initial treatment with any triptan is a reasonable choice when the headache is moderate to severe or in migraine of any severity when nonspecific medication has failed to provide adequate relief in the past (grade C). Patients with nausea and vomiting may be given intranasal or subcutaneous sumatriptan (grade C).

Ergotamine (DHE) by mouth or rectum (and caffeine combination) may be considered in the treatment of selected patients with moderate to severe migraine (grade B). DHE nasal spray is safe and effective for the treatment of acute migraine attacks and should be considered for use in patients with moderate-to-severe migraine (grade A). DHE through non-oral routes may be given to patients with nausea and vomiting (grade C). Non-oral routes of DHE are reasonable initial treatment choices when the headache is moderate to severe, or in migraine of any severity when nonspecific medication has failed to provide adequate relief in the past (grade C). Intravenous DHE in combination with an antiemetic is an appropriate treatment choice for patients with severe migraine (grade B).

Nonspecific medications include antiemetics, NSAIDs, and opiate analgesics. They may be used as adjuncts to treatment with triptans or when these primary agents fail.

Oral antiemetics are an adjunct to treat nausea associated with migraine (grade C). Metoclopramide intramuscular/intravenous is an adjunct to control nausea (grade C) and may be considered as intravenous monotherapy for migraine pain relief (grade B). Prochlorperazine intravenous, intramuscular, and per rectum (PR) may be a therapeutic choice for migraine in the appropriate setting (grade B). Prochlorperazine PR is an adjunct in the treatment of acute migraine with nausea and vomiting (grade C). Chlorpromazine intravenous may be a therapeutic choice for migraine in the appropriate setting (grade B). Serotonin receptor (5-HT3) antagonists are not effective as monotherapy for migraine pain relief (grade B), but may be considered as adjunct therapy to control nausea in selected patients with migraine attacks (grade C).

NSAIDs (oral) and combination analgesics containing caffeine are a reasonable first-line treatment choice for mild-to-moderate migraine attacks or severe attacks that have been responsive in the past to similar NSAIDs or nonopiate analgesics (grade A). Acetaminophen alone is not recommended for migraine (grade B). Intramuscular ketorolac is an option that may be used in a physician-supervised setting, although conclusions regarding clinical efficacy cannot be made at this time (grade C). Butalbital-containing analgesics should be used with careful monitoring for overuse, medication-overuse headache, and withdrawal concerns (grade B).

Butorphanol nasal spray is a treatment option for some patients with migraine (grade A); however, the well-established risk of overuse and dependence with this medication requires special attention. Butorphanol may be considered when other medications cannot be used or as a rescue medication when significant sedation would not jeopardize the patient (grade C). Parenteral opiates are a rescue therapy for acute migraine when sedation side effects will not put the patient at risk and when the risk of abuse has been addressed (grade B).

Preventive Treatment

Table 1 summarizes preventive therapies for migraine. The goals of migraine preventive therapy are to (1) reduce attack frequency, severity, and duration; (2) improve responsiveness to treatment of acute attacks; and (3) improve function and reduce disability. When considering preventive treatment, these consensus-based principles of care will enhance the success of preventive treatment.

1. Medication use:
   a. Initiate therapy with medications that have the highest level of evidence-based efficacy.
   b. Initiate therapy with the lowest effective dose of the drug. Increase it slowly until clinical benefits are achieved in the absence of, or until limited by, adverse events.
   c. Give each drug an adequate trial. It may take 2–3 mo to achieve clinical benefit.
   d. Avoid interfering medications (e.g., overuse of acute medications).
   e. Use of a long-acting formulation may improve compliance.
2. Evaluation:
   a. Monitor the patient's headache through a headache diary.
   b. Re-evaluate therapy. If after 3–6 mo, headaches are well controlled, consider tapering, or discontinuing treatment.
3. Take coexisting conditions into account. Some conditions are more common in persons with migraine: stroke, myocardial infarction, Raynaud's phenomenon, epilepsy, affective and anxiety disorders. These conditions present both treatment opportunities and limitations:
   a. Select a drug that will treat the coexistent condition and migraine, if possible.
   b. Establish that the treatments being used for migraine are not contraindicated for the coexistent disease.
   c. Establish that the treatments being used for coexistent conditions do not exacerbate migraine.
   d. Beware of all drug interactions.

Table 1
Preventive Therapies for Migraine

Group 1[a,b]	Group 2[c]	Group 3[d]	Group 4[e]	Group 5[f]
Amitriptyline	β-blockers	A: Antidepressants	Methysergide	Carbamazepine
Divalproex sodium	Atenolol/ metoprolol/nadolol	Bupropion		Clomipramine
Propranolol/timolol	Ca-blockers	Doxepine		Clonazepam
	Nimodipine/ verapamil	Fluvoxamine		Clonidine
	NSAIDs	Imipramine		Nicardipine
	Indomethacin	Mirtazepine		Nifedipine
	Aspirin	Nortriptyline		Pindolol
	Fenoprofen	Paroxetine		
	Flurbiprofen	Protriptyline		
	Ketoprofen	Sertraline		
	Mefenamic acid	Trazodone		
	Naproxen sodium	Venlafaxine		
	Fluoxetine (racemic)	Other		
	Gabapentin	Topiramate		
	Other	Cyproheptadine		
	Feverfew	Diltiazem		
	Magnesium	Ibuprofen		
	Vitamin B$_2$	B: Side-effect concerns		
		Phenelzine		

[a] Does not include combination products.
[b] Medium-to-high efficacy, good strength of evidence, and mild-to-moderate side effects.
[c] Lower efficacy than those listed in first column, or limited strength of evidence, and mild-to-moderate side effects.
[d] Clinically efficacious based on consensus and clinical experience, but no scientific evidence of efficacy.
[e] Medium-to-high efficacy, good strength of evidence, but with side-effect concerns.
[f] Evidence indicating no efficacy over placebo.

4. Direct special attention to women who are pregnant or want to become pregnant. Preventive medications may have teratogenic effects. If treatment is absolutely necessary, select a treatment with the lowest risk of adverse effects to the fetus.

5. Many migraine patients try nonpharmacological treatment to manage their headaches before they begin or concurrently with drug therapy. Behavioral treatments are classified into three broad categories: relaxation training, biofeedback therapy, and cognitive-behavioral training (stress-management training). Physical treatment includes acupuncture, cervical manipulation, and mobilization therapy.

SOURCES

1. Silberstein, SD. For the US Headache Consortium. Practice Parameter: Evidence-based Guidelines for Migraine Headache (An Evidence-Based Review.) Report of the Quality Standards Subcommittee of the American Academy of Neurology. Neurology 55:754–762, September 2000.
2. The International Classification of Headache Disorders (2004), 2nd ed. Cephalalgia, 24(suppl 1):1–150.

23 Concussion Guidelines in Athletes

David Webner, MD

CONTENTS

INTRODUCTION

Sports, and specifically contact sports, have the potential for serious injury and it is vital to balance the risks of participation with the safety of the participants. It is the role of physicians and health care professionals, to be the objective and unbiased arbiter of decisions relating to the health of athletes under their care. It is the job of the medical staff to allow the participation and return to play of the athletes without compromising their health or safety.

The American Academy of Neurology (AAN) guidelines were based on 71 articles on concussion in athletics, and these consisted of class II (one or more well-developed clinical trials) and class III (expert opinion, unrandomized historical controls, or case studies) evidence *(1)*. A consensus was formulated based on the guidelines developed from the Colorado Medical Society, seminars given by faculty on sports-related concussions, and meetings by physicians and laypeople concerned with this issue. The ultimate goal was to develop guidelines that would help prevent morbidity and mortality related to structural brain

From: *Current Clinical Practice: Essential Practice Guidelines in Primary Care*
Edited by: N. S. Skolnik © Humana Press, Totowa, NJ

damage, second impact syndrome (rare cause of sudden death resulting from repeated concussion in an athlete who is not yet symptom free from the initial concussion), and long-term neurological sequelae from repeated concussions. Neurologists, neurosurgeons, sports medicine physicians, physiatrists, neuropsychologists, athletic trainers, and players all participated in the development of the following clinical guidelines in concussion management in sports.

DEFINITION

Concussion or mild traumatic brain injury is defined as a "trauma-induced altreration in mental status, with or without a loss of consciousness (LOC)." Symptoms can occur shortly after the injury or even minutes later. By closely monitoring the athlete, the medical professional can see the progression or resolution of the patient's concussion symptoms.

The observed features of concussions include a blank expression, inability to accurately answer basic questions and follow commands, difficulty with concentration and generalized confusion, lack of orientation to the surrounding environment, speech and coordination deficits, labile emotional states, memory loss, and at times LOC.

Concussion symptoms can be divided into early and late categories and the severity of the concussion is sometimes related to the length of symptomatology. Initial symptoms include headache, poor recognition of surrounding environment, nausea/vomiting, and vertigo. Symptoms seen days to even weeks later in more severe concussions include continued headaches, concentration deficits, lightheadedness, amnesia, easy fatigability, disrupted sleep–wake cycle, irritability, photo- and phonophobia, diplopia, tinnitus, anxiety, and depression.

GRADING

Concussion grading arrived at by the AAN was developed based on the previous Colorado Medical Society guidelines. There are three grading levels, the final of which is further subdivided into brief and prolonged LOC (Table 1).

Grade I concussion is characterized by transient confusion without LOC and symptoms/mental status changes (e.g., headache, poor concentration, verbal, and motor deficits) that resolve in less than 15 min. Grade I concussion has also been referred to in the literature and vernacular as a "ding" or having one's "bell rung." These milder forms of concussion may be more difficult to identify, given the temporary nature of the symptoms, and the reluctance of the athlete to report them.

Grade II concussion also includes the same symptoms and signs as grade I, but they are present for more than 15 min. In general, symptoms lasting longer than 1 h warrant closer medical attention and follow up.

Table 1
Concussion Grading and Return to Play Guidelines

Concussion	Definition	Return to play: first concussion[a]	Return to play: second concussion[a]
Grade I	No LOC Transient confusion Symptoms <15 min	Same game	1 wk
Grade II	No LOC Transient confusion Symptoms >15 min	1 wk	2 wk
Grade III	LOC Brief or prolonged	Brief: 1 wk Prolonged: 2 wk	1 mo or more (clinical discretion)

[a]Return to play time frame is period without signs or symptoms of concussion with complete rest. Athlete then resumes participation after a normal exercise challenge. LOC, loss of consciousness.

Grade III concussion is distinct from the previous grade by the presence of an LOC. The LOC may be either brief (seconds) or prolonged (minutes) and return-to-play recommendations in grade III injuries are based on this distinction.

SIDELINE ASSESSMENT

Prompt sideline identification of an athlete with concussion symptoms can be invaluable in preventing further injury. The basics of sideline examination include a mental status evaluation and brief neurological assessment. Mental status questions can be divided into three groups: orientation, concentration, and memory. The athlete should first be quizzed regarding time, place, person, and as to the nature of the event that had just occurred. Concentration can be tested using repetition and then reversal of three-, four-, and five-digit sequences and reciting the months backwards. Finally, memory function can be assessed by asking the athlete about current game details: score, play, and overall strategy. Long-term memory can include questions about previous games or current news events. Immediate and 5 min word and object recall is also a useful tool for the presence of post-retrograde amnesia (memory disturbances after the traumatic event).

A brief neurological exam may also be undertaken, especially if the athlete's symptoms fail to resolve quickly. Eyes are assessed by pupillary reaction and symmetry to light and accommodation. Coordination tests including finger–nose–finger testing, and tandem gait forwards and backwards. Sensation and proprioception ability is evaluated with Romberg and finger–nose testing with eyes closed.

All concussed athletes should have a sideline evaluation. In grade I injury, a neurological exam is not mandatory, unless clinically indicated. Athletes with a first grade I concussion need further exercise challenge evaluation on the sidelines in order to return to the game. This testing can be done with sideline sprints, cutting and pivoting, and push-ups/sit-ups. This testing must not produce a recurrence of the player's previously resolved concussion symptoms. Grade 2 and 3 concussion evaluation must include neurological examination. In addition, these athletes cannot return to play the same day under any circumstances.

RETURN-TO-PLAY GUIDELINES

The task of deciding if an athlete is able to resume competition/practice is especially important in concussion injuries. The following standards set up by the AAN are in place to give the health care professional a framework with which to base return-to-play issues (Table 1).

Athletes with their first grade I concussion are able to resume competition provided they have no recurrence of their symptoms after a sideline exercise challenge test. With a second grade I concussion in the same game, the recommendation is that the athlete must be removed from the contest, and may return after 1 wk of complete, asymptomatic rest, provided the exercise challenge does not cause a recurrence of symptomatology.

Grade II concussions are managed by removal of athlete from the field, performance of a complete sideline examination, with a follow-up examination by a health care professional in the next 24 h. Prior to clearance and return to play, a physician must perform a neurological examination of the athlete. If this is within normal limits, the athlete may return after 1 wk of asymptomatic rest and subsequent exercise challenge. A second grade II concussion mandates removal from the contest and return to athletic activity only after the patient is symptom-free at rest for at least 2 wk. General guidelines for head imaging (computed tomography [CT] or magnetic resonance imaging [MRI]) may also be important in athletes suffering a grade II concussion. If their symptoms persist for longer than 1 wk, or increase in intensity, imaging is indicated.

Grade II concussions are delineated by LOC. All athletes with concussion and alteration in consciousness need evaluation in the emergency department. If symptoms dictate, a neurological examination as well as head imaging is performed. The athlete should be admitted to the hospital if his or her symptoms do not improve or acutely worsen. An urgent neurosurgical consult should be obtained for worsening mental status changes, focal neurological deficits, or increasing severity of postconcussion symptoms.

Most athletes with a brief LOC will be discharged if their hospital and sideline evaluations are normal, but it is important to send them home with strict observation by their family/guardian.

Return to play after an initial grade III concussion when the LOC is brief dictates that the athlete be symptom-free for 1 wk at rest and then after an exercise challenge. When the first grade III concussion occurs with longer LOC, the athlete may return to play after 2 wk of symptom-free rest.

A second grade III concussion is followed by at least 1 mo of symptom-free rest, but clinical evaluation and history may dictate that the athlete be withheld from competition for the remaining of the current season. If the CT or MRI shows cerebral edema, hematoma, or additional intracranial pathology, then the athlete is not permitted to return to play for a full year and serious discussion regarding cessation of the contact sport should be undertaken.

ADDITIONAL CONCUSSION INFORMATION

Since the development of the AAN guidelines in 1997, there has been considerable research and further investigation in the field of concussion evaluation and management, and some of these highlights were touched on in a statement from the first International Conference on Concussion in Sport in Vienna in November 2001. The following information is from the summary statement in the *Clinical Journal of Sport Medicine* in January 2002 made by the Concussion in Sport Group (CISG) at the Vienna conference *(2)*.

NEUROPSYCHOLOGICAL TESTING

Over the past few years a number of neuropsychological assessment tools have been developed for use in athletes sustaining concussions. The tests that are written include standardized assessment of concussion and the McGill abbreviated concussion evaluation. Computer-based test examples are IMPACT, CogSport, ANAM, and Headminders.

The CISG commented that these tests were important for concussion evaluation, possibly contributing to understanding concussion injury in the future, and also helping to manage the athlete with a concussion. Baseline neurocognitive testing was recommended for athletes involved in contact sports, but also used the utility in athletes postconcussion who had not received baseline testing. Although the CISG did not make neurocognitive testing mandatory in managing a concussion, they did encourage its use.

FUTURE RESEARCH

The CISG also commented on current and future research ideas in concussion assessment, predisposing factors, and brain function after concussion. The contemporary research includes electroencephalogram assessment, showing reproducible abnormalities in postconcussive states, biochemical blood markers (S-100, neuron-specific enolase, and myelin basic protein), which are markers of neuron cell damage, and genetic phenotyping. The latter involves the ApoE4 gene abnormality, whose presence has been shown to be a risk factor for worse outcomes after moderate to severe head injury. Additionally, researches looking at the various impact forces received/transmitted during a concussion are being studied, with the hopes of understanding more about the pathogenesis of the injury.

PREVENTION AND EDUCATION

Finally, the CISG discussed the various equipment protective devices that have been implemented and should be used in the prevention of brain injury. The most effective interventions thus far have been helmets and the application of rule changes that prohibit blows to the head in many contact sports. They also stressed the importance of continuing to educate athletes, parents, and coaches alike with teaching videos, outreach lectures, support groups, and endorsement by professional sports organizations to make identification and treatment of concussion an important part of contact sports participation.

SOURCES

1. American Academy of Neurology: Practice parameter (1997) The management of concussion in sports (summary statement). Neurology 48:581–585.
2. Summary and Agreement Statement of the First International Conference on Concussion in Sport, Vienna 2001. Clin J Sport Med 12(1):6–11, January 2002.

24 Restless Legs Syndrome

Mathew Clark, MD

CONTENTS

INTRODUCTION

Restless legs syndrome (RLS) has been called "the most common disorder that is never heard of." Although most primary care physicians have developed at least a passing familiarity with RLS in recent years, it remains true that this condition is very much underdiagnosed and undertreated. In an effort to promote more widespread awareness of RLS in the medical community and to share up-to-date knowledge regarding management of this condition, several guidelines, updates, and management algorithms have been published. These are summarized next.

DESCRIPTION

RLS has four essential diagnostic features:

1. An urge to move the legs, usually accompanied by uncomfortable sensations.
2. The urge to move or uncomfortable sensations that begin during periods of rest or inactivity.
3. These sensations are partially or totally—but temporarily—relieved by movement.
4. Symptoms are worse in the evening or at night.

These symptoms may be infrequent, or they may be nearly constant, persisting throughout the day. Symptoms may be quite mild, and only noticeable in

From: *Current Clinical Practice: Essential Practice Guidelines in Primary Care*
Edited by: N. S. Skolnik © Humana Press, Totowa, NJ

certain situations, or they may be experienced as intense and nearly unbearable. Affected patients typically have trouble with sedentary activities, such as sitting through meetings, being a passenger on a long trip, or going to the theater. Insomnia is often a significant problem when the combination of inactivity and time of day may make initiation of sleep very difficult.

Although RLS is by definition a condition that is experienced only during wakefulness, many patients with RLS also experience a related phenomenon, periodic leg movements of sleep (PLMS). PLMS condition causes stereotypical contractions of the legs as the patient sleeps. These contractions are often of sufficient intensity and frequency to significantly disrupt sleep. Accordingly, patients with RLS and PLMS often have trouble with both the initiation and maintenance of sleep, leading to significant daytime sleepiness and fatigue (1–3).

EPIDEMIOLOGY

In the United States, between 5 and 10% of the adult population experiences symptoms of RLS. Not all of these individuals will experience symptoms of sufficient frequency or intensity to warrant treatment. Symptoms tend to become more common with advancing age, and are more common in elderly patients than in young adults. There is a family history of RLS in two-thirds of affected patients.

Most cases of RLS are idiopathic; the cause of these symptoms is currently not well understood. There are some conditions in which RLS is seen with greater frequency. Iron deficiency—even at levels insufficient to cause anemia—is associated with more frequent symptoms of RLS. Pregnancy is associated with RLS, with 19% of pregnant women reporting some symptoms; about one-third of these women describe their symptoms as "severe." Patients with renal failure often experience RLS; studies have reported a prevalence of 20–57% in this population.

DIAGNOSIS

Diagnosis of RLS is by history. Patients should experience all four of the listed diagnostic criteria: the urge to move accompanied by dysesthesias, symptoms brought on at rest, relieved by movement, and worse in the evening or night. There is no role for a polysomnogram in diagnosing RLS, although this may be helpful in diagnosing PLMS. Iron status should be assessed. A serum ferritin is the recommended test; levels less than 50 are associated with a greater prevalence of RLS symptoms, even in the absence of anemia.

TREATMENT

Nonpharmacological

Not all patients with RLS require treatment with medications. Recommended nonpharmacological measures include the following:

- Replacement of iron, if iron deficiency is documented.
- Mental alerting activities, such as video games or crossword puzzles, at times of boredom/physical inactivity.
- Trial of abstinence from alcohol, nicotine, and caffeine.
- Trial of avoidance of medications with potential to worsen RLS symptoms. These medications include antidepressants (except buproprion), neuroleptic agents, dopamine-blocking antiemetics (such as metoclopramide), and sedating antihistamines.

Medications

The following classes of medications have demonstrated efficacy in treating RLS symptoms:

- *Dopaminergic medications:* Medications in this class include levodopa/carbidopa combinations (Sinemet) and the dopamine agonists (DA) such as pergolide (Permax), ropinirole (Requip), and pramipexole (Mirapex). Balancing their excellent track record in relieving RLS symptoms is a tendency to develop unacceptable side effects. These include augmentation (the development of RLS symptoms earlier in the day after a bedtime dose of medication) and rebound (a wearing off of medication with an increased intensity of symptoms). Approximately 70% of patients taking regular levodopa/carbidopa will develop augmentation or rebound. This statistic is considerably smaller for those using DA.
- *Opioids:* Even weak opioids such as codeine or propoxyphene may be helpful in RLS, as may the opioid agonist tramadol. Higher potency opioids such as hydrocodone, oxycodone, or methadone are often helpful in more severe cases when weaker opioids are ineffective. Concerns about side effects and dependence make this a second-line option in most algorithms, yet this class of medications has been shown to maintain efficacy over long periods without a need for dose escalation.
- *Anticonvulsants:* These includes both carbamazepine and gabapentin, which are effective in treating RLS. Use of these agents may be limited by concerns about cost and side effects. They may be particularly helpful in situations involving neuropathy or a painful quality to the RLS symptoms.
- *Benzodiazepines:* These agents have demonstrated efficacy in RLS, particularly in patients for whom sleep-onset insomnia is a primary concern. Use of these medications is limited by concerns about dependence, tolerance, and daytime drowsiness.
- *Clonidine and magnesium:* These medications have demonstrated efficacy in small trials. No specific recommendation is currently made regarding their use.

MANAGEMENT OF RESTLESS LEGS SYNDROME

For purposes of management, the algorithm of the Medical Advisory Board of the RLS Foundation divides RLS into *intermittent, daily*, and *refractory* types.

Intermittent RLS

Patients with *intermittent* RLS have symptoms that are troublesome enough, when present, to require treatment, but that do not occur frequently enough to necessitate daily treatment. Recommendations, in addition to nonpharmacological measures, include the intermittent use of the following medications:

- Carbidopa/levodopa, 25/100 (0.5–1 tablet) or controlled-release (CR) 25/100 (1 tablet) can be used at bedtime or for RLS associated with specific activities, such as airplane or lengthy car rides.
- DA. The nonergot DAs (ropinirole or pramipexole) appear to have fewer troublesome side effects. Because these medications take 90–120 min to begin working, they are of limited usefulness once symptoms have begun.
- Low-potency opioids or opioid agonists, such as propoxyphene (65–200 mg), codeine (30–60 mg), or tramadol (50–100 mg).
- Benzodiazepines or benzodiazepine agonists (temazepam, triazolam, zolpidem, and zaleplon).

Daily RLS

Patients in this category have RLS that is frequent and troublesome enough to require daily therapy. Recommendations, in addition to nonpharmacological measures, include use of the following medications:

- DA are the drugs of choice in most patients with *daily* RLS. Pramipexole (Mirapex) is normally given as 0.125 mg once daily, taken 2 h before major RLS symptoms usually start. This dose may be increased by 0.125 mg for every 2–3 d until symptoms are relieved. Most patients need 0.5 mg or less; doses up to 2 mg may be needed. Ropinirole (Requip) is dosed at 0.25 mg daily, also 2 h before symptoms, and increased by 0.25 mg for every 2–3 d as needed. Most patients require 2 mg or less; doses up to 4 mg may be needed.
- Gabapentin may be an alternative choice, particularly when symptoms are painful as described earlier. The treatment is usually once or twice daily, given late in the afternoon or before sleep. Dosing may start at 100–300 mg per dose; mean daily doses of 1300–1800 mg were used in one trial.
- Low-potency opioids (e.g., codeine or propoxyphene) or tramadol may be an alternative choice.

Refractory RLS

Patients with *refractory* RLS symptoms have daily RLS treated with a DA with one or more of the following: inadequate initial response despite adequate doses, response that has become inadequate with time, intolerable adverse effects, augmentation that is not controllable with additional earlier doses of the drug. In addition to the following approaches, referral to a RLS specialist should be considered:

- Change to gabapentin.
- Change to a different DA.
- Add gabapentin, a benzodiazepine, or an opioid.
- Change to a high-potency opioid (oxycodone 5–15 mg), hydrocodone (5–15 mg), methadone (5–10 mg), or tramadol (50–100 mg).

No specific recommendations address the treatment of RLS in pregnant women or children.

SOURCES

1. Hening W, Allen R, Earley C, Kushida C, Picchietti D, Silber M (1999) The treatment of restless legs syndrome and periodic limb movement disorder: an American Academy of Sleep Medicine Review. Sleep 22:970–999.
2. Hening WA, Allen RP, Earley CJ, Picchietti DL, Silber MH (2004) Restless Legs Syndrome Task Force of the Standards of Practice Committee of the American Academy of Sleep Medicine. An update on the dopaminergic treatment of restless legs syndrome and periodic limb movement disorder. Sleep 27:560–583.
3. Silber MH, Ehrenberg BL, Allen RP, et al. (2004) Medical Advisory Boards of the Restless Legs Syndrome Foundation. An algorithm for the management of restless legs syndrome. Mayo Clin Proc 79(7):916–922.

VII PSYCHIATRY

25   Depression

Pharmacological Treatment

John E. Sutherland, MD

CONTENTS

DIAGNOSES

Major depression is a clinical syndrome lasting at least up to 2 wk, during which the patient experiences either depressed mood or anhedonia (a decrease in interest in things that used to give pleasure) with at least five of the following nine symptoms:

- Depressed mood.
- Anhedonia.
- Appetite disturbance.
- Sleep disturbance.
- Fatigue.
- Psychomotor retardation or agitation.
- Poor self-image or guilt.
- Concentration impairment.
- Suicidal ideation.

EPIDEMIOLOGY

In the United States, the prevalence of depression is about 3% and the life-time incidence is about 17%. The pervasiveness and incidence is approximately

From: *Current Clinical Practice: Essential Practice Guidelines in Primary Care*
Edited by: N. S. Skolnik © Humana Press, Totowa, NJ

twice as common in women as compared with men. Major depression is the fourth leading cause of worldwide disease burden. Depression is seen more frequently than any other disorder except hypertension. Multiple risk factors include family history, substance abuse, chronic illness, chronic pain, adolescence, and advancing age.

NATURAL HISTORY AND PROGNOSIS

An untreated episode of depression usually lasts for about 6 mo or longer. About 50% of patients have a second episode, and a second episode increases the risk of a third episode to 80%. Episodes become longer and more frequent with age. About 15% of severely depressed patients might commit suicide. Outpatient treatment of depression has markedly increased in the United States. Nearly half of all patients stop taking their antidepressant medication within 1 mo of treatment.

THERAPEUTIC OPTIONS AND REFERRAL

Four types of therapy have proven efficacy for depressive disorders: pharmacotherapy, psychotherapy, electroconvulsive therapy, and herbal and nutritional products. Most patients can be treated as outpatients, but inpatient care is recommended for seriously depressed or suicidal patients. Psychiatrist referral is indicated with suicidal ideation, severe depression, aggressive ideation, bipolar disorder, atypical depression, psychotic depression, substance abuse, or treatment resistance.

Pharmacotherapy

Multiple antidepressants are available that exert their therapeutic and adverse effects through three chemical monamine neurotransmission systems (i.e., by increasing the levels of norepinephrine, serotonin, or dopamine in the synapse); and by resultant secondary changes in presynaptic and postsynaptic receptor physiology. Many trials have shown all the categories to be equally efficacious. Selection of antidepressant agents is based in part on such criteria as anticipated tolerance and adverse effects. Newer agents such as the selective serotonin reuptake inhibitors (SSRIs), serotonin and norepinephrine reuptake inhibitors, and dopamine reuptake inhibitors have simpler dosage schedules, different adverse effect profiles, and less likelihood of overdose deaths compared with older tricyclic antidepressants (TCAs) and monamine oxidase inhibitors (MAOIs). Theoretically, choosing a drug is made easier by matching either patient's symptoms to likely medication side effects or by knowing whether the patient or family member responded favorably to a particular antidepressant in the past. Choosing a well-tolerated drug might enhance patient adherence, which will improve the likelihood of achieving and maintaining a full remission *(1,2)*.

RECOMMENDATIONS AND TREATMENT STRATEGY

Physicians should consider treating for acute major depression, including elderly patients without significant combined comorbid conditions, with either TCAs or newer antidepressants, such as SSRIs, as equally efficacious. Antidepressant therapy should be started promptly when depression is diagnosed. The initial dosage should be maintained for at least 3–4 wk before it is increased. A trial of 6–8 wk at the maximum tolerated dosage is necessary to confirm the success or failure of the treatment. Usually an improvement in symptoms will not be noted until after 2–6 wk of therapy. The response rate to initial treatment is only 50–60%, but more than 80% of depressed patients will respond to at least one medication.

The physician with patient input should review the adverse drug profiles so that an agent that fits the clinical needs of the patient can be chosen.

(Note the following, identified in brackets, is not from the guidelines but deemed useful in treatment of patients, from ref. *3*).

For the patient whose depression has specific components, common side effects of drugs can be used to fit the clinical profile:

- With generalized anxiety, agitation, and insomnia, mirtazapine and trazodone are beneficial.
- With desired weight gain, mirtazapine is indicated.
- With a tobacco cessation goal, bupropion is preferred.
- With hypersomnia, cognitive slowing, retarded depression, and pseuodementia, bupropion or venlafaxine are beneficial.
- With more severe depression, moderate-to-high dose venlafaxine, TCAs, or mirtazapine are useful.
- With diabetic neuropathy, duloxetine is indicated.

Specific drugs should be avoided in certain patient profiles:

- With hypersomnia and motor retardation, avoid mirtazapine and trazodone.
- With obesity, mirtazapine and TCAs are not preferred.
- With sexual dysfunction preceding depression, avoid SSRIs and venlafaxine.
- With agitation and insomnia, avoid bupropion and venlafaxine.
- With a seizure disorder, bupropion is contraindicated.
- With hypertension, venlafaxine is relatively contraindicated.

Antidepressant medication should be continued at least 4 mo beyond initial recovery or improvement to decrease the probability of short-term relapse. If full remission is achieved, 6–12 mo of continued pharmacotherapy at the same dose is recommended as it decreases the risk of relapse by 70%. Follow-up visits after remission can be tapered gradually to every 3 mo. Discontinuation of therapy should be done gradually to minimize withdrawal reactions.

If at 6 wk a patient shows no response or a poor response to an adequate dose of antidepressant medication, treatment should be changed. Choices have evolved more by anecdote than by systematic study. It is uncertain whether a change of drug classes or within classes is most effective. The benefits of switching patients to another category and to switch medications within a category have both been demonstrated. Adding a second depressant from a category with a different mechanism of action often enhances clinical efficacy and has been demonstrated. (Note: not explicitly as a part of guidelines. A great deal of evidence supports the use of lithium augmentation. Other augmentation options that have been proven useful include buspirone, triiodothyronine, antipsychotics, and anticonvulsants. For refractory or atypical depression in motivated and compliant patients, monamine oxidase inhibitors might be useful.)

Psychotherapy With Pharmacotherapy

Combining pharmacotherapy and psychotherapy can be more effective than either modality alone. This has been shown with a variety of methods in different settings, both with initial treatment for patients with persistent symptoms and in prevention of relapse. Primary care physicians can also incorporate counseling as adjunctive therapy.

Herbal and Nutritional Products

St. John's Wort (*Hypericum perforatum* L) has been demonstrated to be more effective than placebo for the short-term treatment of mild and moderate depression. Minimal efficacy has been demonstrated in moderately severe depression. This treatment is not approved by the US Food and Drug Administration and preparations may vary substantially from those in randomized trials. St. John's Wort is well tolerated.

Omega-3 fatty acids and *S*-adenosyl-L methionine have both been demonstrated to have possible efficacy in the treatment of depression.

(Note: author's opinion not explicitly addressed in the guidelines. Exercise may play an important role in relieving depression. Evidence of efficacy is limited but promising enough to consider implementation in clinical practice.)

CONCLUSIONS

Acute major depression is a common and debilitating illness. An accurate and early diagnosis is important. Referral to a psychiatrist is important in severe cases and with suicidal ideation. All available antidepressants are equally efficacious. Selecting a medication by matching its side-effect profile to patient characteristics is supported by case reports and likely enhances compliance. Although many patients settle for partial improvement, the goal of the treatment should be complete remission. Patients whose symptoms do not improve with therapy should be switched to a different monotherapy or multiple drugs. Once full remission has been achieved, 4–12 mo of continued pharmacotherapy of the same dose is recommended as it decreases the risk of relapse. Discontinuation of therapy should be done gradually to minimize withdrawal reactions. Nearly half of the patients stop taking their antidepressant prescription medication within the 1 mo of treatment. Education of patients regarding daily dosing, delayed onset of effect, side effects, and dose titration is very important. Future studies are necessary on functional status, quality of life, relapse prevention, long-term maintenance, and combine pharmacotherapy and psychotherapy.

SOURCES

1. Snow V, Lascher S, Mottur-Pilson C (2000) For the American College of Physicians— American Society of Internal Medicine Pharmacological treatment of acute major depression and dysthymia: clinical guideline, Part 1. Ann Intern Med 132:743–756.
2. Williams JW, Jr, Mulrow CD, Chiquette E, Noel P, et al. (2000) A systematic review of newer pharmacotherapies for depression in adults: evidence report summary: clinical guidelines, Part 2. Ann Intern Med 132:743–756.
3. Sutherland JE, Sutherland SJ, Hoehns JD (2003) Achieving the best outcome in treatment of depression. J Fam Pract 52:201–209.

26

Diagnosis, Evaluation, and Treatment of the School-Aged Child With Attention Deficit Hyperactivity Disorder

Richard Neill, MD

CONTENTS

INTRODUCTION

Two guidelines issued by the subcommittee on attention deficit hyperactivity disorder (ADHD) of the Committee on Quality Improvement for the American Academy of Pediatrics provide guidance for primary care clinicians interested in diagnosing and treating ADHD in school aged children. The 11 recommendations in these two guidelines encompass the spectrum of care for children suspected of or diagnosed with ADHD in the primary care setting.

The guidelines were developed using well-defined methodology for evidence review and included collaboration with interested primary care and specialty groups. Three levels of evidence (good, fair, and poor) and three levels of recommendations (strong, fair, and weak) reflect the data and consensus underlying each recommendation. Clinical options are made where the evidence or consensus supports multiple potential management paths. The guidelines were developed and issued over overlapping development cycles of 2 and 3 yr, respectively, from 1997 to 2001. Ongoing review and updated resources related to these two guidelines can be found at the American Academy of Pediatrics website *(1–3)*.

From: *Current Clinical Practice: Essential Practice Guidelines in Primary Care*
Edited by: N. S. Skolnik © Humana Press, Totowa, NJ

DIAGNOSIS AND EVALUATION OF THE CHILD WITH ADHD

Recommendation 1: In a child 6–12 yr old who presents with inattention, hyperactivity, impulsivity, academic underachievement, or behavior problems, primary care clinicians should initiate an evaluation for ADHD (strength of evidence: good; strength of recommendation: strong).

The high prevalence of ADHD in school-aged children requires vigilance on the part of clinicians. Presentations of ADHD may vary widely, including many behaviors not evident to the clinician observing children in an office setting. Common presentations include referral from school for academic underachievement and failure, disruptive classroom behavior, inattentiveness, problems with social relationships, parental concerns regarding similar phenomena, poor self-esteem, or problems with establishing or maintaining social relationships.

The following questions may be useful at visits for school-aged children as an initial screen for ADHD or as a measure of school performance.

1. How is your child doing in school?
2. Are there any problems with learning that you or the teacher has seen?
3. Is your child happy in school?
4. Are you concerned with any behavioral problems in school, at home, or when your child is playing with friends?
5. Is your child having problems completing class work or homework?

Recommendation 2: The diagnosis of ADHD requires that a child meet *Diagnostic and Statistical Manual* (DSM-IV) criteria (strength of evidence: good; strength of recommendation: strong). DSM-IV identifies three types of ADHD based on the predominance of symptoms in three domains: inattention, hyperactivity, and impulsivity. Importantly, symptoms must be present in two or more settings (e.g., home and school) and the behaviors must adversely affect function in school or social settings for a diagnosis of ADHD to be made. DSM-IV criteria are listed in Table 1.

Problems with using DSM-IV criteria for the diagnosis of ADHD include its development and testing in psychiatric rather than primary care settings, its lack of accounting for gender-based differences or developmental variations in behavior, and inherent subjectivity in behavior interpretation.

Recommendations 3 and 4 are parallel guidelines for behavior observation in the home and school settings, respectively. For this reason, they are discussed together.

Recommendation 3: The assessment of ADHD requires evidence directly obtained from parents or caregivers regarding the core symptoms of ADHD in various settings, the age of onset, duration of symptoms, and degree of functional impairment (strength of evidence: good; strength of recommendation: strong).

Recommendation 4: The assessment of ADHD requires evidence directly obtained from the classroom teacher (or other school professional) regarding the core symptoms of ADHD, the duration of symptoms, the degree of functional impairment, and coexisting conditions. The physician should review any reports from a school-based multidisciplinary evaluation, where they exist, which will include assessments from the teacher or other school-based professional (strength of evidence: good; strength of recommendation: strong). Behavior rating may be performed by parents or guardians using a variety of methods including open-ended questions, focused questions about specific behaviors, semistructured interviews, questionnaires, or rating scales. Regardless of the method used to obtain data, behavior should focus on evaluation of DSM-IV domains of attentiveness, hyperactivity, and impulsivity. A global impression of behavior within any domain is insufficient.

Because the diagnosis of ADHD requires observation of behaviors in more than one setting, school-based observations are critically important. Because teachers have the most contact with children, they are the logical observer in school. As with home observation, a variety of methods of teacher reporting are acceptable.

Children who are home-schooled or who spend a significant portion of their day in nonschool settings (such as day care), should have their behaviors monitored in at least one other non-home setting.

Recommendation 3A: Use of scales is a clinical option when evaluating children for ADHD (strength of evidence: strong; strength of recommendation: strong).

Recommendation 4A: Use of these scales is a clinical option when diagnosing children for ADHD (strength of evidence: strong; strength of recommendation: strong). Specific behavior rating scales for use by parents or teachers to monitor specific behaviors within the three domains of ADHD have been shown to have modest ability to differentiate children with ADHD from normal, age-matched community controls. However, most of these have been validated in ideal circumstances. As a result, their performance in less than ideal circumstances is likely less predictive of ADHD. The behaviors observed are also subject to observer bias. All these issues reinforce the notion that results from any behavior rating scale should be interpreted within the overall clinical setting.

Commonly used behavior rating scales include the Connors Teacher (or Parent) Behavior Rating Scale or Barkley's School Situations Questionnaire. Whether these scales provide additional benefit beyond narratives or descriptive interviews informed by DSM-IV criteria is not known.

Recommendation 3B: Use of broadband scales is not recommended in the diagnosis of children for ADHD, although they might be useful for other purposes (strength of evidence: strong; strength of recommendation: strong).

Recommendation 4B: Use of teacher global questionnaires and rating scales is not recommended in the diagnosing of children for ADHD, although they might be useful for other purposes (strength of evidence: strong; strength of recommendation: strong). Behavior rating scales that measure global behavior do not distinguish well between children with and without ADHD. Additional

Table 1
DSM-IV Diagnostic Criteria for ADHD

A. Either 1 or 2

(1) Six (or more) of the following symptoms of inattention have persisted for at least
6 mo to a degree that is maladaptive and inconsistent with developmental level:

Inattention

   (a) Often fails to give close attention to details or makes careless mistakes
       in schoolwork, work, or other activities

   (b) Often has difficulty sustaining attention in tasks or play activities

   (c) Often does not seem to listen when spoken to directly

   (d) Often does not follow through on instructions and fails to finish school-
       work, chores, or duties in the workplace (not because of oppositional
       behavior or failure to understand instructions)

   (e) Often has difficulty organizing tasks and activities

   (f) Often avoids, dislikes, or is reluctant to engage in tasks that require
       sustained mental effort (such as schoolwork or homework)

   (g) Often loses things necessary for tasks or activities (e.g., toys, school
       assignments, pencils, books, or tools)

   (h) Is often easily distracted by extraneous stimuli

   (i) Is often forgetful in daily activities

(2) Six (or more) of the following symptoms of hyperactivity-impulsivity have
persisted for at least 6 mo to a degree that is maladaptive and inconsistent with
developmental level:

Hyperactivity

   (a) Often fidgets with hands or feet or squirms in seat

   (b) Often leaves seat in classroom or in other situations in which remaining
       seated is expected

   (c) Often runs about or climbs excessively in situations in which it is
       inappropriate (in adolescents or adults, may be limited to subjective
       feelings of restlessness)

   (d) Often has difficulty playing or engaging in leisure activities quietly

   (e) Is often "on the go" or often acts as if "driven by a motor"

   (f) Often talks excessively

Impulsivity

   (a) Often blurts out answers before questions have been completed

   (b) Often has difficulty awaiting turn

   (c) Often interrupts or intrudes on others (e.g., butts into conversations or games)

(Continued)

Table 1 *(Continued)*

B. Some hyperactive-impulsive or inattentive symptoms that caused impairment were present before 7 yr of age

C. Some impairment from the symptoms is present in two or more settings (e.g., at school [or work] or at home)

D. There must be clear evidence of clinically significant impairment in social, academic, or occupational functioning

E. The symptoms do not occur exclusively during the course of a pervasive developmental disorder, schizophrenia, or other psychotic disorder and are not better accounted for by another mental disorder (e.g., mood disorder, anxiety disorder, dissociative disorder, or personality disorder)

Code based on type:

314.01 Attention deficit hyperactivity disorder, combined type: if both criteria A1 and A2 are met for the past 6 mo

314.00 Attention deficit hyperactivity disorder, predominantly inattentive type: if criterion A1 is met but criterion A2 is not met for the past 6 mo

314.01 Attention deficit hyperactivity disorder, predominantly hyperactive, impulsive type: if criterion A2 is met but criterion A1 is not met for the past 6 mo

314.9 Attention deficit hyperactivity disorder not otherwise specified

research is needed to determine whether they are useful in differentiating other behavior disorders in the setting of ADHD. As a result their use in the diagnosis of ADHD is discouraged.

Discrepancies in behavior reporting between home, school, or other settings can and does occur in either direction and do not preclude a diagnosis of ADHD. In some instances observation from additional settings can shed light on discrepancies.

Recommendation 5: Evaluation of the child with ADHD should include assessment for coexisting conditions (strength of evidence: strong; strength of recommendation: strong). A diagnosis of ADHD requires assessment for (although not exclusion of) other psychological and medical comorbidities such as oppositional defiant disorder, mood disorders, anxiety disorders, and learning disabilities. The coexistence of ADHD and of these individual conditions ranges from estimates of 35% for oppositional-defiant or conduct disorders and 18% for mood disorders.

Diagnostic features separating ADHD from oppositional-defiant or conduct disorders include in the latter two, a pattern of negativistic, defiant, or disobedient behaviors, outright violations of the basic rights of others, or major age-appropriate social norms or rules are violated. These conditions may be more highly associated with ADHD with predominant hyperactivity-impulsivity behaviors.

Assessment of mood or anxiety symptoms through history can be adequate to establish one of these diagnoses. A family history of mood or anxiety disorders is common in children with either of these conditions.

Rates of learning disabilities that coexist with ADHD in settings other than primary care have been reported to range from 12 to 60%. Unfortunately, there is little data on their coexistence in the primary care setting.

Recommendation 6: Other diagnostic tests are not routinely indicated to establish the diagnosis of ADHD (strength of evidence: strong; strength of recommendation: strong). There is no evidence to support the use of thyroid, lead, or other blood work or imaging studies on an indiscriminate basis. Continuous performance tests of vigilance or distractibility have been studied but found to have low odds ratios for differentiating ADHD from normal children.

TREATMENT OF CHILDREN WITH ADHD

Recommendation 1: Primary care clinicians should establish a management program that recognizes ADHD as a chronic condition (strength of evidence: good; strength of recommendation: strong). The high prevalence of ADHD in primary care settings means clinicians will see children with ADHD. Therefore, they should have a strategy in place for diagnosis and management that includes attention to the principles of care for children with chronic illness like ADHD, such as the following:

- Provide information about the condition.
- Update and monitor family knowledge and understanding on a periodic basis.
- Counsel about family response to the condition.
- Provide developmentally appropriate education to the child about ADHD, with updates as the child grows.
- Be available to answer family questions.
- Ensure coordination of health and other services.
- Help families set specific goals in areas related to the child's condition and its effects on daily activities.
- Link families with other families that have children with similar chronic conditions as needed and as available.

A comprehensive care plan for the child with ADHD is likely to improve parent and child adherence to treatment recommendations. Care provided within the context of a supportive environment that includes community-based resources outside the physician's office increases the likelihood of thorough family understanding of the condition, treatment options, and common concerns. Physicians should be aware of community resources and know how to make referrals when needed to ensure the family's access to the needed information.

Recommendation 2: The treating clinician, parents, and the child, in collaboration with school personnel, should specify appropriate target outcomes to guide management (strength of evidence: good; strength of recommendation: strong).

The primary goal of ADHD treatment is minimizing dysfunction arising from impulsive, hyperactive, or inattentive behaviors. Focusing on three to six behaviors and desired changes prior to initiation of treatment improves chances for success at treatment. Behaviors might be identified within a number of functional areas:

- Improvements in relationships with parents, siblings, teachers, and peers.
- Decreased disruptive behaviors.
- Improved academic performance, particularly in volume of work efficiency, completion, and accuracy.
- Increased independence in self-care or homework.
- Improved self-esteem.
- Enhanced safety in the community, such as crossing streets or riding bicycles. Target outcomes should follow from the key symptoms that the child manifests and the specific impairments caused by these symptoms.

The goals should be realistic, attainable, and measurable. The methods of treatment and monitoring change will vary as a function of the target outcomes.

Recommendation 3: The clinician should recommend stimulant medication (strength of evidence: good) and/or behavior therapy (strength of evidence: fair), as appropriate, to improve target outcomes in children with ADHD (strength of recommendation: strong).

Both stimulant medication and behavioral intervention have been shown to improve outcomes.

Stimulant Medication

Core symptoms of hyperactivity, inattentiveness, and impulsivity are improved by appropriate stimulant use. Effects on achievement or intelligence tests are more modest.

Methylphenidate and dextroamphetamine (short, intermediate, and long-acting versions of each) are the most commonly used stimulants, with no clinical difference seen between them in effectiveness or side effects among groups. Individual children, however, may show differential responses to one compared with the other. Pemoline, a long-acting stimulant, is rarely used now because of its rare but potentially fatal hepatotoxicity. Methylphenidate and dextroamphetamine require no serological, hematological, or electrocardiogram monitoring in otherwise healthy children.

Tricyclic antidepressants and bupropion have also been studied for use in ADHD with effects comparable to stimulants; however, their use is recommended as a second-line agent after stimulant use owing to the higher risk of adverse events in children.

Stimulant dosages are not weight-dependent, therefore, clinicians should begin with a low dose of medication and titrate upward, recognizing that the first dose at which a response is achieved may not be the best dose to improve function. Dosing schedules vary depending on target outcomes, allowing for 5- or 7-d schedules as well as single or multiple dosing on any individual day. The best dose of medication for a given child is the one that leads to optimal effects with minimal side effects.

Common side effects from stimulants tend to occur early and are short-lived, including jitteriness, decreased appetite, stomach ache, headache, delayed sleep onset, or social withdrawal. Most can be managed with dose or schedule adjustment. Stimulants should be used with caution in children with seizure disorders or those who are on other chronic medications. Concerns over growth delay with stimulant use have proved ill-founded. Many clinicians continue to recommend summer "medication holidays," although their benefit is unclear.

Recommendation 3A: If stimulant is prescribed and it does not work at the highest feasible dose, the clinician should recommend another.

About 80% of children will respond to a stimulant if tried in systematic fashion. Children who fail to respond to one stimulant often have a positive response to alternative stimulants. Those who fail two stimulants can be tried on a third type or formulation, although as indicated in recommendation 4, lack of response to treatment should lead the clinician to assess the diagnosis and/or the possibility of undiagnosed coexisting conditions.

Behavior Therapy

Several techniques have been studied and shown to be effective at minimizing ADHD behaviors, although not always to the point of normal function in school and social settings (*see* Table 2). Behavioral interventions are distinct from psychological interventions that attempt to address the child's emotional status (i.e., via play therapy) or thought patterns (i.e., via cognitive-behavior therapy).

Where available, clinicians should offer or refer parents for training in behavioral therapy techniques. Schools may sometimes offer parent training as part of educational rehabilitation services or may recommend an individual education plan. Use of behavioral therapies in the classroom and monitoring through periodic reports can guide treatment based on agreed on behavioral outcomes.

Recommendation 4: When the selected management for a child with ADHD has not met target outcomes, clinicians should evaluate the original diagnosis, use of all appropriate treatments, adherence to the treatment plan, and presence of coexisting conditions (strength of evidence: weak; strength of recommendation: strong). A lack of response to treatment may reflect (1) unrealistic target symptoms; (2) lack of information about the child's behavior; (3) an incorrect diagnosis; (4) a coexisting condition affecting the treatment of the ADHD; (5) lack of adherence to the treatment regimen; or (6) a treatment failure.

Table 2
Effective Behavioral Techniques for Children
With Attention Deficit Hyperactivity Disorder

Technique	Description	Example
Positive reinforcement	Providing rewards or privileges contingent on the child's performance	Child completes an assignment and is permitted to play on the computer
Time out	Child hits sibling impulsively and is required to sit for 5 min in the corner of the room	Removing access to positive reinforcement contingent on performance of unwanted or problem behavior
Response cost	Withdrawing rewards or or privileges contingent on the performance of unwanted or problem behavior	Child loses free time privileges for not completing homework
Token economy	Combining positive reinforcement and response cost. The child earns rewards and privileges contingent on performing desired behaviors and loses the rewards and privileges based on undesirable behavior	Child earns stars for completing assignments and loses stars for getting out of seat. The child cashes in the sum of stars at the end of the week for a prize

As discussed previously, treatment of ADHD, while decreasing a child's level of impairment, may not fully eliminate the core symptoms of inattention, hyperactivity, and impulsivity. Similarly, children with ADHD may continue to have difficulties with peer relationships despite adequate treatment, and treatment for ADHD frequently shows no association with improvements in academic achievement as measured by standardized instruments.

Evaluation of treatment outcomes requires a careful collection of information from appropriate sources, including parents, teachers, other adults in the child's environment (e.g., coaches), and the child. Re-evaluation for coexisting conditions, assessment of reasons for nonadherence (e.g., side effects, cost, perceived lack of response) and consideration of true treatment failure should all occur.

Recommendation 5: The clinician should periodically provide a systematic follow-up for the child with ADHD. Monitoring should be directed to target outcomes and adverse effects by obtaining specific information from parents, teachers, and the child (strength of evidence: fair; strength of recommendation: strong).

A comprehensive plan for monitoring therapy including measures of targeted outcomes, medication side effects, and communicating with parents and teachers at periodic intervals can improve the likelihood of treatment success. The frequency of monitoring will vary depending on stage of treatment, degree of dysfunction, complications, and adherence. Changes in educational or home expectations of performance will also influence monitoring of treatment. Once stable, an office visit every 3–6 mo allows for assessment of learning and behavior.

SOURCES

1. Committee on Quality Improvement and Subcommittee on Attention-Deficit/Hyperactivity Disorder (2000) *Clinical Practice Guideline: Diagnosis and Evaluation of the Child with Attention-Deficit/Hyperactivity Disorder.* Pediatrics 105:1158–1170.
2. Subcommittee on Attention-Deficit/Hyperactivity Disorder and Committee on Quality Improvement (2001) *Clinical Practice Guideline: Treatment of the School-Aged Child With Attention-Deficit/Hyperactivity Disorder.* Pediatrics 108:1033–1044.
3. Diagnosis and Evaluation of ADHD http://www.pediatrics.org/cgi/content/full/105/5/1158. Treatment of School Age Children with ADHD http://www.pediatrics.org/cgi/content/full/108/4/1033.

27 Practice Guidelines for the Treatment of Patients With Delirium

Mary Hofmann, MD, FACP
and Doron Schneider, MD

CONTENTS

SUMMARY OF RECOMMENDATIONS

In general, the treatment of delirium is broken down into three parts—psychiatric management, environmental and supportive interventions, and somatic interventions. In the broadest terms, the underlying cause of the delirium should be sought and treated if possible. Behavioral and environmental intervention should be optimized and instituted first. If necessary, to prevent patient distress or harm, pharmacological interventions should be instituted, the mainstay of which is haloperidol therapy.

DISEASE DEFINITION, EPIDEMIOLOGY, NATURAL HISTORY, AND DIFFERENTIAL DIAGNOSIS

Definition

Delirium is a disturbance of consciousness, attention, cognition, and perception that develops over a short period of time and tends to fluctuate

From: *Current Clinical Practice: Essential Practice Guidelines in Primary Care*
Edited by: N. S. Skolnik © Humana Press, Totowa, NJ

during the course of the day. This usually represents a sudden and significant decline from a previous level of functioning and cannot be better accounted for by an evolving dementia. As *inattention* is a hallmark of delirium, cognitive function (for dementia evaluation) is difficult to assess clinically during periods of delirium.

Common Clinical Features

Common clinical features include dysarthria, dysnomia, dysgraphia, illusions, hallucinations, disturbances in sleep–wake cycles, and disturbances in emotion. Two subtypes of delirium are described based on changes in psychomotor activity. Agitation is seen in "hyperactive" delirium and lethargy is seen in "hypoactive" delirium. Additionally, a number of nonspecific neurological abnormalities such as tremor, myoclonos, asterixis, and reflex changes may be seen.

Prevalence

Delirium is found in 10–40% of all elderly, hospitalized patients, up to 51% of postoperative patients, and 80% of patients with terminal illnesses. Often, prodromal symptoms such as anxiety, restlessness, irritability, or sleep disturbances are seen 1–3 d before overt delirium. Episodes of delirium may last 1 wk to 2 mo with the typical episode resolving in 10–12 d. Longer courses and incomplete recovery characterize delirium in the elderly hospitalized patients. Indeed, delirium is a harbinger of poor long-term prognosis. Delirium in elderly, hospitalized patients has been associated with 22–76% chance of dying during the hospitalization and 25% death rate within 6 mo of discharge.

Differential Diagnosis

The most common differential diagnosis is whether the patient's clinical condition is owing to delirium alone, worsening of a pre-existing dementia alone, or a delirium superimposed on a pre-existing dementia. Careful history with a focus on temporal onset of symptoms and fluctuations during a 24-h period are helpful in clarifying the diagnosis. Patients with dementia usually do not have the fluctuations in consciousness that are seen in delirium.

Causes of Delirium

When delirium occurs as a result of a medical illness, careful and comprehensive assessment must be undertaken to determine its etiology. General medical conditions that commonly cause delirium are represented in Table 1.

Common causes of delirium include substances of abuse, prescription medications, and toxins (Table 2). Half-life of the drug/toxin is an important

Table 1
Underlying Conditions Commonly Associated With Delirium

Type	Disorder
Central nervous system disorder	Head trauma
	Seizures
	Postictal state
	Vascular disease (e.g., hypertensive encephalopathy)
	Degenerative disease
Metabolic disorder	Renal failure (e.g., uremia)
	Hepatic failure
	Anemia
	Hypoxia
	Hypoglycemia
	Thiamine deficiency
	Endocrinopathy
	Fluid or electrolyte imbalance
	Acid–base imbalance
Cardiopulmonary causes	Myocardial infarction
	Congestive heart failure
	Cardiac arrhythmia
	Shock
	Respiratory failure
Systemic illness	Substance intoxication or withdrawal
	Infection
	Neoplasm
	Severe trauma
	Sensory deprivation
	Temperature dysregulation
	Postoperative state

determinant of rapidity of onset and duration of delirium during exposure and withdrawal periods.

Due to multiple etiologies, fully 44% of elderly hospitalized patients have multiple causes of delirium.

USE OF FORMAL ASSESSMENT MEASURES

1. Several *screening* instruments are available to screen for dementia. These are mostly tailored for the usage of nurses.
2. Several formal *diagnostic* tools are available. For example, the confusion assessment method is utilized in many care settings.

Table 2
Substances That Cause Delirium Through Intoxication or Withdrawal

Category	Substance
Drugs of abuse	Alcohol
	Amphetamines
	Cannabis
	Cocaine
	Hallucinogens
	Inhalants
	Opioids
	Phencyclidine
	Sedatives
	Hypnotics
	Other
Medications	Anesthetics
	Analgesics
	Antiasthmatic agents
	Anticonvulsants
	Antihistamines
	Antihypertensive and cardiovascular
	Medications
	Antimicrobials
	Antiparkinsonian medications
	Corticosteroids
	Gastrointestinal medications
	Muscle relaxants
	Immunosuppressive agents
	Lithium and psychotropic medications
	with anticholinergic properties
Toxins	Anticholinesterase

3. Several instruments are available for rating *severity* of delirium. These are usually based on behavioral symptoms, confusion, and cognitive impairment.
4. No laboratory test is available with sufficient operating characteristics (sensitivity/specificity) to assist in the rule in or rule out of delirium.

ASSESSMENT AND TREATMENT

The treatment principles of delirium include psychiatric treatment, behavioral and environmental treatment, and somatic or pharmacological treatment.

Psychiatric treatment includes coordination of care with other clinicians, identifying causes and initiating immediate interventions, and treatment for reversible causes. The etiology of delirium is ascertained by careful history, physical examination, and evaluation of laboratory data. These are summarized in Table 3.

Table 3
Assessment of the Patient With Delirium

Domain	Measure
Physical status	History
	Physical and neurological examinations
	Review of vital signs and anesthesia record if postoperative
	Review of general medical records
	Careful review of medications and correlation with behavioral changes
Mental status	Interview
	Cognitive tests, for example, clock face, digit span, trail making tests
Basic laboratory tests—consider for all patients with delirium	Blood chemistry: electrolytes, glucose, calcium, albumin, blood urea nitrogen, creatinine, SGOT, SGPT, bilirubin, alkaline phosphatase, magnesium, PO_4
	Complete blood count
	Electrocardiogram
	Chest X-ray
	Measurement of arterial blood gases or oxygen saturation
	Urinalysis
Additional laboratory tests—ordered as indicated by clinical condition	Urine culture and sensitivity (C and S)
	Urine drug screen
	Blood tests, for example, venereal disease research laboratory, heavy metal screen, Vitamin B_{12} and folate levels, lupus erythematosus prep, antinuclear antibody, urinary porphyrins, ammonia, human immunodeficiency virus
	Blood cultures
	Measurement of serum levels of medications, for example, digoxin, theophylline, phenobarbital, and cyclosporine
	Lumbar puncture
	Brain computed tomography or magnetic resonance imaging

Initiate Interventions for Acute Conditions

As patients with delirium may have life-threatening medical illnesses, frequent monitoring of vital signs, fluid intake and output, and levels of oxygenation is essential *(1)*. The medication regimen should be carefully reviewed with unnecessary medications withdrawn and doses of necessary medications

Table 4
Examples of Reversible Causes of Delirium and Their Treatments

Condition	Treatment
Hypoglycemia or delirium of unknown etiology in which hypoglycemia is suspected	Tests of blood and urine for diagnosis Thiamine hydrochloride, 100 mg i.v. 50% glucose solution, 50 mL i.v.
Hypoxia or anoxia, for example, resulting from pneumonia, obstructive or restrictive pulmonary disease, cardiac disease, hypotension, severe anemia, or carbon monoxide poisoning	Immediate oxygen
Hyperthermia, for example, temperature	Rapid cooling
Above 40.5°C or 105°F Severe hypertension, for example, blood pressure of 260/150 mmHg, with papilledema	Prompt antihypertensive treatment
Alcohol or sedative withdrawal	Appropriate pharmacological intervention Thiamine, i.v. glucose, magnesium phosphate, and other B vitamins
Wernicke's encephalopathy	Thiamine hydrochloride, 100 mg i.v. thiamine daily, either intravenously
Anticholinergic delirium	In severe cases, physostigmine unless contraindicated

minimized. Medical disorders such as hypoglycemia, hypoxia, hyperthermia, hypertension, and substance-induced disorders should be rapidly corrected. Examples of reversible causes of delirium are found in Table 4.

Monitor and Ensure Safety

Suicidality, violence potential, fall risk, and wandering risk, inadvertent self-harm risk should all be assessed with appropriate measures taken to ensure safety. Use of restraints should be minimized as they may increase agitation and hence decrease safety.

Patients should also be monitored for hallucinations, delusions, aggressive behavior, agitation, affective liability, and sleep disturbances.

Environment and Supportive Intervention

There is some evidence that environmental interventions can reduce the severity of delirium and improve outcomes. Visual impairment, auditory impairment, and sensory overstimulation (such as an intensive care unit) and understimulation should be assessed and, when possible, corrected. Reorientation efforts such as the introduction of clocks, calendars, and family pictures or other familiar household items can be beneficial. Family education about delirium and its cause cannot be overstressed. Constant reorientation to time and place and reassurance that the delirium is both reversible and temporary by caregivers and family alike is helpful.

Somatic/Pharmacological Interventions

Antipsychotics have been the medication of choice in the treatment of delirium. Evidence for their efficacy has come from case reports and uncontrolled trials in comparison. There are no published randomized, double-blind, and placebo-controlled trials for drug treatment either for choice of drug or optimal dosing.

HALOPERIDOL

It is generally believed that haloperidol is the first drug choice for the treatment of delirium. It is a high-potent dopamine-blocking agent with few or no anticholinergic side effects, minimal cardiovascular side effects, and no active metabolites. It can be given orally, intramuscularly (i.m.) or intravenously (i.v.), which is an advantage in a patient unable or unwilling to take it orally. Generally, low starting doses of 0.25–0.5 mg of haldol every 4 has needed are suggested for the elderly patients and this can be titrated up to 1–2 mg every 2–4 h as needed. Higher doses of haloperidol, including continuous infusions, have been studied and can be safe and effective in selected patients.

OTHER ANTIPSYCHOTICS

Droperidol has a rapid onset of action and relatively short half-life. It is more likely to cause sedation and hypotension than haloperidol. It has been found to be an effective treatment for hospitalized patients with agitation, although not necessarily delirium.

There has been very little study of the newer antipsychotic medications (risperidone, olanzapine, and quetiapine) in the treatment of delirium. These agents, however, are increasingly being used for the treatment of delirium. Note because guideline was issued; the Food and Drug Administration (FDA) issued a warning that a typical antipsychotic drugs used to treat behavioral disorders in elderly patients with dementia have shown a higher death rate associated with their use compared with patients receiving a placebo. The FDA stated that in analyses of 17 placebo-controlled studies of four drugs in the atypical antipsychotic class, the rate of death for those elderly patients with dementia was about 1.6–1.7 times that of placebo. Over the course of these trials averaging about 10 wk in duration, the rate of death in drug-treated patients was about 4.5%, compared with a rate of about 2.6% in the placebo group. Whether this issue also applies to the traditional

antipsychotics is a matter of ongoing review (http://www.fda.gov/cder/drug/
infopage/antipsychotics/default.htm, accessed 6/25/05).

Side Effects

Antipsychotics can increase the QTc interval and have been associated with
torsades de pointes and ventricular fibrillation. A baseline electrocardiogram and
cardiac monitoring is suggested for patients receiving high doses or intravenous
dosing of haloperidol. All antipsychotics may be associated with sedation, anticholinergic effects, and α-adrenergic blockade effects causing hypotension. In
addition, extrapyramidal side effects such as tardive dyskinesia and neuroleptic
malignant syndrome can also occur. As with all pharmacological therapy, the
risks and benefits of drug intervention should be weighed carefully.

OTHER PHARMACOLOGICAL TREATMENTS

Multiple other medications have been studied in the treatment of delirium, but
are not recommended except in certain circumstances. Opioid analgesia may be
indicated in the treatment of delirium in which pain is an aggravating factor.

Benzodiazepenes are recommended when withdrawal from benzodiazepines
or alcohol is suspected. When used for nonwithdrawal-associated delirium,
low-dose and short-acting benzodiazepines in combination with antipsychotics
may increase efficacy and decrease side effects better than when either agent is
used alone. As some patients may experience a worsening of delirium with benzodiazepines, antipsychotics, specifically haloperidol, remain the pharmacological treatment of choice. Cholinergic medications (cholinesterase inhibitors)
have been used in a limited fashion to treat delirium.

Any patient with delirium who has a reason to be vitamin-B deficient (alco-
holic, etc.) should be given multivitamin replacement. Electroconvulsive therapy has not been shown to be an effective treatment for delirium.

SPECIAL CONSIDERATIONS

The presence of delirium does not in itself mean that a patient is incompe-
tent or lacks capacity to give informed consent.

CLINICAL FEATURES INFLUENCING TREATMENT

Comorbid Psychiatric Conditions

Treatment of comorbid psychiatric conditions such as dementia or depression should be minimized during episodes of delirium as medications to treat
these conditions might exacerbate delirium.

Comorbid General Medical Conditions

AIDS/HIV

Approximately 30–40% of hospitalized AIDS patients develop delirium. AIDS patients may be more sensitive to extrapyamidal side effects from antipsychotics.

LIVER DISEASE

When benzodiazeopines are required in the treatment of the delirious patient with liver disease, temazepam, oxazepam, or lorazepam should be used. These agents undergo glucuronidation and not p450 metabolism in the liver.

SOURCES

1. American Psychiatric Association Practice Guideline For the Treatment of Patients with Delirium (1999);(http://www.psych.org/psych_pract/treatg/pg/Practice%20Guidelines8904/Delirium.pdf accessed Oct. 14, 2005).

28 Panic Disorder

Diane Dietzen, MD, FACP
and Doron Schneider, MD

CONTENTS

PROCESS OF DEVELOPMENT OF GUIDELINE

The Practice Guideline for the Treatment of Patients with Panic Disorder was initially published in 1998 *(1)*. A committee of the American Psychiatric Association (APA) performed a literature review and drafted a document, which was then revised by the members and other organizations, and approved by the APA assembly and Board of Trustees. The intent was to revise this guideline at 3- to 5-yr intervals, but as yet no revision is in process. The committee categorized the strength of its endorsement for each recommendation on a scale of I–III:

I. Recommended with substantial clinical confidence.
II. Recommended with moderate clinical confidence.
III. May be recommended on the basis of individual circumstances.

From: *Current Clinical Practice: Essential Practice Guidelines in Primary Care*
Edited by: N. S. Skolnik © Humana Press, Totowa, NJ

These numbers are referenced in parentheses throughout this chapter as they were designated in the original text.

DEFINITION, DEMOGRAPHIC DATA, AND EPIDEMIOLOGY

Panic disorder, as described in the Diagnostic and Statistical Manual, 4th edition (DSM-IV) criteria consists of periodic episodes of intense fear or discomfort, combined with fear or worry about recurrent attacks with symptoms present for more than 1 mo. Of the 13 symptoms listed in the DSM-IV, 4 must be present. Symptoms include dyspnea, tachycardia, palpitations, headaches, dizziness, paresthesias, choking, smothering feelings, nausea, fear of losing control, fear of dying, and sweating. Attacks generally are abrupt in onset and peak after about 10 min. They can be associated with a trigger situation, or be nocturnal or unexpected. Patients will describe an "urge to escape" during an attack or a feeling of impending doom. The differential diagnosis of panic disorder includes posttraumatic stress disorder, separation anxiety, substance abuse or withdrawal, or a number of medical illnesses.

Panic disorder has a lifetime prevalence in the US population of 1.6–2.2%. The risk is twofold higher in females, and eightfold higher in first-degree relatives of patients with panic disorder. Age at first onset is usually between ages 20 and 30, but the diagnosis can be made in other age groups. About 33–50% of patients with panic disorder will also have agoraphobia, and 50–60% will develop major depression during their lifetime. The depression can present before or after the diagnosed panic disorder.

MORBIDITIES OF PANIC DISORDER

Patients with panic disorder may also have increased the use of emergency medical services, more frequent hospital admissions for physical symptoms, suicide (if depression is also present), substance abuse, or impaired social or occupational function.

INITIAL CONSIDERATIONS IN DIAGNOSIS

Diagnostic Evaluation

The initial elements of the diagnostic evaluation are a thorough history (including specific symptoms) of the episodes, past general medical history, a past psychiatric history, and a history of any substance abuse. Family, occupational, social history, review of systems, mental status examination, physical examination, and lab testing as indicated by the history are also warranted. It is important to assess the impact on activities of daily life and whether any life-threatening behavior is present (grade I). The guideline recommends that the treating physician guide the ordering of lab and diagnostic testing (grade I).

Evaluating Particular Symptoms

A symptom diary may be helpful in understanding the frequency of attacks, the symptom constellation, and associated internal and external stimuli that may have precipitated the attacks.

Evaluating Functional Impairment

The impact of panic attacks on the patient and the family should be addressed. Phobic avoidance often leads to significant changes in activities but may have become routine for patient and family. If family members find the phobic behaviors beneficial, support for those behaviors may increase and be counterproductive to treatment. It is important to ascertain the patient's criteria for a good outcome with treatment of the disorder.

Monitoring Psychiatric Status

Comorbid illness such as substance abuse and depression should be assessed initially and during ongoing treatment. The patient will require monitoring with the expectation that the course of the illness may fluctuate. The physician or other caregivers are advised to establish a therapeutic alliance with the patient, and to anticipate plans for separations from the provider during care.

Patient and Family Education

The patient and the family, if appropriate, should be educated about the nature of the disorder, the plan for treatment, and the fluctuating, chronic course of the illness. Patients often need reassurance that there is no underlying medical disorder exists. Patients also require reassurance that the symptoms they experience are physiological and therapy will be beneficial. Effects of the illness on the function of the patient should be reviewed.

Enhancing Compliance

Interaction with other health professionals is often required to improve patient compliance with therapy. Education of other providers and family may resolve frustrations with patient behaviors and is beneficial to all. Enlisting the aid of the family in therapy is helpful. Addressing common patient fears about medication and cognitive therapy directly will also enhance compliance.

Working to Address Signs of Relapse

The fluctuating and recurrent nature of panic disorder is an important part of patient education. The relationship with the physician should be continued after initial treatment, and the patient should be encouraged to contact the provider with any increased symptoms of panic, as well as symptoms of depression or anxiety.

Choosing Site of Treatment

A decision about initial in-patient or outpatient therapy can be made after the earlier mentioned factors are addressed. Most patients can be managed on an outpatient basis without hospitalization (grade I). Patients with coexisting substance abuse or depression may require admission. Patients with severe medical illness or symptoms not clearly related to panic disorder may also require admission. Each of the above areas of evaluation carries a grade I recommendation.

ISSUES TO BE EVALUATED
IN CHOOSING INITIAL TREATMENT

Suicidality

About 20% of patients with panic disorder, or 12% of those with panic attacks alone, will attempt suicide at some time in their life. It is unclear whether this is directly related to their panic disorder or to other comorbid psychiatric disorders such as depression. Screening for suicidal thoughts or plans is important at diagnosis of panic disorder and during treatment.

Substance Abuse

Patients with substance abuse and panic disorder have a poorer prognosis than those with panic disorder alone. Cocaine, alcohol, and sedatives are common substances of abuse. Initial evaluation should determine if substance abuse is the primary diagnosis, as this may alter treatment. Withdrawal syndromes resulting from substance abuse should be treated first. Benzodiazepines should be avoided in the treatment of patients with substance abuse disorders.

Mood Disorder

Mood disorders, especially depression, are common with panic disorder. The depression can be unipolar or bipolar. Similar to substance abuse, concomitant depression leads to greater morbidity, including hospitalizations and suicide attempts. Patients with depression and panic disorder often complain of overstimulation when treated with antidepressant medications and should be started on low doses with slow upward titration.

Other Anxiety Disorder or Personality Disorder

Other anxiety disorders to be identified in panic disorder patients include posttraumatic stress disorder, obsessive-compulsive disorder, and generalized anxiety disorder. These may change the relationship of the provider to the patient, either to create more avoidance of treatment, or more dependence on therapy.

UNCOMPLICATED PANIC DISORDER, WITHOUT ANY OF THE EARLIER MENTIONED COMORBIDITIES IS UNCOMMON

Medical Issues to be Considered in Treatment

MEDICAL ILLNESS

Panic disorder may exist with other medical illnesses. Evaluation for underlying medical causes of panic symptoms, such as withdrawal from medication or hyperthyroidism should be excluded. Panic is also more common in patients with other illness not directly related to symptoms. For example, panic disorder is more commonly diagnosed in patients with irritable bowel syndrome, migraine headache, and pulmonary disease. Some studies suggest that anxiety may increase mortality in patients with cardiovascular disease. If treatment of underlying medical problems fails to resolve symptoms of panic, or if panic attacks are felt to be a separate and unrelated condition, treatment targeting panic symptoms should be commenced. Treatment of panic disorder with medical illness does not change unless drug doses need to be altered for renal or hepatic disease. Conversely, symptoms of medical illness may improve with anxiety or panic therapy.

Pediatric and Geriatric Populations Gender and Cultural Influences on Treatment

Separate guidelines exist for treatment of panic disorder in the pediatric population. Treatments have been poorly studied in the pediatric population. In the geriatric population the authors recommend a thorough search for underlying medical illness with any psychiatric medications initially administered at lower doses.

The prevalence of panic and anxiety disorders is higher in women. Although panic diagnosis is not more common in the African-American population it may present with more somatic symptoms and the specific symptoms and include isolated sleep paralysis and possibly hypertension. No studies of panic in other cultures or ethnic populations have been described.

Formulation of Treatment Plan

A treatment plan should be devised only after a comprehensive medical and psychiatric evaluation (including inquiries about substance abuse) has been performed. Psychiatric therapy, medical therapy, or a combination may be part of the treatment plan. Goals of therapy include decreasing frequency of attacks, decreased anticipatory anxiety, and the treatment of depressive symptoms. Choices of therapeutic modality should be individualized for each patient and guided by efficacy and with consideration of comorbidities.

PSYCHOTHERAPY

Cognitive Behavioral Therapy

The panel reviewed 12 available trials of cognitive-behavioral therapy (CBT) for panic disorder and designated it as a grade I. Trials were heterogeneous in treatment duration and clinical endpoints. The follow-up period ranged from 6 mo to 8 yr. An average 88% of patients were "panic free" (not meeting the DSM criteria) at 1 yr and 50% were panic free at 2 yr. Significant placebo effect (up to 75% response rate) was seen in many trials.

The elements of CBT are psychoeducation, symptom monitoring, anxiety management, cognitive restructuring, and in vivo exposure to fear cues. CBT is usually done in an individual setting but can be done in a group. Psychoeducation is the initial period of educating the patient about the disorder symptoms and the treatment plan. Patients are subsequently asked to monitor symptoms and triggers, often by keeping a diary. Anxiety management is taught by teaching a method for control of symptoms such as abdominal breathing. Cognitive restructuring encourages the patient to examine alternative outcomes of cues to panic, and their likelihood. In vivo exposure is usually done by asking the patient to create a hierarchy of anxiety-provoking situations, then entering these situations daily, increasing the duration and difficulty of exposures over time. "Flooding" the immediate exposure to the most fear inducing cues, is an alternative method. CBT may help ease benzodiazepine withdrawal.

About 10–30% of patients are unwilling to perform tasks central to CBT such as keeping symptom diaries and being exposed to fear-inducing situations. Adverse effects of CBT are increased anxiety during treatment, development of dependence on the therapist, and ineffectiveness in addressing comorbid psychiatric disorders if they exist.

Other Psychotherapy

All other available psychotherapies for panic disorder have a level grade III rating.

Psychodynamic therapy is usually long-term therapy, directed at resolution of core lifelong conflicts. Courses about using this method for shorter-term treatment of panic disorder are available and supported with one small nonrandomized study and case reports, which describe effectiveness. There are no randomized control trials (RCTs) of psychodynamic therapy.

Mindfulness, meditation, marital therapy, and support groups are described as adjuncts to panic disorder therapy.

Length of Psychotherapy

The length of therapy is about 12 wk. After 6–8 wk, the therapy should be assessed for benefit. If therapy is effective, tapering can begin at 12 wk.

PHARMACOLOGICAL THERAPY

Classes of Drug Therapy

SELECTIVE SEROTONIN REUPTAKE INHIBITORS

Four selective serotonin reuptake inhibitors (SSRIs) were approved for therapy at the time the guideline was written fluoxetine (Prozac), sertraline (Zoloft), paroxetine (Paxil), and fluvoxamine (Luvox). The authors briefly reviewed the trial data for each.

Fluoxetine was studied in one double-blind, placebo-controlled trial, and several open trials, and was shown to decrease symptoms. A dose of 20 mg was more effective than 10 mg. Response rates were 44–76% (similar to CBT and other agents). Median dose reported was 20–30 mg.

Sertraline was studied in two reported RCTs. One trial demonstrated a 79% rate of decreased symptoms, with a 59% placebo response. The second RCT demonstrated a 77% decrease in panic attacks vs 51% with placebo. Dose ranges for these trials were not reported.

Paroxetine has also been shown to be effective in double-blind, placebo-controlled trials with an 80% response rate in one trial vs 50% placebo. The most effective dose in two of the trials was 40 mg. One trial compared paroxetine with clomipramine and placebo, and found the two drugs to be superior to placebo and equally effective.

Fluvoxamine response rates, again from a small number of trials, were in the 61–81% range with 30–40% placebo responses. Dose ranges were not described.

Citalopram was not approved for therapy in the United States when the guideline was published, but trial data from Europe indicated that at a dose of 20–30 mg daily the drug was superior to placebo and comparable with clomipramine.

All drugs in this class are felt to have similar short-term efficacy. A meta-analysis of 27 studies demonstrated similar effect sizes. It is unclear whether the effect sizes are greater than those reported for alprazolam or imipramine, although this is suggested by one meta-analysis. Because of a more tolerable side-effect profile, the SSRI class is initial choice of therapy. SSRIs are not lethal in overdose, and anticholinergic side effects are not present. Headache, irritability, nausea, insomnia, sexual dysfunction, increased anxiety, drowsiness, and tremor are possible side effects. SSRIs reviewed here are hepatically metabolized, and doses should be adjusted with liver disease. At the time of guideline publication, no concerns about an increased risk of suicide was present with these agents. More recently, SSRIs have been shown to increase the risk of suicide in children and adolescents. There is a syndrome of withdrawal from SSRIs characterized by dizziness, incoordination, headache, and irritability. These symptoms can last up to 2 wk after the drug is discontinued. When implementing SSRI therapy, an increase in anxiety at the beginning of therapy should be anticipated. Therapy should be commenced with low doses (10 mg of fluoxetine or paroxetine, or 50 mg of fluvoxamine). An increase to a therapeutic dose should take place over days, and then should be titrated up as needed over several weeks. A clinical response may not be seen in the initial 4 wk and the length of therapy needed to assess effect ranges from 6 to 12 wk. Therapy should be continued for an unclear period. Studies indicate 36 wk is effective, but other lengths have not been studied. SSRI therapy should be tapered over the course of weeks to avoid withdrawal syndrome.

TRICYCLIC ANTIDEPRESSANTS

Imipramine was first reported as a treatment in 1964. The authors reviewed 15 trials of this drug. Generally, patients were treated for at least 4 wk, and assessed at 8–12 wk. Between 40 and 70% of patients were reported to be panic free with imipramine, and 15–50% with placebo. Anticipatory anxiety and phobic avoidance were decreased in some trials also. Other tricyclic antidepressants (TCAs) have been poorly evaluated. One trail with desipramine and two with clomipramine showed efficacy similar to imipramine. Side effects of TCAs are predominantly anticholinergic, and include sweating, orthostasis, sleepiness, urinary retention, and exacerbation of narrow-angle glaucoma. Patients with cardiac conduction abnormalities can have fatal arrhythmias with TCAs. Fatigue, weakness, weight gain, and sexual dysfunction are also reported. Increased doses are associated with increased side effects and drop-out rates. Up to 36% of patients drop out at imipramine doses of 200 mg.

TCAs should also be implemented at low dose, for example, 10 mg/d of imipramine, and titrated over weeks to a dose of about 100 mg. Optimum dose is between 150 and 300 mg. For clomipramine, the optimal dose is lower, 25–150 mg. Length of therapy is 4 wk to first response, about 8 wk to dose adjustment, and continued therapy for 8–12 wk if response is evident. Few trials evaluate longer use, but some describe 6–8 mo of therapy.

BENZODIAZEPINES

Benzodiazepine therapy represents the most rapidly acting drug class. Symptom reduction can be seen within just a few days of therapy. Alprazolam was the only benzodiazepine approved by the Food and Drug Administration for panic disorder therapy at the time of guideline publication. Two meta-analyses have reviewed alprazolam therapy. In six of seven double-blind, placebo-controlled trials, 55–75% of patients were panic free with alprazolam vs 15–50% with placebo. Twelve studies evaluated other benzodiazepines, including clonazepam, diazepam, lorazepam, and chloradiazepoxide. These trials did not indicate inferiority or superiority to alprazolam.

Side effects of benzodiazepines include sedation, fatigue, ataxia, and memory impairment. It should not be used in the elderly and in patients with a history of substance abuse. Despite concern, studies have failed to demonstrate dose escalation by patients. Patients with panic disorder may be especially prone to symptoms with benzodiazepine taper. About 33–100% of patients in trials report withdrawal or recurrent panic symptoms during the tapering phase of therapy. Long-acting benzodiazepines may decrease the likelihood of withdrawal. Tapering should be slow and focus on a 10% reduction in dose per week. The APA has a separate task force focused on benzodiazepine therapy.

Patients may require up to 10 mg/d of alprazolam. Clonazepam doses of 1–2 mg/d are an alternative. Optimal doses of other benzodiazepines are unclear. In summary, benzodiazepines allow the most rapid control and should be considered initially (grade III). These agents should be avoided in those with a history of substance abuse or dependence. Optimal treatment duration is not defined. Withdrawal or panic symptoms should be anticipated during tapering.

MONOAMINE OXIDASE INHIBITORS

Monoamine oxidase (MAO) inhibitors are reserved for cases of panic disorder that are unresponsive to other types of therapy. Because of the serious nature of the side effects, including tyramine reactions and drug interactions, hypotension, weight gain, paresthesia, sleep disturbances, myoclonus, dry mouth, and edema, MAO inhibitors should be used only by experienced physicians. Doses would be 45–90 mg of phenelzine, titrated for several weeks to effect. No recommendations about maintenance or taper are provided. Reversible inhibitor of MAO-A, a related class of drugs not available in the United States, have shown efficacy in overseas trials. The authors felt that all four of the classes above have good evidence of effectiveness (grade I) and are roughly equal in efficacy (grade II).

OTHER AGENTS

Velnefaxine, trazodone, bupropion, and nefazodone have all been found to be effective in small or single trials. Anticonvulsants such as carbamazepine and valproate have been studied in a few trials without clear conclusions. There is no evidence that conventional antipsychotics have a role in the treatment of panic disorder. β-blockers are not primary therapy but may be used adjunctively. Calcium channel blockers have no documented role. Clonidine has been shown to be some efficacy in panic disorder but its use is limited secondary to its side-effect profile. Buspirone has some activity in panic disorder but information provided is limited.

DURATION OF THERAPY

Acute therapy with either CBT or medication lasts about 12 wk at which point, frequency and severity of attacks should be markedly reduced. Frequency of CBT appointments can be diminished and patients may expect many months to years of reduced symptomatology. Duration of medication therapy may be more protracted (often 12–18 mo) resulting from symptom recurrence during tapering. Optimal duration of medical treatment has not been defined. Failure to respond to medical therapy within 6–8 wk necessitates re-evaluation of diagnosis and treatment plan (grade III). Booster treatment or longer treatment with relapse can be considered. CBT and medication for panic disorder are both effective with no evidence of superiority of either modality. Selection of modality should be in collaboration with an informed patient (grade I). Issues of costs, adverse effects, therapist availability, and comorbid illnesses may influence choice (grade I).

COMBINATION THERAPY

Combination medication and psychotherapy may be important for poor responders of single modality therapy or for those with severe agoraphobia.

PROGNOSIS

About 4–6 yr after diagnosis, 30% of patients will be without symptoms of panic disorder, 40–50% will be improved but still symptomatic, and 20–30% will be the same or worse than at diagnosis.

RESEARCH DIRECTIONS

The authors listed the following goals for future research:

1. To look epidemiologically at panic disorder and coexisting anxiety disorders.
2. To evaluate whether panic disorder implies a higher rate of long-term cardiovascular morbidity and mortality.
3. To study the management of panic disorder in childhood.
4. To evaluate the length of treatment or role of booster treatment.
5. To evaluate how to identify treatment responders to CBT or medication.
6. To study relative efficacy of medications or combinations.

SUMMARY

Panic disorder requires a complete evaluation of diagnosis to investigate comorbid psychiatric and medical disorders and to assess functional impairment. The relationship of the therapist is important to educate, encourage follow-up, and prevent relapse. Psychotherapy or medication therapy are both standard of care and either can be chosen after risks and benefits, costs, and availability have been explored with the patient. Panic disorder is an often recurrent illness and continued symptoms or treatment for other psychiatric disorders over time is not uncommon.

SOURCES

1. (1998) Am J Psychiatry May 155(5 Suppl):1–34.

Index